Fitness For Dummies

Ten Keys to a Successful Fitness Program

1. **Set goals.**

   Rather than say, "I want to get in shape," say, "I'm going to walk for 20 minutes three times a week" or "I'm going to lose 10 pounds in four months." Make your goals specific and realistic.

2. **Reward yourself.**

   If you lose those 10 pounds, buy yourself that watch you've been wanting. Sure, it's bribery, but it works. Just don't reward yourself with a seven-layer fudge cake.

3. **Keep a log.**

   Record the details of your workouts in a daily exercise diary. Your log will help you track your progress and stay motivated.

4. **Pace yourself.**

   Don't do three hours of exercise your first time out. You'll burn out fast and probably get injured. Always keep yourself hungry for more.

5. **Find a buddy.**

   Working out with a friend or a group can push you to new heights — or get your butt off the couch when you'd rather stay home and watch reruns of "Bewitched."

6. **Get your fitness tested.**

   Don't worry — you can't flunk! A fitness evaluation will pinpoint the areas you need to work on, such as your aerobic conditioning, strength, flexibility, and body fat.

7. **Expect to work hard.**

   Exercise shouldn't be painful, but if you've neglected your body, don't expect a free ride.

8. **Buy the right equipment.**

   You don't need to blow your retirement savings, but investing in the right exercise gizmos or health club membership will increase your chance of success.

9. **Find a hero.**

   Your hero can be your grandma who walks a mile every day — or a coworker who used to have a beer gut and now runs 10k races. Find someone who makes you think, "If *that* person can do it, I sure as heck can."

10. **Educate yourself.**

    The more you know about fitness, the more fun you'll have working out. You can keep up with exercise trends and techniques in magazines, newsletters, and books — even on the Internet.

BUSINESS AND
GENERAL
REFERENCE
BOOK SERIES
FROM IDG

Fitness For Dummies™

Quick Reference Card

Ten Fitness Myths Debunked

1. **You don't have to exercise for 30 consecutive minutes.**

   Nowhere is it written — in the U.S. Constitution or the Five Books of Moses — that in order to benefit from aerobic exercise, you need to do it for a half hour. If your goal is to improve your health, three 10-minute sessions per day will suffice.

2. **You *can* get fat eating fat-free foods.**

   One Reduced Fat ChipsAhoy! cookie has 50 calories; a regular ChipsAhoy! has 53. Fat-free doesn't mean calorie-free.

3. **Lifting weights won't turn you into Amazon Woman or the Incredible Hulk.**

   Virtually all women and most men can't develop huge muscles without spending hours a day in the gym lifting very heavy weights.

4. **If you stop exercising, your muscles won't turn to fat.**

   They'll just shrink. Fat and muscle are two different entities; you can't turn one into the other.

5. **Don't start your workout by stretching your muscles.**

   Stretch *after* you have warmed up with at least five minutes of light exercise, such as walking. Stretching a cold muscle can lead to injury.

6. **The best personal trainers aren't necessarily the ones who look best in their Lycra.**

   Look for trainers who have a professional certification or a degree in exercise physiology or a related field.

7. **You can't "spot reduce."**

   In other words, you can't selectively zap fat off a particular part of your body, such as your thighs or your stomach.

8. **Those neoprene "waist trimming" belts won't help you lose fat.**

   At best, you'll lose water weight, which you'll regain when you drink. At worst, these products leave you dangerously dehydrated.

9. **Exercise during pregnancy does not increase the rate of miscarriage or cause birth defects.**

   Prenatal exercise is perfectly safe for most women — as long as they use common sense and don't try to set a world record in the high hurdles. Be sure to get a doctor's approval, however.

10. **Eating spicy foods will not speed up your metabolism or help you lose fat.**

    No food has special fat-burning powers — not even the long-revered grapefruit or the amino acid shakes that bodybuilders gulp down by the gallon.

. . . For Dummies: Bestselling Book Series for Beginners

Praise for Fitness For Dummies

"Hey, who are you guys calling a Dummy? When it comes to fitness, like most male American slugs, I'm actually more of a complete blathering moronic idiot. This book will come in handy for those of us who don't know a fat gram from Phil Gramm or a donut from a bagel. Now all I need to know is how to look cool and studly in the gym while sweating profusely."

— Steve Elling, *Raleigh News & Observer*

"This book is a joy to read — written with wit and style, it comes as a welcome reassurance that both razor sharp accuracy and first-rate writing can co-exist in the same package."

— Jonathan Bowden, M.A. C.S.C.S., Senior Faculty, Equinox Fitness Training Institute and Contributing Editor, *Fitness* magazine

"*Fitness For Dummies* is a smart buy for the exercise enthusiast. It's the fitness equivalent of carbo-loading!"

— Karen Crouse, Sports Writer, *Orange County Register*

"This is one of the most comprehensive, authoritative — and entertaining — fitness books I've ever seen."

— Sharon Cohen, Executive Editor, *Men's Fitness* magazine

"Many popular fitness books don't have 'Dummies' in the title, but they seem to be written by dummies. This book, however, is an all inclusive reference that doesn't push a particular method, but instead will be useful no matter whether you are a highly resistant couch potato, a former athlete, or an average Joe or Joanna. It is thorough, informative, clear, concise, and *very, very* funny."

— Katie Schmitz, M.S.Ed., author of the *Weight Watchers Activity Plan*

"No one is more of a dummy when it comes to exercise than I am. Until I read *Fitness For Dummies,* I thought taking a book like this off the shelf counted as a workout. Now I know better. It's only a warm-up!"

— Phil Rosenthal, Columnist, *Los Angeles Daily News*

"The exercise content and evaluations in this book are outstanding. Liz and Suzanne are the ultimate professionals, and *Fitness For Dummies* will help all exercisers maximize their potential."

— Nicole Dorsey, Fitness Director, *Fitness* magazine

"*Fitness For Dummies* is the definitive book for people who would like to achieve a stronger, healthier body."

— Mark Allen, Six-Time Ironman Champion

"Suzanne and Liz have created an insider's guide through the maze of misinformation about fitness. Before you buy an exercise gadget, a gym membership, or a fitness video, read this book!"

— Mary Duffy, Editor-in-Chief, *Women's Sports + Fitness* magazine

"*Fitness For Dummies* is a real rarity: a fitness book written by fitness writers — two of the best. It's full of smart, jargon-free, common-sense advice for anyone whose interested in fitness. These two are not afraid to tell the truth. It's like getting the word from a trusted friend."

— Peg Moline, Editorial Director, *Shape* magazine

"I am duly impressed with this newest entry into the ...*For Dummies* series. From dispelling myths such as how we really burn fat to a comprehensive look at every choice of equipment on the market today, this book becomes a trustworthy, truly helpful guide to getting in shape."

— Diana Nyad, World Record Holder, Longest Swim in History & TV Broadcaster

"A great source of information for anyone beginning a fitness program — complete, but simple enough to understand, without having a degree in exercise physiology."

— Charlie Cherny, ACSM Health/Fitness Instructor

"Finally, a comprehensive guide that takes the intimidation out of fitness."

— Heidi Dvorak, Editor-in-Chief, *Living Fit* magazine

"As a guide to healthier living, from helpful nutrition tips to a sensible daily exercise routine, *Fitness For Dummies* is enough to lift you right up off the LA-Z-BOY!"

— Jerry Crowe, Reporter, *Los Angeles Times*

"*Fitness For Dummies* is like a security blanket for workout beginners. It's so good at demystifying the fitness world that you can't possibly feel intimidated anymore. If I had it when I started working out, I wouldn't have felt like I'd landed on Saturn the first time I walked into the gym."

— Terri Troncale, *The Birmingham News*

"*Fitness For Dummies* is terrific!"

— Rich Tosches, syndicated columnist

"*Fitness For Dummies* speaks to fools everywhere who want a fun workout — not a lesson in exercise physiology. The book helps you get fit without numbing your brain!"

— Gordon Monson, Columnist, *The Salt Lake Tribune*

"Unlike most fitness books, this one washes down with the ease of chewable vitamins. *Fitness For Dummies* teaches with humor. Sofa slugs beware: Laughing aloud will strengthen your abdomen."

— Sam Farmer, staff writer, *San Jose Mercury News*

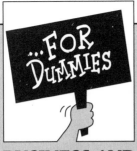
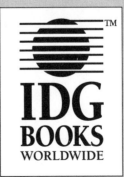

FITNESS
FOR
DUMMIES™

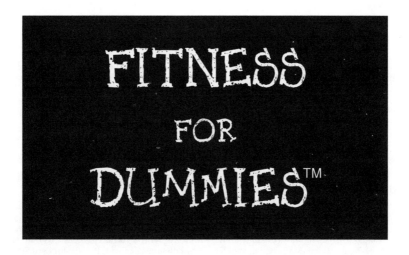

FITNESS FOR DUMMIES™

by Suzanne Schlosberg
and
Liz Neporent

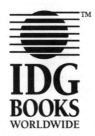

IDG Books Worldwide, Inc.
An International Data Group Company

Foster City, CA ♦ Chicago, IL ♦ Indianapolis, IN ♦ Southlake, TX

Fitness For Dummies™

Published by
IDG Books Worldwide, Inc.
An International Data Group Company
919 E. Hillsdale Blvd.
Suite 400
Foster City, CA 94404
http://www.idgbooks.com (IDG Books Worldwide Web site)
http://www.dummies.com (Dummies Press Web site)

Library of Congress Catalog Card No.: 96-76255

ISBN: 1-56884-866-8

Printed in the United States of America

10 9 8 7 6 5 4 3 2

1O/QU/RS/ZW/IN

Distributed in the United States by IDG Books Worldwide, Inc.

Distributed by Macmillan Canada for Canada; by Transworld Publishers Limited in the United Kingdom and Europe; by WoodsLane Pty. Ltd. for Australia; by WoodsLane Enterprises Ltd. for New Zealand; by Longman Singapore Publishers Ltd. for Singapore, Malaysia, Thailand, and Indonesia; by Simron Pty. Ltd. for South Africa; by Toppan Company Ltd. for Japan; by Distribuidora Cuspide for Argentina; by Livraria Cultura for Brazil; by Ediciencia S.A. for Ecuador; by Addison-Wesley Publishing Company for Korea; by Ediciones ZETA S.C.R. Ltda. for Peru; by WS Computer Publishing Company, Inc., for the Philippines; by Unalis Corporation for Taiwan; by Contemporanea de Ediciones for Venezuela. Authorized Sales Agent: Anthony Rudkin Associates for the Middle East and North Africa.

For general information on IDG Books Worldwide's books in the U.S., please call our Consumer Customer Service department at 800-762-2974. For reseller information, including discounts and premium sales, please call our Reseller Customer Service department at 800-434-3422.

For information on where to purchase IDG Books Worldwide's books outside the U.S., please contact our International Sales department at 415-655-3172 or fax 415-655-3295.

For information on foreign language translations, please contact our Foreign & Subsidiary Rights department at 415-655-3021 or fax 415-655-3281.

For sales inquiries and special prices for bulk quantities, please contact our Sales department at 415-655-3200 or write to the address above.

For information on using IDG Books Worldwide's books in the classroom or for ordering examination copies, please contact our Educational Sales department at 800-434-2086 or fax 817-251-8174.

For press review copies, author interviews, or other publicity information, please contact our Public Relations department at 415-655-3000 or fax 415-655-3299.

For authorization to photocopy items for corporate, personal, or educational use, please contact Copyright Clearance Center, 222 Rosewood Drive, Danvers, MA 01923, or fax 508-750-4470.

is a trademark under exclusive license to IDG Books Worldwide, Inc., from International Data Group, Inc.

About the Authors

Suzanne Schlosberg

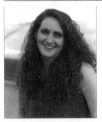

Suzanne Schlosberg's writing career began with a fluke assignment her freshman year in college. She happened into the college newspaper office one afternoon to find the sports editor frantic: An NBA game was about to start and the scheduled reporter had called in sick. Three hours later, Suzanne was conducting post-game interviews with a half dozen naked, 7-foot basketball players. She decided she liked this writing stuff.

Suzanne went on to become a features reporter for the *Daily News* of Los Angeles and a senior editor at *Shape* magazine. She is currently a contributing editor to *Health*. Suzanne has bicycled across the United States twice and has chronicled these and other fitness adventures in newspapers and national magazines. She is the author of *The Ultimate Workout Log* and co-author of *Kathy Smith's Fitness Makeover*. She also is known for her humor pieces that appear in the *Los Angeles Times*.

Suzanne lives in Orinda, California, where she lifts weights and rides her bike regularly. Although she enjoys Northern California, she has remained true to her Los Angeles roots, which means that she drives her sport utility vehicle to her health club — a .8 mile roundtrip.

Liz Neporent

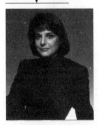

Liz Neporent is a certified trainer and president of Frontline Fitness, a corporate fitness consulting company in New York City. Her job is to make sure the fitness centers for such prestigious companies as Salomon Brothers Inc., Scholastic Inc., and Prudential Securities have the right kind of weight machines, the best classes, and the appropriate number of toilets.

Liz holds a Master's degree in exercise physiology and is certified by the American Council on Exercise, the American College of Sports Medicine, and the National Strength and Conditioning Association. She is the co-author of *Buns of Steel: Total Body Workout, Abs of Steel,* and *Crunch Fitness.* She's also a frequent contributor to *Shape, Fitness,* and *Family Circle.* She appears regularly on TV and radio as an authority on exercise.

Liz has run exactly 48 miles a week for twenty-two years and has competed in more than 20 marathons and ultra-marathons. At one point Liz had 40 jump ropes, 32 dumbbells, four stationary bikes, and a VersaClimber crammed into her New York apartment. She recently whittled this down to 16 dumbbells, two jump ropes, one bike, one dog, and one husband, Jay Shafran.

ABOUT IDG BOOKS WORLDWIDE

Welcome to the world of IDG Books Worldwide.

IDG Books Worldwide, Inc., is a subsidiary of International Data Group, the world's largest publisher of computer-related information and the leading global provider of information services on information technology. IDG was founded more than 25 years ago and now employs more than 8,500 people worldwide. IDG publishes more than 275 computer publications in over 75 countries (see listing below). More than 60 million people read one or more IDG publications each month.

Launched in 1990, IDG Books Worldwide is today the #1 publisher of best-selling computer books in the United States. We are proud to have received eight awards from the Computer Press Association in recognition of editorial excellence and three from *Computer Currents'* First Annual Readers' Choice Awards. Our best-selling *...For Dummies*® series has more than 30 million copies in print with translations in 30 languages. IDG Books Worldwide, through a joint venture with IDG's Hi-Tech Beijing, became the first U.S. publisher to publish a computer book in the People's Republic of China. In record time, IDG Books Worldwide has become the first choice for millions of readers around the world who want to learn how to better manage their businesses.

Our mission is simple: Every one of our books is designed to bring extra value and skill-building instructions to the reader. Our books are written by experts who understand and care about our readers. The knowledge base of our editorial staff comes from years of experience in publishing, education, and journalism — experience we use to produce books for the '90s. In short, we care about books, so we attract the best people. We devote special attention to details such as audience, interior design, use of icons, and illustrations. And because we use an efficient process of authoring, editing, and desktop publishing our books electronically, we can spend more time ensuring superior content and spend less time on the technicalities of making books.

You can count on our commitment to deliver high-quality books at competitive prices on topics you want to read about. At IDG Books Worldwide, we continue in the IDG tradition of delivering quality for more than 25 years. You'll find no better book on a subject than one from IDG Books Worldwide.

John J. Kilcullen

John Kilcullen
President and CEO
IDG Books Worldwide, Inc.

Eighth Annual Computer Press Awards ≥1992

Ninth Annual Computer Press Awards ≥1993

Tenth Annual Computer Press Awards ≥1994

Eleventh Annual Computer Press Awards ≥1995

IDG Books Worldwide, Inc., is a subsidiary of International Data Group, the world's largest publisher of computer-related information and the leading global provider of information services on information technology. International Data Group publishes over 275 computer publications in over 75 countries. Sixty million people read one or more International Data Group publications each month. International Data Group's publications include: **ARGENTINA:** Buyer's Guide, Computerworld Argentina, PC World Argentina; **AUSTRALIA:** Australian Macworld, Australian PC World, Australian Reseller News, Computerworld, IT Casebook, Network World, Publish, Webmaster; **AUSTRIA:** Computerwelt Osterreich, Networks Austria, PC Tip Austria; **BANGLADESH:** PC World Bangladesh; **BELARUS:** PC World Belarus; **BELGIUM:** Data News; **BRAZIL:** Annuário de Informática, Computerworld, Connections, Macworld, PC Player, PC World, Publish, Reseller News, Supergamepower; **BULGARIA:** Computerworld Bulgaria, Network World Bulgaria, PC & MacWorld Bulgaria; **CANADA:** CIO Canada, Client/Server World, ComputerWorld Canada, InfoWorld Canada, NetworkWorld Canada, WebWorld; **CHILE:** Computerworld Chile, PC World Chile; **COLOMBIA:** Computerworld Colombia, PC World Colombia; **COSTA RICA:** PC World Centro America; **THE CZECH AND SLOVAK REPUBLICS:** Computerworld Czechoslovakia, Macworld Czech Republic, PC World Czechoslovakia; **DENMARK:** Communications World Danmark, Computerworld Danmark, Macworld Danmark, PC World Danmark, Techworld Denmark; **DOMINICAN REPUBLIC:** PC World Republica Dominicana; **ECUADOR:** PC World Ecuador; **EGYPT:** Computerworld Middle East, PC World Middle East; **EL SALVADOR:** PC World Centro America; **FINLAND:** MikroPC, Tietoverkko, Tietoviikko; **FRANCE:** Distributique, Hebdo, Info PC, Le Monde Informatique, Macworld, Reseaux & Telecoms, WebMaster France; **GERMANY:** Computer Partner, Computerwoche, Computerwoche Extra, Computerwoche FOCUS, Global Online, Macwelt, PC Welt; **GREECE:** Amiga Computing, GamePro Greece, Multimedia World; **GUATEMALA:** PC World Centro America; **HONDURAS:** PC World Centro America; **HONG KONG:** Computerworld Hong Kong, PC World Hong Kong, Publish in Asia; **HUNGARY:** ABCD CD-ROM, Computerworld Szamitastechnika, Internetto online Magazine, PC World Hungary, PC-X Magazin Hungary; **ICELAND:** Tolvuheimur PC World Island; **INDIA:** Information Communications World, Information Systems Computerworld, PC World India, Publish in Asia; **INDONESIA:** InfoKomputer PC World, Komputek Computerworld, Publish in Asia; **IRELAND:** ComputerScope, PC Live!; **ISRAEL:** Macworld Israel, People & Computers/Computerworld; **ITALY:** Computerworld Italia, Macworld Italia, Networking Italia, PC World Italia; **JAPAN:** DTP World, Macworld Japan, Nikkei Personal Computing, OS/2 World Japan, SunWorld Japan, Windows NT World, Windows World Japan; **KENYA:** PC World East African; **KOREA:** Hi-Tech Information, Macworld Korea, PC World Korea; **MACEDONIA:** PC World Macedonia; **MALAYSIA:** Computerworld Malaysia, PC World Malaysia, Publish in Asia; **MALTA:** PC World Malta; **MEXICO:** Computerworld Mexico, PC World Mexico; **MYANMAR:** PC World Myanmar; **NETHERLANDS:** Computer! Totaal, LAN Internetworking Magazine, LAN World Buyers Guide, Macworld Netherlands, Net, WebWereld; **NEW ZEALAND:** Absolute Beginners Guide and Plain & Simple Series, Computer Buyer, Computer Industry Directory, Computerworld New Zealand, MTB, Network World, PC World New Zealand; **NICARAGUA:** PC World Centro America; **NORWAY:** Computerworld Norge, CW Rapport, Datamagasinet, Financial Rapport, Kursguide Norge, Macworld Norge, Multimediaworld Norge, PC World Ekspress Norge, PC World Nettverk, PC World Norge, PC World ProduktGuide Norge; **PAKISTAN:** Computerworld Pakistan; **PANAMA:** PC World Panama; **PEOPLE'S REPUBLIC OF CHINA:** China Computer Users, China Computerworld, China InfoWorld, China Telecom World Weekly, Computer & Communication, Electronic Design China, Electronics Today, Electronics Weekly, Game Software, PC World China, Popular Computer Week, Software Weekly, Software World, Telecom World; **PERU:** Computerworld Peru, PC World Profesional Peru, PC World SoHo Peru; **PHILIPPINES:** Click!, Computerworld Philippines, PC World in Asia; **POLAND:** Computerworld Poland, Computerworld Special Report Poland, Cyber, Macworld Poland, Networld Poland, PC World Komputer; **PORTUGAL:** Cerebro/PC World, Computerworld/Correio Informático, Dealer World Portugal, Mac*In/PC*In Portugal, Multimedia World; **PUERTO RICO:** PC World Puerto Rico; **ROMANIA:** Computerworld Romania, PC World Romania, Telecom Romania; **RUSSIA:** Computerworld Russia, Mir PK, Publish, Seti; **SINGAPORE:** Computerworld Singapore, PC World Singapore, Publish in Asia; **SLOVENIA:** Monitor; **SOUTH AFRICA:** Computing SA, Network World SA, Software World SA; **SPAIN:** Communicaciones World España, Computerworld España, Dealer World España, Macworld España, PC World España; **SRI LANKA:** Infolink PC World; **SWEDEN:** CAP&Design, Computer Sweden, Corporate Computing Sweden, Internetworld Sweden, it.branschen, Macworld Sweden, MaxiData Sweden, MikroDatorn, Nätverk & Kommunikation, PC World Sweden, PCaktiv, Windows World Sweden; **SWITZERLAND:** Computerworld Schweiz, Macworld Schweiz, PCtip; **TAIWAN:** Computerworld Taiwan, Macworld Taiwan, NEW ViSiON/Publish, PC World Taiwan, Windows World Taiwan; **THAILAND:** Publish in Asia, Thai Computerworld; **TURKEY:** Computerworld Turkiye, Macworld Turkiye, Network World Turkiye, PC World Turkiye; **UKRAINE:** Computerworld Kiev, Multimedia World Ukraine, PC World Ukraine; **UNITED KINGDOM:** Acorn User UK, Amiga Action UK, Amiga Computing UK, Apple Talk UK, Computing, Macworld, Parents and Computers UK, PC Advisor, PC Home, PSX Pro, The WEB; **UNITED STATES:** Cable in the Classroom, CIO Magazine, Computerworld, DOS World, Federal Computer Week, GamePro Magazine, InfoWorld, I-Way, Macworld, Network World, PC Games, PC World, Publish, Video Event, THE WEB Magazine, and WebMaster; online webzines: JavaWorld, NetscapeWorld, and SunWorld Online; **URUGUAY:** InfoWorld Uruguay; **VENEZUELA:** Computerworld Venezuela, PC World Venezuela; and **VIETNAM:** PC World Vietnam. 10/22/96

Acknowledgments

From Suzanne:

Extra-special thanks to Dana Sullivan, Nancy Kruh, and Hayes Jackson for their fast and brilliant editing; to Judy Schlosberg and Teri Breuer for their careful proofreading; and to Tina Gerson and Chris Grisanti for graciously donating photos to this book. You guys deserve the big bucks. In the meantime, I hope dinner and a movie will suffice.

I'm grateful to my agent, Felicia Eth, for her persistence. Thanks, also, to Grace Garne, Brad Kearns, Richard Motzkin, and Laurie Muggee for sharing their knowledge and advice. I'm lucky to have such a loving family and helpful friends. I especially want to thank my parents, my grandparents, my sister, and Alec Boga for their constant encouragement and Nancy Gottesman for always being available when I wanted to procrastinate.

I reserve my greatest thanks for Liz Neporent, who had no idea what she was getting into when she agreed to be my co-author. Thanks, Liz, for your great ideas, your long hours, and your wake-up calls. Stick to being a trainer and writer; you will not cut it as a concierge.

From Liz:

Many thanks to my two Frontline partners, Jay Shafran and Bob Welter, for picking up the slack and spurring me on during the writing of this and previous books. In fact, many thanks to the entire Frontline gang, with special emphasis to Holly Byrne, Nancy Ngai, Terry Certain, and Terry King, the terrific managers who leave me with (almost) nothing to worry about, except for an occasional mouse in the aerobics room. I'm also indebted to photographers Dan Kron and Richard Lee for going way beyond the call of duty.

My terrific parents, grandmother, mother-in-law, and various brothers and sisters have also been extremely encouraging and helpful, and so has my good friend Patty Buttenheim. Eli Jacobson has been kind enough to impart to me everything he knows about exercise and tax law — he knows a great deal about one of those subjects.

Finally, special thanks to Suzanne Schlosberg, my co-author, some-time editor, and friend who drags me kicking and screaming through every assignment yet somehow manages to make me look good.

Publisher's Acknowledgments

We're proud of this book; please send us your comments about it by using the Reader Response Card at the back of the book or by e-mailing us at feedback/dummies@idgbooks.com. Some of the people who helped bring this book to market include the following:

Acquisitions, Development, & Editorial

Project Editor: Bill Helling

Acquisitions Editor: Sarah Kennedy, Executive Editor

Copy Editor: Suzanne Packer

Technical Reviewers: Edmund R. Burke, Ph.D.; Holly Anne Byrne; Ralph LaForge, M.S.; Susan Taman Levy, M.S., R.D.; Timothy J. Moore; Lloyd R. Hines, M.S.; Patricia M. Buttenheim, R.N., M.A.

Editorial Manager: Mary C. Corder

Editorial Assistant: Ann Miller

Production

Project Coordinator: Debbie Sharpe

Layout and Graphics: E. Shawn Aylsworth, Brett Black, Elizabeth Cárdenas-Nelson, J. Tyler Connor, Cheryl Denski, Todd Klemme, Jenny Shoemake, M. Anne Sipahimalani, Michael Sullivan, Gina Scott, Angela F. Hunckler, Kate Snell, Tricia R. Reynolds

Proofreaders: Betty Kish, Christine Meloy Beck, Nancy Price, Carl Saff, Robert Springer, Carrie Voorhis

Indexer: Liz Cunningham

Special Help: Jamie Klobuchar

General and Administrative

IDG Books Worldwide, Inc.: John Kilcullen, CEO; Steven Berkowitz, President and Publisher

Dummies, Inc.: Milissa Koloski, Executive Vice President and Publisher

Dummies Technology Press and Dummies Editorial: Diane Graves Steele, Vice President and Associate Publisher; Judith A. Taylor, Brand Manager

Dummies Trade Press: Kathleen A. Welton, Vice President and Publisher; Stacy S. Collins, Brand Manager

IDG Books Production for Dummies Press: Beth Jenkins, Production Director; Cindy L. Phipps, Supervisor of Project Coordination; Kathie S. Schutte, Supervisor of Page Layout; Shelley Lea, Supervisor of Graphics and Design; Debbie J. Gates, Production Systems Specialist; Tony Augsburger, Reprint Coordinator; Leslie Popplewell, Media Archive Coordinator

Dummies Packaging and Book Design: Patti Sandez, Packaging Assistant; Kavish+Kavish, Cover Design

◆

The publisher would like to give special thanks to Patrick J. McGovern, without whom this book would not have been possible.

◆

Contents at a Glance

Cartoons at a Glance

By Rich Tennant • Fax: 508-546-7747 • E-mail: the5wave@tiac.net

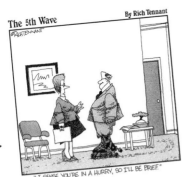

page 225

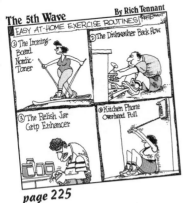

page 263

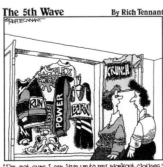

page 71

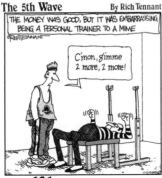

page 131

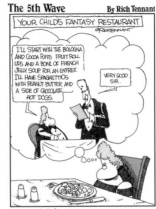

page 326

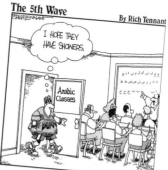

page 181

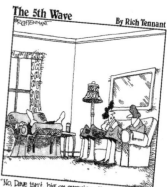

page 7

Table of Contents

Foreword

· ·

*W*hen it comes to staying in shape, top athletes think they know everything. At least I did. Back when I was playing college ball, I figured that
the best way to pack on muscle was to eat a lot of fat. My idea of the Food
Pyramid was to stack a cheeseburger on top of a double cheeseburger.

As soon as I was drafted into the NBA, the trainers set me straight on a lot of
things. Now, I'm more of a chicken and turkey man. Not only that, but I actually
stretch after every workout, and I use the StairMaster to increase my stamina.
All of this enlightenment has improved my game from a conditioning standpoint.

But the truth is, I still have a lot to learn about fitness. That's why I'm so excited
that Suzanne Schlosberg and Liz Neporent have created *Fitness For Dummies.*
Not only is this book remarkably comprehensive, but it's a lot of fun, too.
Suzanne and Liz have a light, easy style that grabs your attention and makes
you want to keep reading.

Fitness For Dummies couldn't have been published at a better time. Consumers
are more overwhelmed than ever with fitness choices: exercise gadgets, health
clubs, diet plans, workout programs, and so on. People tell me all the time that
they feel confused by all of the options. This is why *Fitness For Dummies* is so
valuable. Suzanne and Liz cut right to the chase about what works and what
doesn't. Fitness novices will be grateful to own this book, but fitness veterans
have plenty to gain from it, too. I learned something new in just about every
chapter. (Now I know what the Food Pyramid really is.)

It has truly been an honor for me, as a guard, to write the foreword for this
book. Remember, the best thing you can do when you feel a little dumb is to
educate yourself!

Charlie Ward

Heisman Trophy winner and NBA point guard

Introduction

• •

*W*hen you saw *Fitness For Dummies* on the shelf, you probably thought, *"Another* fitness book? This country needs another fitness book like it needs another daytime talk show."

But you picked up this book, sensing it was different. And it is. You already know that exercise will make you look better, feel better, and live longer, so we don't spend a whole lot of time telling you that. With *Fitness For Dummies,* we do something more important: We tackle your fears. Maybe you're afraid of struggling to lift a 3-pound weight when the guy next to you is hoisting a 70-pound dumbbell like it's a beer mug. Maybe you worry that operating a stairclimber requires a degree in mechanical engineering. Maybe you're afraid that no matter what exercise routine you start, sooner or later you'll end up back in the recliner.

Fitness For Dummies gives you the tools to ease these fears. You won't find a 30-day exercise routine here. Instead, you'll learn how to spot a good routine when you see one — whether it's at a health club, on TV, or in a book, magazine, or video. You'll learn how to find a qualified exercise instructor and how to choose the right equipment to meet your goals. You'll learn strategies to combat exercise boredom and to keep going when it would be easier to just put your feet up.

This book tells you the stuff you really want to know, such as

- How do you know if you have too much body fat?
- Does exercise really have to hurt?
- Are those infomercial gadgets worth "three easy payments of $19.95"?
- Can you fit exercise into a life already filled with a job and kids?
- Are celebrity videos any good?
- Is it true that exercise can speed up your metabolism?
- Can you actually become "Rock Solid in 6 Weeks," like the magazines say?
- Is it better join a health club or work out at home?
- Can you get fat on fat-free foods?
- Will exercise ever be fun?

We don't want you to become a fitness statistic. The fact is, among people who start an exercise program, half quit within eight weeks. *Fitness For Dummies* will give you the knowledge to make sure that *you* stick with fitness for the rest of your life.

How to Use This Book

You can use this book in two ways:

- If you want a crash course in fitness, read the book cover-to-cover. You'll get a thorough understanding of what it takes to get in shape. And you'll come across topics you might not have thought to look up, such as proper etiquette in the gym and how to judge the accuracy of fitness reports in the media.

- If you want to learn about a specific topic, such as choosing a health club or buying an exercise bike for your home, you can flip to that section and get your answers right away. Use the book as a reference every time you boldly enter uncharted territory, like a body-sculpting class or the exercise aisle at your video store. *Fitness For Dummies* is basic enough for the fitness rookie to understand, but this book is also useful for workout veterans who want to learn about the latest fitness concepts, gadgets, or training techniques.

How This Book Is Organized

Fitness For Dummies is divided into six parts. The chapters within each part cover specific topic areas in detail. You can read each chapter or part without having to read what came before, although we may refer you to other sections for more information about certain topics. Here's a brief look at the six parts.

Part I: Getting Your Butt off the Couch

In this part, we give you the tools — and the inspiration — to get started on a fitness program. We explain the important first steps, such as getting your fitness tested, pinpointing *why* you want to get in shape, and setting realistic goals. Then we offer strategies for sticking with your exercise plan. This part also includes a chapter on nutrition basics, so you know from the get-go that revamping your eating habits is a crucial step toward getting fit.

Part II: Working Your Heart

This part is devoted to *aerobic* exercise—the type of exercise that strengthens your heart and lungs, burns lots of calories, lowers your stress level, and gives you the energy to chase down your cat for his monthly bath. We tell you how long, how often, and how hard you need to work out in order to lose fat and live longer. We cover your major aerobic options, both indoor and outdoor, and offer tips on how to combat boredom when you're walking, climbing, or pedaling in place.

Part III: Building Strength

In this part we explain why everyone—whether you're 18 years old or 80, male or female—ought to be lifting weight. We give you the know-how to get started and answer questions such as, What's the difference between weight machines, dumbbells, and barbells? How much weight should I lift? How many exercises should I do? What's a deltoid, and why should I care?

Part IV: Braving the Gym

Walking into a health club can be a terrifying proposition, sort of like landing cold in some foreign country where you don't know a soul, don't speak the language, don't know the customs, and feel like everyone's staring at you. This part gives you the information you need to enter a gym with confidence. We explain how to choose a good club and a qualified trainer, we fill you in on locker room etiquette, and we tell you how to get through an exercise class when you feel like you have two left feet that are tied together.

Part V: Exercising at Home

Health clubs aren't for everyone, so we devote this part of the book to helping you choose the best fitness equipment for your budget, your goals, and the size of your living room. We cover a wide range of equipment, from space-age stairclimbers to $3 rubber exercise tubes. We offer tips for designing your home gym so that you'll actually use the stuff you buy, and we warn you about the schlocky gizmos out there in TV-land.

Part VI: The Part of Tens

Every ...*For Dummies* book has a Part of Tens. These chapters give you a different spin on some of the information already presented in the other parts. For instance, scattered throughout the book are mentions of excellent, low-priced fitness products; in Chapter 22, "Ten Great Fitness Investments under $100," we tell you which of these products we consider to be the *best* bargains. In Chapter 23, "Ten Fitness Rip-Offs," we give you our picks for the *worst* fitness products. The Part of Tens also includes topics we don't discuss elsewhere, such as how to stay fit when you travel, how to exercise safely when you're pregnant, and how to nurse yourself back from a pulled muscle.

Icons Used in This Book

This icon signals the use of fancy fitness terminology, like "target training zone" and "body composition." We think it should be a felony for fitness instructors to use terms like "contraindicated joint action," but some exercise jargon is actually useful to know about.

This icon highlights first-rate fitness products, from treadmills to water bottles to nutrition newsletters. The phone numbers for these products are listed in Appendix A.

This icon warns you about hucksters who offer false promises, sell bogus products, or try to snare you with slimy sales tactics. We also use this icon to caution you about common exercise mistakes, such as neglecting to adjust the seat on an exercise machine.

We use our Myth Buster superhero to dispel popular fitness myths. For instance, in Chapter 5, we explain that exercise doesn't have to hurt in order to be good for you. In Chapter 16, we explain that you can't sweat off excess fat by wearing vinyl workout suits.

We use this icon when we tell a story about our own adventures in fitness or recount the experiences of people we know. The anecdotes range from the wacky to the inspirational to the just plain helpful.

This icon flags great strategies for getting in shape, such as recording your workouts in a daily log. We also use the target for money-saving tips, such as asking your health club to waive its initiation fee.

This icon appears beside discussions that aren't critical if you want to learn exercise basics. But reading these sections will deepen your fitness knowledge and will come in handy if you find yourself at a dinner party with a bunch of personal trainers.

Part I
Getting Your Butt off the Couch

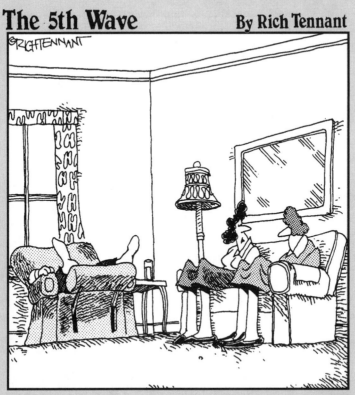

The 5th Wave   By Rich Tennant

"No, Dave isn't big on exercise. About once every 3 years we take him to the doctors and have his pores surgically opened."

In this part . . .

We help you get going on a fitness program — no matter what shape you're in. Chapter 1 explains the important first step: getting your fitness evaluated, either at home or by a professional. Chapter 2 helps you devise a game plan: You learn to set goals, track your progress, and use strategies to make exercise a habit. Chapter 3 covers one of the best of these strategies: educating yourself through magazines, books, and the Internet. Chapter 4 fills you in on nutrition basics. You get the lowdown on fat, protein, carbohydrates, vitamins, and minerals — and you learn whatever happened to the Four Food Groups.

Chapter 1

Testing Your Fitness

- -

In This Chapter

▶ How healthy are you?

▶ What is your heart rate and blood pressure?

▶ How much of you is fat?

▶ How strong are your muscles?

▶ How flexible are your joints?

▶ How fit are your heart and lungs?

- -

*W*e've never been fond of tests that you can't study for, or at least cheat on. Nevertheless, we think the first step toward getting in shape is having your fitness evaluated. Don't panic. This test isn't like your driver's license renewal exam: You can't flunk, and you don't have to stand in line for three hours listening to people rant and rave about government bureaucracy. A fitness test simply gives you key information about your physical condition.

We constantly hear people say, "I'm so out of shape. I need to lose weight." But that's like telling a travel agent, "I'm in Europe. I need to go to Africa." Your travel agent needs to know the specifics: Are you in Rome? Berlin? Moscow? Do you want to go to Cairo? Cape Town? The Kalahari desert? Before you embark on a fitness program, you need to know your starting point with the same sort of precision. A *fitness evaluation* gives you important departure information, such as your heart rate, body fat, strength, and flexibility. Armed with these facts, you or your trainer can design an intelligent plan to get you to your fitness destination. And when you get there, you'll have the numbers to prove just how far you've come.

In this chapter, we describe what to expect when you get your fitness tested by a professional so that you can evaluate your tester while he's evaluating *you*. We also explain how to test your fitness on your own. However, even if you do most of the testing yourself, consider getting certain aspects of your fitness tested at a sports medicine clinic or fitness center. As you complete the various fitness tests, record your results on the chart found in Appendix B.

Questions about Your Health

When you join a gym, one of the first things that you should be asked to do — after signing your check, of course — is to fill out a "health history questionnaire." This is a list of questions designed to give a snapshot of your overall well-being, including your eating and exercise habits, your risk for developing cardiovascular disease, and any orthopedic limitations or significant medical conditions that you might have. Typical questions include: Do you have any chronic joint problems such as arthritis? Do you have a high stress level? Are you currently taking any over-the-counter or prescription medications?

If you don't belong to a gym, ask yourself the following questions, which are designed to indicate your risk of developing heart disease:

- Are you inactive?
- Do you have a history of heart disease?
- Do you have diabetes or high blood sugar?
- Do you have a history of high blood pressure?
- Did your mother, father, sister, or brother develop any form of heart disease before age 50?
- Do you smoke cigarettes or have you quit within the last two years?
- Do you have high cholesterol, either total cholesterol higher than 200 mg/dl or HDL less than 35 mg/dl?

If you answered "yes" to at least one question and you're over age 35, see a physician for a complete *medical* evaluation before you even pursue a *fitness* testing session. A physician is the only one who can accurately determine if exercising puts you in any danger. If you answered yes to two or more questions, get a check up no matter how old you are.

Some gyms may request that you be tested by a physician if a staff member feels you may have a medical problem. Don't look upon this request as a giant pain in the butt. In fact, a request like this should tell you that your gym is on the ball. Some health clubs, including many of the larger chains, just want your money. They may require no testing at all — other than the test that determines whether you can sign your name on a credit-card slip. If that's the case, you need to take responsibility for getting tested.

After you fill out your questionnaire, your tester should discuss the answers with you and ask for more information if necessary. If you're a smoker, for instance, he might ask you how much you smoke. Respond honestly and thoroughly. Don't say that you run five miles a day if you haven't run since high school — or if you *intend* to run every day but just haven't gotten around to it.

Let your tester be the judge of what's important. We know two men who neglected to tell their tester that they'd each had a lung removed. Another man we know somehow forgot to mention the minor heart attack he'd suffered the week before. Hey, these things matter.

Measuring Your Heart Rate

Your *heart rate,* also known as your *pulse,* is the number of times your heart beats per minute. Your fitness evaluation should include a measure of your *resting heart rate,* which, logically enough, is your heart rate at rest — when you're sitting still. Ideally, your resting heart rate should be between 60 and 90 beats per minute. It may be slower if you're athletic or genetically predisposed to a low heart rate; it may be faster if you're nervous or have recently downed three double cappuccinos. In addition to caffeine, stress and certain over-the-counter medications can speed up your heart rate.

After a month or two of regular exercise, your resting heart rate usually drops. This means that your heart has become more efficient. It may need to beat only 80 times per minute to pump the same amount of blood (or more) than it used to pump in 90 beats. This is good because in the long run, you'll save wear and tear on your heart.

The simplest place to take your own pulse is at your wrist. Rest your middle and index fingertips lightly on your opposite wrist, directly below the base of your thumb. Most people can see the faint bluish line of their *radial artery;* place your fingertips here. Count the beats for a full minute. Or if you have a short attention span, count for 30 seconds and multiply by 2.

Taking Your Blood Pressure

Your blood pressure is a measurement that you should have tested by a professional. Home blood pressure equipment tends to be inaccurate — and so do those machines in the mall that cost a quarter.

Blood pressure is a measurement of how open your blood vessels are. Low numbers mean that your heart doesn't have to work very hard to pump the blood through your blood vessels. Ideally, your blood pressure should read 120/80 or below. If your blood pressure is slightly higher, don't get stressed (that'll only increase it even more). However, if your blood pressure is higher than 145/95, you are considered *hypertensive,* a fancy term for having high blood pressure. In case you're wondering, the top number, called your *systolic* blood pressure, measures pressure as your heart ejects blood. The bottom number, your *diastolic* blood pressure, measures pressure when your heart relaxes and prepares for its next pump.

If you get a high blood pressure reading, ask your tester to try again. The numbers can be affected by many factors, such as illness, caffeine, nervousness, or racing into your test because you were late. But if you repeatedly get high readings, see a doctor.

How Fit Is Your Heart?

Most reputable clubs perform something called a *submax* test. That's short for submaximal test, which is fitness jargon for a test that evaluates your heart rate when you're working at less than your maximum effort. Typically, this takes you to about 75 to 85 percent of your maximum. A maximal test — in which you go all-out — should only be performed by a physician or in the presence of a physician.

Submaximal tests are usually given by a trainer, exercise physiologist, or physician and are performed on a stationary bicycle. Some gyms may perform these tests on a treadmill or on a stairclimber. (If you're a runner, request a treadmill test; if you're a cyclist, take the test on a stationary bike. You're best at what you practice most.) The test usually lasts about 15 minutes. During this time, you increase your intensity every 3 or 4 minutes while the tester monitors your heart rate and blood pressure.

Overall, the test shouldn't be very hard. On a bike, the worst it should feel like is pedaling up a moderately steep hill for a few minutes. The hardest part is keeping the bike at the exact speed the tester asks you to keep it at.

A conscientious tester will help you use the results of your submax test to customize a whole aerobic training program (for more tips on designing an aerobic program, see Chapter 5). Some gyms make a big fanfare of testing, but then they just file away the results without using them as a tool to help fine-tune your workout program.

Here's a simple way to test your aerobic fitness on your own. All you need is a watch with a second hand and a course that's exactly one mile long. Warm up with a slow walk for 5 to 10 minutes, and then time yourself as you walk the mile as briskly as you can. (Walking one mile should take between 10 and 25 minutes.) Take your pulse right before you stop, and make a mental note of it. Also note your time as you complete your mile.

One minute after you finish the mile, take your pulse again (this number is called your *recovery heart rate*). See how far your pulse has dropped from the pulse check you did right at the end of your walk. Try this test again in two months and see how much faster you can walk the mile and how much more quickly you recover. If a mile sounds like too much for you right now, do a half mile or even walk around the block. Just make it a distance that you can remeasure at a later date.

How Much of You Is Fat?

During your evaluation, your tester will — and should — weigh you. Just realize that knowing your weight is of limited value. When you hop on a scale, you learn the grand total weight of your bones, organs, blood, fat, muscle, and other tissues. This number can be misleading because muscle weighs more per square inch than fat.

For instance, let's consider two men who stand 5-foot-8 and weigh 190 pounds. One guy might be a lean bodybuilder who happens to have a lot of muscle packed onto his frame. Another guy might be a couch potato whose gut hangs four inches over his belt buckle. Even a low weight doesn't necessarily indicate good health or fitness. It may simply mean that you have small bones and very little muscle.

Because your weight can be misleading, knowing your *body composition* is helpful. This is the not-so-exact science of determining how much of your body is composed of fat and how much of it is composed of *lean body tissue,* the sum of everything else. Your body composition is also called your *body-fat percentage.* If you score a 20 percent on a fat test, this means, naturally, that 20 percent of your weight is composed of fat.

What to do with your results

At the end of your fitness evaluation, make sure your tester doesn't just file away the results in a drawer. He should sit down with you and explain what the results *mean*. It's not enough for him to say, "Well, your resting heart rate is 72, you did 23 sit-ups, and your body fat is 28 percent." He should explain how your results stack up against other people who are your age and your gender, and he should tell you which areas need the most improvement.

All of this information should be detailed on a piece of paper (sort of like a report card) that you can take home. Save this piece of paper so you can see how much you've improved later. One day, it might mean more to you than your high school diploma.

Schedule a second fitness evaluation in six weeks. Those first weeks of training can bring about some dramatic changes, and it's really motivating to see how well you've done. After that, changes are steady but somewhat slower. Get tested again every three to six months. Don't go longer than a year without reevaluating your progress. You don't want to waste time with a workout program that's not getting results.

Your body fat percentage is not necessarily a measure of your health. It's true that cardiovascular disease, diabetes, and certain cancers are more prevalent among overweight people — men who have more than 20 percent body fat and women who have more than 30 percent. However, some researchers now believe that, in many cases, these health problems are not caused by the extra fat itself but rather by a lack of exercise and a poor diet. In other words, if you exercise regularly and eat well, extra body fat won't compromise your health. This is an area of controversy, but researchers do seem to agree on one issue: a fat belly carries more of a health risk than hefty thighs. (In fact, some experts maintain that below-the-belt fat poses no disease risk at all, even if a woman far exceeds the 30 percent fat mark.)

Despite the controversy, we think it's worth getting your body fat tested as part of your fitness evaluation. More than your weight, your body fat results can let you know how your fat-loss and exercise program is coming along. For instance, your scale can tell you that you lost 7 pounds. But a body fat test can tell you that a 7-pound loss might mean you lost 10 pounds of fat and gained 3 pounds of muscle — results that are probably more motivating.

Body fat testing also can tell you if you have too little fat. Maybe you can never be too rich, but you definitely can be too thin. For women, super-low body fat can lead to problems such as irregular menstrual periods, permanent bone loss, and a high rate of bone fractures.

Don't become neurotic about the results of your body fat test the way people become obsessed with their weight. Your tester probably will tell you that the ideal score for a woman is between 16 percent and 26 percent, and for a man the ideal range is 12 percent to 18 percent. (Much of the extra fat in women is used to pad reproductive organs.) However, if you score above this range, don't assume that you're unfit or in poor health. Body fat is just one tool you can use to assess your progress. Later in this chapter, we discuss several other indicators of health and fitness. You need to consider all of these indicators together.

Keep in mind that every body fat testing method has room for error. Even the best methods aren't extremely precise. In other words, if you're getting audited by the IRS, you'd better hope that your financial records are more accurate than your body fat test results. You might score a 24 percent using one method and a 29 percent using another. You might even get wildly different readings using the *same* test, depending on the skill of the tester or the condition of the equipment. The only way you can measure body fat with complete accuracy is to burn yourself up and take a carbon count of the ashes. Because that technique doesn't draw too many volunteers, scientists have developed a number of other methods. Here's a look at ones you're most likely to come across.

Pinch an inch

The most common body fat test uses the *skinfold caliper,* a gizmo that resembles a stun gun with salad tongs attached (see Figure 1-1). When your tester fires, the tongs pinch your skin, pulling your fat away from your muscles and bones. (You feel moderate discomfort, like when your great aunt pinches your cheek on the holidays.) A gauge on the caliper measures the thickness of the this hunk of fat. Typically, the tester pinches three to seven different sites on your body, such as your abdomen, the back of your arm, your thigh, your hip, and the back of your shoulder. The numbers from each pinch are plugged into a formula to determine your body fat percentage. Your tester should pinch each site two or three times to verify the measurement.

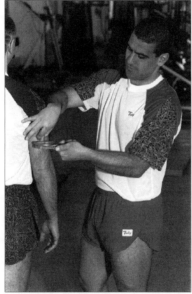

Figure 1-1:
Getting
pinched
with
calipers.

(Photo courtesy of Dan Kron.)

So many things can go wrong with a caliper test. The tester might not pinch exactly the right spot, or he might not pull all of the fat away from the bone. Or he might pinch too hard and accidentally yank some of your muscle. Experts give this test a margin of error of 4 points, meaning your actual body fat percentage could be 4 points higher or lower even when the test is performed properly. Again, don't get too hung up on the specific numbers. Instead, try to focus on *changes* in these numbers from one time to the next. To make the test more reliable, have the same tester perform it each time. Also, get tested *before* your workout. When you exercise, blood travels to your skin to cool you down. This can cause your skin to swell, and you may test fatter than you really are.

A couple of easy home tests

Here's another way to estimate your body fat: Measure your height to the nearest half inch, wrap a tape-measure around the widest part of your hips, and write down the number. Get a ruler and, using the chart in Figure 1-2, run a diagonal line between your hip girth and your height. The point at which the ruler crosses the center line estimates your body fat percentage. If you measure carefully, this number should be fairly close to the results you get from calipers.

Estimating your body fat

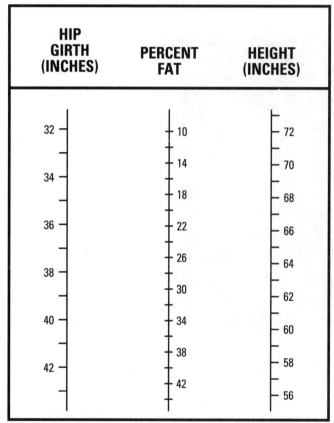

Figure 1-2:
A home test
to measure
body fat.

Human Kinetics Publishers, Inc.
Sensible Fitness, 2nd Edition
Jack Wilmore, Ph.D. CR-1986

A less precise but also helpful way to keep track of your body composition is to take your measurements. You don't get a percentage, but you can use the numbers to keep track of inches lost (or gained, if you're trying to bulk up), which can be motivating in and of itself. If you're losing inches, chances are, you're dropping body fat. Some common places to measure: across the middle of your chest, the center of your upper arm, the smallest part of your waist, the widest part of your hips, the widest part of your thigh, and the widest part of your ankle. You can write these numbers on the chart in Appendix B, "Your Fitness Test Results."

Getting zapped

Another common method of body fat testing is called *bioeletrical impedance*. You lie on your back while a signal travels from an electrode on your foot to an electrode on your hand. The slower the signal, the more fat you have. This is because fat *impedes*, or blocks, the signal. The signal travels quickly through muscle because muscle is 70 percent water and water conducts electricity. Fat, on the other hand, is just 5 percent to 13 percent water.

This test can have a huge margin of error, especially if you're extremely fat or extremely lean. In one study, world-class female distance runners were found to average 20 percent body fat, when actually they were closer to 10 percent. Dehydration also can skew the results wildly. If your body contains less water than usual, the signal will slow down, and you'll appear to have more fat than you really do. Don't drink alcohol or caffeine for at least 24 hours before the test because they can lead to dehydration.

Gyms, hospitals, and health fairs often use variations of this technique. Don't use bioelectrical impedance as your only gauge. Have a caliper test done by an experienced professional, such as a certified trainer or registered dietitian.

Getting dunked

Underwater weighing is the most cumbersome method of body fat testing, but it's also the most accurate. You sit on a scale in a tank of warm water about the size of a Jacuzzi. You basically feel like a giant piece of tortellini floating in a big pot. Then comes the unnerving part: You have to blow *all* the air out of your lungs and bend forward until you're completely submerged. If there's any air trapped in your lungs, the test makes you appear fatter than you really are. Knowing this fact makes you try really, really hard to blow out your air, which makes you feel like you're about to explode. You stay submerged for about five seconds, while your underwater weight registers on a digital scale. The only good part about this whole procedure — for Americans, anyway — is that the scale registers your weight in kilograms, so you have no idea what any of those numbers mean.

Your underwater weight is then plugged into a mathematical equation that determines your body fat. This method of testing is based on the premise that muscle sinks and fat floats. Fat is less dense than water, whereas muscle is more dense. The more fat you have, the more your body wants to float when dunked under water. The denser you are, the more you sink and the more water your body displaces.

The margin of error for this test is 2 percent to $2^1/_2$ percent for young to middle-aged adults. The results are less accurate for children, older adults, and extremely lean people. This is because lean body tissue is made up of other things besides muscle. Bone, for instance, isn't fully formed in children, and it may be somewhat porous in older adults and somewhat denser in superfit people. You can get this test done only at sophisticated sports medicine clinics or labs. It costs about $50 to $100.

Body fat update: The mod pod

Underwater weighing has long been the standard for body fat testing, but a sophisticated new contraption called the BOD POD may one day replace it. The BOD POD is a 5-foot-tall fiberglass chamber that looks like a giant egg with a tinted window. You sit in the chamber for 20 seconds while computerized pressure sensors determine how much air your body displaces — in other words, how much space you take up. (Under water weighing determines the same information, just in a way that's more inconvenient.)

Research suggests that the BOD POD may be as accurate as underwater weighing, but the technology is so new that only a few studies have been conducted. So far the $32,000 machine, manufactured by Life Measurement Instruments, has been sold to a handful of university labs and personal training centers. Some owners are transporting the BOD POD to local health clubs, setting up shop for the day and charging $50 to $100 per test.

How Strong Are You?

Even if the heaviest thing you've lifted lately is a mug of beer, don't worry about strength testing. You're not going to have to do one-arm push-ups or lift some barbell that weighs more than your dad. Strength tests, like the other tests we describe in this chapter, are simply designed to give you a starting point. The results of your strength tests can help you design an appropriate weight-lifting program. You'll find out how much weight you should start with and which muscles need the most attention. For reasons we explain in Chapter 10, most people can gain strength very quickly. If you get started on a good weight-lifting program and stick to it, you're likely to see dramatic changes when you get tested again in two or three months.

Most health clubs don't take true, raw strength measurements; in other words, they don't measure the absolute maximum amount of weight you're capable of lifting. Going for your "max" can be dangerous and can cause more than a little muscle soreness. Instead, health clubs test your muscular endurance: how many times you can move a much lighter weight. You can do many of these tests at home, including the push-up and crunch tests. It helps to have a friend count for you and make sure you're doing the exercise correctly. Here's a look at some of the more common muscular endurance measures.

Your upper body strength

Count how many push-ups you can do without stopping or completely losing good form. For this test, men do the so-called military push-ups, with their legs out straight and toes on the floor. Women do non-military (or modified) pushups, with their knees bent and on the floor; these have been traditionally called female push-ups, but due to the sexist nature of this label, we're not going to use it. Lower your entire body at once until your upper arms are parallel to the floor. Prevent your back from sagging by pulling your abdominals in. We've seen some wacky versions of the push-up. One guy we watched didn't have the strength to lower his body all the way, so he just bobbed his head up and down.

Use the following chart to find out how you stack up against other people of your age and gender. But don't worry if you don't score well. It doesn't really matter where you're starting from as long as you improve. Use the numbers in Tables 1-1 and 1-2 as ballpark figures to aim for.

Table 1-1		Push-Ups—Men			
Age:	**20-29**	**30-39**	**40-49**	**50-59**	**60+**
Excellent	55+	45+	40+	35+	30+
Good	45-54	35-44	30-39	25-34	20-29
Average	35-44	25-34	20-29	15-24	10-19
Fair	20-34	15-24	12-19	8-14	5-9
Low	0-19	0-14	0-11	0-7	0-4

Table 1-2		Push-Ups — Women			
Age:	20-29	30-39	40-49	50-59	60+
Excellent	49+	40+	35+	30+	20+
Good	34-48	25-39	20-34	15-29	5-19
Average	17-33	12-24	8-19	6-14	3-4
Fair	6-16	4-11	3-7	2-5	1-2
Low	0-5	0-3	0-2	0-1	0

Some health clubs also measure upper body strength either on a free-weight bench press or a chest-press machine. (In Chapter 12, we explain the difference between free weights and machines.) Men typically start with 80 pounds, women with 35. But the amount of weight doesn't matter, as long as you use the same weight every time you get tested. You simply do as many repetitions as you can.

Your middle body strength

The strength of your abdominal muscles is usually measured by a sit-up test or a crunch test. A *sit-up test* measures how many *full* sit-ups you can do in one minute. You have your knees bent, and your tester holds your feet down. This test is losing favor among experts, because sit-ups are not a true measure of abdominal strength. (In fact, this test measures abdominal, lower back, *and* hip strength.) Also, full sit-ups can be hard on your lower back. Strength tests are designed to see where you're starting from, *not* to injure you so that you can't even make it to the first workout. If you have a back or neck problem, don't do the sit-up test.

The *crunch test,* which doesn't have a time limit, is more popular because it does measure abdominal strength. However, it's very easy to cheat on and not recommended if you have a history of lower back problems (see Figure 1-3).

Place two pieces of masking tape about half way down the length of a mat, one directly behind the other, about $2\frac{1}{2}$ inches apart. Lie on your back on the mat with your arms at your sides, your finger tips touching the rear edge of the back piece of tape. Bend your knees and place your feet flat on the floor. Curl your head, neck, and shoulder blades upward, sliding your palms along the floor until your finger tips touch the front edge of the front piece of tape. Return to the starting position and keep going until you're too tired to continue or you can't reach the tape. Don't cheat by sliding your arms without moving your body or by moving only one side of your body.

Use Tables 1-3 and 1-4 to gauge the results of your crunch test.

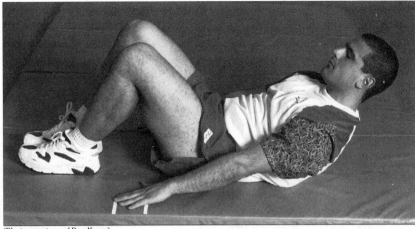

Figure 1-3:
The crunch
test.

(Photo courtesy of Dan Kron.)

Table 1-3		Crunches — Men		
	Age:	Under 35	36-45	Over 45
Excellent		60	50	40
Good		45	40	25
Marginal		30	25	15
Needs work		15	10	5

Table 1-4		Crunches — Women		
	Age:	Under 35	36-45	Over 45
Excellent		50	40	30
Good		40	25	15
Marginal		25	15	10
Needs work		10	6	4

Your lower body strength

The strength of your lower body muscles is often measured on a leg extension
machine, a common health club contraption used to strengthen your front
thigh muscles. (This machine is sort of like a big chair with a high back.) Some
clubs test lower-body strength on other machines. Other clubs skip lower body
testing altogether because it can lead to extreme muscle soreness. We think it's

a good idea to test your leg strength, as long as you don't have knee problems. However, if a club skips this test, there's no need to cancel your membership and storm out of the club in an outrage.

You can test the strength of your thigh and butt muscles at home by doing an exercise called a squat. Women can try this test holding a 5-pound dumbbell in each hand, arms hanging down at their sides. Men can use 15-pound dumbbells. If you're a novice exerciser, you may want to skip the weight and simply place your hands on your hips.

To do a squat, place your feet about hip-width apart and stand up as tall as you can. Bend your knees until your thighs are parallel to the floor and then stand up to the starting position. Make sure you don't "lock" your knees when you stand back up. Do as many squats as you can while maintaining good form. Stop if you start to lose your balance, if you can't keep your heels on the floor, or if you start bending forward.

How Flexible Are You?

How come gymnasts can wrap their legs around their shoulders while you have trouble touching your toes? Because gymnasts are more *flexible* than you are. Flexibility refers to how *far* you can move a joint (your *range of motion*) and how easily you can move it. Because your muscles attach to your joints and are responsible for moving them, flexibility also refers to the mobility of your muscles. If your joints and muscles are inflexible, you are considered *tight*. (In Chapter 7, we explain why this is not good.) The joints most commonly measured during a health club test are the lower back and hips. Many clubs also measure the flexibility of your shoulders, thighs, ankles, wrists, and butt muscles.

Flexibility tests sometimes feel like a cross between circus tryouts and IQ testing. The tester asks you to twist yourself into some strange positions, and you have to figure out what he's talking about. Then you have to see if your body agrees to follow along. Sometimes testers are so used to giving directions that they use confusing shorthand. They might say, "Okay, raise your right leg up, keeping your left leg down and flat against the mat while not allowing your butt to lift off or your back to arch. Now the other side." Huh? Don't be embarrassed to ask for a translation in English.

A really sophisticated way to test flexibility is with an instrument called a *goniometer*. It's a semi-curved ruler that measures in degrees, much like an oversized version of the protractor that you used in high school geometry. To measure your hamstring (rear thigh muscle) flexibility, the tester has you lie on your back and straighten one leg up off the floor as much as you comfortably can. He then holds the goniometer near your butt and measures the number of degrees between the floor and your leg.

Another common and helpful test is the *sit and reach* test, which measures the flexibility of your lower back and rear thigh muscles. You sit with your legs out straight and place your feet flat on the side of a special metal box. Keeping your legs straight, you lean forward and reach toward the box as far as you can. Along the top of the box, there's a scale in inches, which the tester uses to measure how far you reached forward. We find it amusing that the special box costs $200. You could do this same test with the carton that the box comes in.

Some clubs don't get that sophisticated with flexibility measurements; don't hold it against them. As a measure of low back and hamstring flexibility, they may simply ask you to bend over and try to touch your toes. You can also do this test at home. It's okay to estimate your flexibility rather than measure it to the exact degree. At least you'll find out which joints are tight, so you can put extra emphasis on them when you stretch. For details about how to stretch properly, see Chapter 7.

The chart on the next page describes flexibility tests you can do at home (Figure 1-4 shows you one of these tests). You might also encounter these tests during a health club evaluation.

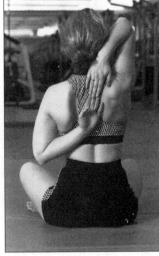

Figure 1-4:
You can do many flexibility tests at home. The test pictured measures shoulder flexibility.

(Photo courtesy of Dan Kron.)

Testing Your Flexibility

The Test	What To Do	You Have Good Flexibility if . . .	Your Flexibility Needs Work if . . .	Your Flexibility Needs *A Lot* of Work if . . . .
Rear thigh and lower back (Toe Touch)	Take off your shoes and stand with your feet together and your knees straight but not locked. Bend forward and reach for the floor.	You can touch the floor with little effort and no discomfort in your rear thighs or low back.	You can just touch your toes with little or no discomfort.	You can't touch your toes, or you feel considerable pain when you try. You may be susceptible to lower back problems.
Shoulder	Reach your right hand behind your back and your left hand across your back toward your right shoulder blade. Try to clasp your hands together behind your back.	You can clasp your hands together.	Your fingertips almost touch.	You aren't within an inch of touching your fingertips together. This means you're susceptible to shoulder and neck pain.
Calf and ankle	Sit on the floor with your legs straight out in front of you. Flex your foot so your toes move toward you.	Your toes move enough towards you so that they are beyond perpendicular to the floor.	Your toes bend so they are just in line with your ankles (exactly perpendicular to the floor).	You can barely bend your toes toward you. You may be susceptible to ankle injuries.
Shin	Sitting in the same position as the calf and ankle test, point your toes and stretch them toward the floor.	Your toes touch or nearly touch the floor.	Your toes come to within an inch or so of the floor.	Your toes barely move toward the floor. You may be susceptible to shin splints (see definition, Chapter 24).
Top, front of hip; buttocks	Lie on your back and hug one knee to your chest; clasp your hands around your shin just below your knee. Keep the other leg straight.	Your straight leg rests on the floor directly in line with your hip, and you can easily hug your bent knee to your chest.	Your leg, when straight, rests along the floor but to the outside of your hip, and you can almost hug your knee to your chest.	Your straight leg doesn't touch the floor, and you can't bring your knee to within a few inches of your chest. You may be susceptible to hip and back pain.
Upper back	Lie on your back with your legs out straight, and lift your arms straight overhead. Now drop your arms back behind you towards the floor.	Your arms easily fall to the floor without your lower back arching up.	Your hands almost touch and your lower back remains in contact with the floor.	Your arms don't come within an inch of touching the floor, and your back arches up. You may be susceptible to upper back and shoulder pain.
Front thigh	Lie on your stomach with one leg straight and bend the other knee so that your heel moves toward your buttocks.	Your heel easily touches your buttocks.	Your heel comes close to but doesn't quite touch your buttocks.	Your heel doesn't come within a few inches of touching your buttocks. You may be susceptible to knee pain.

Chapter 2

Your Plan of Attack

*Y*ou wouldn't start a business without a *plan* — a clear-cut idea of where you want to take your company and how you propose to get there. You'd assess your cash flow and expenses, decide on your hours of operation, and develop strategies to overcome obstacles.

Your workout program deserves the same type of attention. This chapter helps you develop your plan of attack. We show you how to set realistic goals and track your progress, and we offer strategies for sticking to your plan so that your workout program is as successful as any business venture.

Setting Your Goals

Before you embark on an exercise program, clarify *why* you want to get fit. Maybe heart disease runs in your family, and you want to avoid carrying on that tradition. Maybe you can't keep up with your grandkids. Maybe your pants split as you got up to greet your blind date and you thought, "I really ought to do something about this." Whatever the reason, make sure you're doing this for yourself — not simply to please your doctor or to lure back the spouse who left you for someone much younger.

Then once you have your fitness evaluated (see Chapter 1 for details about fitness testing), start setting specific goals. Research shows that goal-setting works. In typical studies, scientists give one group of exercisers a specific goal, such as doing 60 sit-ups. Meanwhile, they tell a second group of exercisers simply, "Do your best." In most cases, the exercisers with specific goals have more success than the comparison groups.

When you start on an exercise program, you need to set a few different types of goals. Look at the big picture while giving yourself stepping stones to get there. Having mini-goals makes your long-term goal seem more feasible. Here's a look at the different types of goals you should set.

Long-term goals

Give yourself a goal for the next three to six months. Some people get really creative with their long-term goals. Melissa Ebie, of Akron, Ohio, has a long-term goal to walk to a friend's house — in Birmingham, Alabama. No, she's not going to literally hoof it 697 miles. Melissa has charted the route on an automobile club map, and for every 20 minutes that she spends doing an aerobic exercise video, she gives herself credit for one mile. At the end of each week, she adds up her "mileage" and uses a yellow highlighter to mark the ground she has covered on the map.

Melissa figures the "walk" to Birmingham will take her more than a year; her six-month goal is to reach the half-way point — Shepherdsville, Kentucky. Last we spoke to Melissa, she was somewhere outside of Sunbury, Ohio.

Make sure your long-term goals are realistic. If you start your swimming program today, traversing the English Channel is not exactly what we'd recommend for a six-month goal. On the other hand, don't be afraid to dream. Choose a goal that really sparks you — something that may be out of reach at the moment but is not out of the realm of possibility. People are often surprised by what they can accomplish. Ellen Halliday, a 64-year-old grandma from southern California, rode her bicycle across the United States, covering 80 miles a day. The first few weeks she was so worn out that she barely had the energy to crawl into her sleeping bag. By the end of the trip, Ellen was sailing into camp with a smile on her face — and a six-pack of beer strapped to her bike. The first thing she did upon crossing the finish line at the end of her trip was pop open a can of Budweiser. "I earned it," she said. "I'm in better shape than most of my children."

Judge for yourself what's realistic. Some people rise to the occasion when they set goals that seem virtually impossible. Other people get discouraged by setting extremely high expectations. We recommend that beginners set moderately challenging goals. If you reach your goals earlier than expected, choose more ambitious ones. Here are some other concrete examples of long-term goals:

- ✔ Lose 8 pounds in 16 weeks.
- ✔ Complete a 5-mile walk or run that's four months away (see Figure 2-1).
- ✔ Do one full push-up and one full pull-up.
- ✔ Walk one mile in under 15 minutes.
- ✔ Bench press 65 pounds.

Short-term goals

Six months is a long time to wait for feelings of success. In order to stay motivated, you need to feel a sense of accomplishment along the way. When Ellen Halliday was bicycling from the West Coast of the United States to the East Coast, she didn't dream about the Atlantic Ocean every day; she'd focus on a goal that seemed more manageable, like getting across Texas. Set short-term goals for one week to one month. Here are some examples.

- ✔ Make it all the way through a step aerobics class without stopping.
- ✔ Improve last week's one-mile walk time by 10 seconds.
- ✔ Use the stairclimber four times this week for 30 minutes each time. At work and at the mall, take the stairs instead of the elevator.
- ✔ Eat a piece of fruit every day for lunch this week and substitute low-fat frozen yogurt for ice cream.
- ✔ Bicycle 60 miles a week for the next four weeks.

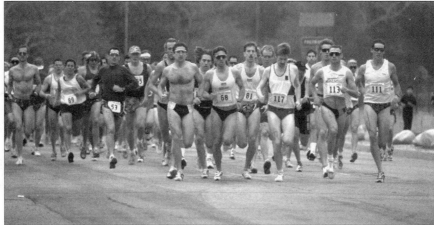

Figure 2-1:
Imagine
yourself at
the starting
line of a
5-mile run.

(Photo courtesy of Christopher Grisanti.)

Immediate goals

Now we're talking about goals for each day or each workout. This way, when you walk into the gym, you won't waste any time figuring out which exercises to do. Here are examples of immediate goals:

- ✔ Spend a full 10 minutes stretching at the end of a workout.
- ✔ Do upper body weight exercises and 20 minutes on the stairclimber.
- ✔ Run two miles.
- ✔ Eat a low-fat turkey burger for lunch instead of a hamburger.
- ✔ Bicycle a hilly course.

Back-up goals

You always need a Plan B, in case something happens and you're not able to reach your primary goal as soon as you want to. By setting back-up goals, you'll have a better chance of achieving *something,* and you won't feel like a failure if your long-term goal doesn't work out. Let's say that your long-term goal is to lose 10 pounds by eating healthier and walking 3 miles a day. Your back-up goal could be increasing your stamina enough to walk 3 miles in less than an hour. Or say that you're training for a 10k run in the spring, but you sprain an ankle and have to stop running. If one of your back-up goals is to strengthen your upper body, you can still keep on track while your ankle heals.

Reward Yourself

You let your kids watch their favorite video when they bring home good grades. You give your golden retriever a doggy treat when he fetches the Frisbee. Be nice to yourself, too. Attach an appropriate reward to each of your long-term, short-term, and immediate goals. If you lose the 15 pounds over 6 months, buy yourself that watch you've been wanting. If you stopped drinking Coke for a whole week, let yourself watch some trashy TV movie. Sure, it's bribery, but it works. Short-term rewards are particularly important because there's always a chance that you might not make it all the way to your long-term goal. You need to give yourself credit for making it even halfway. By the way, triple-decker fudge cake isn't what we have in mind for a reward.

As with your goals, you can get pretty creative with your rewards. We know a guy who asked a friend to hold $500. If he reached his goal of losing 25 pounds, he'd get the money back and buy new clothes. If he *didn't* reach his goal, the money would become a charitable contribution to the Young Republicans. Considering that this guy made Jesse Jackson look like Jesse Helms, this was a very good incentive, indeed. The guy lost his 25 pounds.

Write Everything Down

It's easy to set goals and rewards; it's even easier to forget what they are. You can keep yourself honest — and motivated — by tracking your goals and accomplishments on paper. Our friend Melissa from Ohio prints out a graph of her achievements every week and sticks it to her bathroom mirror. Another friend tapes his goals to the inside of his gym locker. Some people program their computer to flash their goals on-screen twice a day. Here are some other ways that you can monitor your progress.

Make a goal sheet

Write down your goals on a large piece of paper and put it somewhere so that you can see it every day, like next to your desk or on your refrigerator. Next to every goal, write down the corresponding reward. This strategy isn't just for amateurs. Many world-class athletes use it, too. Figure 2-2 is a sample goal sheet that you can fill out each week. Underneath each heading, write down your goal and your target date.

Keep a workout log

Whatever your goals are, a training diary can help you get better results. You'll look back at the end of each week and say, "I did *that?*" And you'll be inspired to do more. Our friend Melissa from Ohio not only tracks her "mileage" on a map, but she also records her exercise video and weight-lifting workouts in a daily diary. "My log keeps me going from week to week," she says. "It's really satisfying to see your accomplishments build up. When I see what hill I tackled that week, it makes me want to try another one."

YOUR GOAL SHEET

Long-term Goals	Long-term Rewards
Back-up Long-term Goals	
Short-term Goals	Short-term Rewards
Weekly Goals	Weekly Rewards
Daily Goals	Daily Rewards

Figure 2-2:
Make a goal
sheet like
the one
here.

Keeping a log shows you whether your goals are realistic and gives you insight into your exercise patterns. If you're losing weight, building strength, or developing stamina, you won't have to wonder what works, because you'll have a blow-by-blow description of everything you've done to reach your goals.

On the other hand, if you get injured or stuck in a rut, you can turn to your diary for clues as to why. You might discover that if you don't eat before you cycle, you cover your usual route 5 minutes slower. Maybe you pull a hamstring every time you run over a certain hilly course. Maybe you get sick if you don't rest at least one day each week.

A workout diary keeps you honest. You might *think* that you're working out four times a week. But when you flip through your log, you might learn that you've been overestimating your efforts.

Bookstores and sporting goods stores carry a variety of logs. You also can buy nifty computer software to track your progress. Some logs are aimed specifically at walkers, others at weight lifters, and some logs have space to chart virtually any activity you can think of. You can use Figure 2-3 and see whether you enjoy tracking your workouts on paper. (Keeping a workout log is not everyone's idea of fun.)

Here are some suggestions for filling in the blanks.

Date and day

Don't forget to note the date and day. This information helps you assess what you've done in a week; when you look back, you'll know whether you ran those 20 miles in one week or two. Also, you might learn that you always have a bad workout on Fridays because you stay up late Thursday nights to watch "ER." Maybe Friday is the day for you to take off. Note the day and dates of your *rest* days as well. This way you know how much rest you're giving yourself.

Goals for the day

Write down what you hope to accomplish during your workout, like completing the 20-minute Roller Coaster program on the stairclimber or swimming a half mile. Rather than scribble a few lines while you're running from the locker room into an aerobics class, fill in this section the night before or, better yet, immediately following your last workout. This will make you stop and think about just what it *is* that you're trying to achieve. If you keep your goals in mind, you'll have more enthusiasm for your workout.

Day of the week	Date			Difficulty Rating ☐
Goals				
Cardiovascular Training	Time			Distance
Strength Training	Weight	Sets	Reps	Notes
Stretching				
Notes				

Figure 2-3:
Here's a sample workout log.

Cardiovascular training

Write down the type of activity, whether it's stationary cycling, walking, skating, or step aerobics. In the "Time/Distance" section, note how long your aerobic session lasted and (when applicable) how far you went—for instance, "jogged 20 minutes on treadmill, 1.8 miles."

Next to "Difficulty Rating," rate your workout on a scale from 1 to 10. Don't base this assessment simply on the number of miles you walked or the number of calories you burned. Instead, rate your workouts according to how *hard* you pushed yourself. A 1 rating would be an extremely easy day; a 10 would be an all-out workout. The purpose of the Difficulty Rating is to remind you to aim for a healthy mix of numbers. If you rate a 9 on Monday, Tuesday is a good day for a 2 workout. Log a 0 for the days you don't exercise.

You might also want to note the weather conditions, including the wind and the temperature, because you work much harder when it's raining or hot. Describe the course you covered (was it hilly or flat?); who you worked out with ("Marge talks too much"); and how you felt before, during, and after your workout. All of these notes may help you trace the root of training problems that crop up. Or they may get you to realize that you always feel great when you work out with a certain friend.

Strength training

Jot down the name of each exercise, the amount of weight you lifted, and the number of sets you did. (If you need any of these terms defined, see Chapter 13.) If you don't know the name of an exercise, make it a point to find out. Writing down "bicep curl" will reinforce the idea that this exercise strengthens your biceps. If you're not sure where your biceps are, see Chapter 10.

You may also want to note what changes you need to make during your next weight-lifting session. Let's say you used 50 pounds on the leg press machine and had a pretty easy time of it. Write down in your diary that next time you want to try 60 pounds. Also note which exercises are particularly easy, and which need more attention.

Stretching

Simply note whether you stretched or not. You can also jot down a few words about which muscles felt the tightest and which stretches felt the best.

Notes

Here's your chance to record any details that don't seem to fit into the other categories. Note that you substituted mustard for mayo on your roast beef sandwich at lunch — and it actually tasted good! Or you might describe a new leg exercise you tried today. Write down whatever you feel is important.

Making Exercise a Habit

As we mentioned in the introduction to this book, 50 percent of new exercisers quit within eight weeks. Of course, we want to make sure that you're among the *other* 50 percent. The following tips can help you get over the hump and boost the odds that you will stick with your new program. We discuss several of these topics in detail throughout the book, but we want you to keep them in mind from the start.

Expect to feel uncomfortable at first

Exercise definitely doesn't need to be painful, but if you've neglected your body, don't expect a free ride. Despite what you hear on infomercials — "just five minutes a day, and you can do this on the couch while watching TV!" — exercise is a serious commitment. You can't get into shape without exerting some real effort and, perhaps, without experiencing some (but not a lot of) discomfort.

Pace yourself

Don't buy every exercise video on the market or try every weight machine in the gym the first day. You'll kill your enthusiasm and flame out fast. Always keep yourself hungry for more.

Work out with friends or join a club

An exercise buddy can push you to new heights — or get your butt outside for a walk on the days when you'd rather stay home and watch reruns of "Bewitched." If you make a date to meet a friend at the gym, you're a lot more likely to show up than if you make a date with yourself.

It's pretty impressive what people can accomplish when they have support from friends. Consider the employees at Bayer Corporation in New Martinsville, West Virginia, who signed up for a 10-week program at the office called "Dump Your Plump." The employees divided themselves into teams of 10. Each week, they earned points for exercising, and at the end of the program, they earned points for meeting their goal weight. "The team concept was the reason we all stuck with it," Kathy Schneider, captain of the winning team (Porky's Revenge), told us. "No one wanted to come into the office and say that they had let the team down by not exercising." Dump Your Plump is a nationwide program offered through businesses, government agencies, churches, and schools. The phone number is listed in the back of this book under "Resources."

What if your company doesn't have a program like Dump Your Plump? What if your friends and family members aren't interested in breaking a sweat? Take the initiative to find workout buddies by joining an exercise class at your community center, a Sierra Club hike, or a charity event or race that has a training program. The Leukemia Society of America has an excellent walking, running, and cycling program geared toward beginners. Some running clubs will find you a buddy who runs at your pace and covers the same weekly mileage.

You can even find workout "partners" on the Internet. We know three women — one in New Mexico, one in Massachusetts, and one in Michigan — who exercise alone but motivate each other by sending e-mail messages about their workouts. "Hearing about someone else's great day helps me have a great day, too," one of them told us. "I actually like to work out by myself — it's my private time away from the kids. But it's nice to compare notes with someone about how much weight you lifted or how many Girl Scout cookies you ate."

Find a hero

Model yourself after someone who's been a fitness success. We've been inspired by many people, including a marathon runner and ocean swimmer who has only one leg. We also know a 65-year-old woman who was hit by a car while bicycling and suffered serious internal injuries in addition to breaking nearly every bone in her body; two years later, she was back on her bike.

These are extreme examples. Your hero can be your grandma who walks a mile in the park every day. It can be some guy at the office who wears size 42 pants but has started going to the gym four times a week. Or maybe your hero is a woman who walks to work instead of taking the train. Just find someone about whom you can say, "If *that person* can do it, I sure as heck can."

Mix it up

If you fall in love with the StairMaster, fine, do it every day for the rest of your life. But most people need variety to stay motivated, so try several different activities. Expect to change or modify your workout every couple of months. There's an unlimited number of ways to get you back into your favorite pants.

Buy the right equipment

Cycling isn't going to be fun if you're riding an old clunker. Walking isn't going to be comfortable or safe if you're doing it in sandals. You don't need to spend megabucks on top-of-the-line pro-quality equipment, but investing in the right equipment and clothing will pay you back several times over. (See Chapter 9 for equipment information and Chapter 22 for tips on buying athletic shoes.)

Don't compare yourself to anyone else

Recognize that people come in all shapes and sizes, and everyone improves at a different pace. It's great to get inspiration from other people, but don't let anyone else's accomplishments diminish your own. Be proud that you've worked up to walking 3 miles every other day, even if your neighbor runs 10 miles a day.

Be forgiving

Don't get mad at yourself if you miss a few days—or even a few months—of exercise. If you fall off the wagon, just try again. You have the rest of your life to get this right.

Chapter 3

Educating Yourself

· ·

· ·

*A*ny subject is less intimidating if you know something about it. Consider home repair. This we know nothing about. When we want to renovate the bathroom and the plumber says, "Looks like the green board is shot and your shut-off valves need replacing," we shrug and make out a check. Our ignorance makes us feel a bit foolish, and it probably costs us big bucks. On the other hand, if we took the time to read up on this topic, we might not have to call a plumber to replace every wing nut. We might even think it's fun to join Internet arguments about the merits of linoleum. And who knows — we might not have those homicidal urges when certain boyfriends and husbands postpone Valentine's Day dinner to watch "This Ol' House" rate weather-proof paints.

In other words, it always pays to educate yourself, whether you're talking about ceiling tiles or stairclimbers. You'll have more confidence and more fun with your workouts if you read about fitness in magazines, newsletters, and books — even on the Internet. You can keep abreast of the latest exercise techniques, workout gadgets, and nutrition controversies. And you can get inspirational tips from folks who overcame their inertia.

Of course, you also can get completely confused. One book we own says, "walking will never get you fit." Another book on our shelf says, "walking provides top-notch aerobic training." Both sides cite scientific research to support their view. Because so much conflicting and misleading information is published about fitness, it's important to read exercise publications with a critical eye. This chapter helps you wade through the garbage and choose the publications that can best educate and inspire you.

Sifting Through Scientific Research

It seems like every day on the news you hear about some new study that seems to contradict the one you heard the month before. First, beta carotene protects against cancer; then it's useless. A daily glass of red wine reduces your risk of heart disease; then scientists say *any* type of alcohol has the same effect. Moderate exercise makes you live longer; then only vigorous exercise can increase your life span. How do you find out the truth?

First, realize that there may not actually *be* a truth, at least not yet. We all want to know the bottom line now, yet it may take decades for scientists to reach a legitimate conclusion. That "startling new report" you hear about on TV might simply be one minuscule piece in a gigantic puzzle — one scientist's best guess. But because of the way news is generated and reported, you might not get the full picture. Scientists sometimes overstate their findings because they want media attention or grant money. Journalists often hype ambiguous results because they need a big story. Or they may get the facts wrong because they had only two hours to decipher a 20-page study full of phrases like "deuterium oxide concentration was measured by using a fixed-filter single-beam infrared spectrophotometer."

Here's a good example of what can go wrong: When a Harvard University study found that vigorous exercise was associated with longer life, the media jumped on the story; press reports gave the idea that high-intensity workouts were better than moderate workouts after all. The problem was, most of the news reports didn't define "vigorous." The actual study used the term "vigorous" so loosely as to include brisk walking, an activity most people would consider moderate. One magazine article was so confused that it referred to "walking briskly" as vigorous exercise and "brisk walking" as nonstrenuous.

Stuff like this happens all the time. So to get a good handle on the facts, you've got to pay attention to the way studies are reported. The following tips will help you sort through the research that you read and hear about.

Look for context

Does the news report mention how the latest research compares to the studies that came before it? The results of a single study might be a complete aberration. A while back, the media hyped a couple of studies suggesting that yo-yo dieting (repeatedly losing and gaining weight) slows your metabolism. But what they failed to report was that more than 40 other studies found that yo-yo dieting *didn't* affect metabolic rate. Don't alter your lifestyle on the basis of one study. Many theories are later proven to be wrong. And don't jump on any bandwagon if a study's recommendations don't sit well with you. We hate red wine and wouldn't drink it even if science proved it could make you live to 150.

Consider the source

A health study is more likely to be legit if it comes out of a major university or government agency rather than some mysterious, private institute. Some private companies and foundations do valid research, but many organizations with impressive-sounding names, like Sportlife Exercise Health Sciences Institute, are just facades for companies promoting their products. Look for the term *independent research*. A tobacco study done by RJ Reynolds or a rating of treadmill brands done by a treadmill manufacturer should fall under the category of *things that make you go "Hmmmm."* On the other hand, just because a study was conducted at an Ivy League university, doesn't mean it's the gospel.

Don't assume cause and effect

If a study says that eating oat bran is *linked to* or is *associated with* low blood cholesterol levels, this doesn't mean eating oat bran *causes* low cholesterol levels. Maybe the oat bran eaters are health conscious and get a lot of exercise. You have to ask, "Was it the oat bran or the exercise?"

Look for comparison groups

We recently came across a magazine article touting the benefits of a powdered food replacement. As evidence, the article cited a study of 28 overweight women who cut their daily calories by taking the powder twice a day instead of food; the subjects also exercised three times a week. After two months, the article states, "an astounding one hundred percent" of the women lost weight and felt better. Astounding? *Any* overweight person who cuts calories and exercises regularly is going see results after two months. For the study to have any validity, the researchers should have compared the group taking the powder with a control group of similar subjects who ate the same number of calories and followed the same exercise program but didn't use the product.

Do some math

You often read that a certain habit "doubles" the risk of death or "increases the risk of disease by 50 percent." These figures can be misleading. In a study that followed 115,000 nurses for 16 years, researchers found that gaining 11 to 18 pounds in middle age raised the nurses' heart disease risk by 25 percent. But the number of deaths in the study was so small that a 25 percent increase would mean the difference between 10 deaths in 10,000 people and 12 or 13 deaths.

Notice the length of the study

Pay attention to how many subjects were included and *who* those subjects were. A four-week study on six 20-year-old women doesn't tell you that a weight-loss pill or exercise regimen is or is not safe or effective. Maybe a pill stops working after two months. Maybe 20-year-old women react differently to the pill than does the rest of the population.

For the same reasons, don't make too much of animal studies. The way an obese mouse responds to a diet drug may not be the same way that you respond. Chromium picolinate, a diet supplement touted on bottles as a "Super Reducer!", has received tons of good press. What you may not hear is that most of the fat-loss studies have been performed on pigs. There's virtually no evidence suggesting the pills help burn extra fat on humans. In fact, most of the human studies show no benefit at all.

Recognize that people lie in surveys

Large studies usually rely on written questionnaires or phone surveys, a method that can lead to very misleading results. Subjects might not remember how many leafy green vegetables they ate last month, or they might exaggerate their exercise habits. The President's Council on Physical Fitness recently reported that 50 percent of Americans exercise vigorously at least twice a week. But virtually all other studies have found the percentage to be much lower, even as low as 5 percent of the adult population. How to account for the discrepancy? The Council relied on random phone surveys to gather its data.

According to the *New England Journal of Medicine,* nearly half of all research participants overestimate how much they exercise and an equal percentage underestimate how much they eat.

Fitness Magazines

Just when the fitness magazine industry seems to be saturated, along comes yet another magazine devoted to exercise, health, and nutrition. This is good news — we welcome more choices. Even better, fitness magazines are becoming more specialized, so you have an excellent chance of finding a magazine that speaks to you. There's at least one fitness magazine to suit every type of exerciser: pregnant women, African-American women, Christian women, men over 40, walkers, runners, high school girls, home exercisers, and cooking enthusiasts who want to be fit.

But the stiff competition makes some magazines resort to underhanded marketing tactics, including sensational headlines and misleading articles. Ask a trainer or fitness-minded friends for magazine recommendations. Also, keep in mind the following tips for judging the fitness information that you read in magazines.

Check out specialty magazines

You're more likely to get good fitness information from magazines that specialize in fitness than from general interest or beauty magazines that mix in an occasional exercise article. This isn't a hard-and-fast rule: Some mainstream magazines run perfectly good fitness stories, and some fitness magazines run perfectly lousy ones. But women's fashion and beauty magazines are notorious for unrealistic promises like "Permanent Weight Loss! A revolutionary three-week plan."

Be especially wary of magazine pieces that offer fitness advice from celebrities; being a movie star doesn't make you an exercise expert. *Cosmopolitan* magazine recently ran a story titled "Energy Secrets from 20 Top Dynamos," in which Jane Fonda weighs in with advice to drink iced carbonated water three times a day. "The cold bubbles rush into your system, plumping up red blood cells. It's the best way to feed your brain and muscles throughout the day." Enough said.

Beware of sensational headlines

Stay away from magazines whose cover lines seem way too good to be true, such as "Drop 9 lbs. in 7 Days," which is the fitness equivalent of "Elvis lives." And if the fitness article is next to a story about Burt Reynolds' ghost having a secret rendezvous with a two-headed man, you're probably not getting your information from the right source. Tabloid rags have caught on to the fact that the American public is obsessed with weight loss, so what's one more story about an alien diet or Jeane Dixon predicting the health regimens that work?

Look for reputable sources

Keep your eyes open for magazine articles that don't even attempt to back up their claims with quotes from at least a couple of experts. (For a definition of *expert,* see Chapter 15.) And forget publications that espouse a single exercise theory that's at odds with everything else you read. One fitness magazine promotes a strength-training program designed to reduce your hips and thighs by training these muscles so much that they shrink. The magazine devotes 25 of its 96 pages to articles and advertisements for this *overtraining* method, repeatedly citing testimonials from the guy who created it and the women who are his disciples. Not surprisingly, the magazine offers no opinions from any respected professional fitness organizations (see Chapter 15 for a list) and no evidence of the method's safety.

Pay attention to the ads

Virtually all fitness magazines, including the reputable ones, accept advertisements that make bogus claims. The quality of the ads isn't necessarily a good reason to dismiss a magazine. Typically, the writers and editors have no control over what advertisements are run.

Still, certain ads should raise a red flag. It's hard to take a magazine's health advice seriously if the publication accepts cigarette ads, as many women's magazines do. Surprisingly, you even find cigarette ads in *Self,* an otherwise fine publication that offers plenty of accurate fitness advice. Magazine editors do their best to steer clear of advertiser influence, but sometimes the powers that be force editors to censor articles. One of us called a fitness-related magazine to pitch a story about a U.S. Army study suggesting that smokers have a higher injury rate than nonsmokers. The editor said she had to reject the story idea because the magazine didn't want to offend its cigarette advertisers.

One last point about advertisements: Don't confuse them with articles. Advertisers often use layouts, typeface, and photos that are very similar to the magazine's editorial style so that readers won't make the distinction. The more manipulative ads even have *bylines* (for instance, "By Joe Schmo") so that the ads look like articles that have been written by regular reporters. Most magazines require advertisers to include the word *advertisement* at the top or bottom of the page, but sometimes the type is so small that it's easy to miss.

Newsletters

If you like your fitness and health information in small doses, we recommend subscribing to one of the many excellent newsletters out there, particularly those affiliated with prominent universities or respected nonprofit organizations. These publications don't have the glossy photos or fancy layouts, but they get right to the point. Many do a good job of setting the record straight when the mainstream media misreport a study.

A fitness beginner might want to start with a newsletter that covers a broad range of health, nutrition, and exercise topics. You can learn about everything from heartburn drugs, to soy protein, to how many calories you burn while playing the cello. Informative newsletters include the *University of California at Berkeley Wellness Letter,* the *Penn State Sportsmedicine Newsletter, Harvard Women's Health Watch,* the *Harvard Heart Letter,* and the *Mayo Clinic Health Letter.*

Among the nutrition newsletters that we recommend: *Tufts University Diet & Nutrition Letter* and *Nutrition Action,* published by the Center For Science in the Public Interest (the activist organization that called fettuccine alfredo "a heart attack on a plate"). On the exercise front, we like *Running and FitNews, Running Research News,* and *Fitness Matters.* If you subscribe to fitness magazines, chances are you'll get newsletter offers in the mail. Take them up on a free issue and judge for yourself.

Newspapers

We're glad daily papers have stepped up their fitness coverage, but don't use the dailies as your only source of fitness information. Newspaper reporters tend to be very responsible about attributing information to experts. The problem is, given the reporters' tight deadlines, they often have no choice but to interview the first available expert, who may not necessarily be the best expert (and may not be an expert at all). Magazine writers sometimes run into this problem, too.

Also, newspaper reporters tend to be jack-of-all-trades types who may not have the fitness experience to distinguish a real expert from a charlatan. Only the largest newspapers can afford to have reporters who cover the fitness beat exclusively. If you're looking for articles about fitness trends, training techniques, and exercise equipment, mainstream fitness magazines tend to be better sources than newspapers.

Books

Maybe it's the thickness or maybe it's the binding, but sitting there on the shelf, books seem to have an aura of authority — much more so than magazine articles flanked by diet pill advertisements. In reality, most fitness books undergo *less* editorial scrutiny than newspaper and magazine articles, so you really have to watch what you buy. Many book publishers do not have the budget to hire fact checkers, so the writers are contractually responsible for the accuracy of the information. At magazines and newspapers, the editors — not just the writers — are responsible for the accuracy of a story. *Fitness For Dummies,* of course, is a safe bet.

These days the fitness shelves are packed with workout programs designed or ghost-designed by celebrity trainers or trainers with celebrity clients. Some of these books are helpful — you can get good tips on proper weight-lifting form and ideas for designing your own workout. And some of the trainers are motivating and earnest; they genuinely want the public to get in shape.

Then you have the so-called experts whose sole purpose is to sell their image. Beware of authors who claim to know something that nobody else does. Typically, their *secrets* and *special techniques* are common knowledge glorified with a fancy name. One author says her secret is the *interset technique:* doing a set of weight-lifting repetitions for one muscle group followed by an exercise set that works another muscle group. If this is considered a secret, then so is the fact that airplanes fly.

In general, take the information you want from fitness books and discard anything that doesn't seem to work for you. You don't need to follow anybody's entire program.

The Internet

Surfing the Internet for fitness information is a bit like entering into telephone multiple mailbox hell — you press one key after another, and pretty soon, you're either totally lost or back where you started. You might have the intention of finding out how to train your abdominals and with a few unwitting clicks of the mouse, you're downloading porn. Still, if you have the time and patience to look around, you can get some great up-to-the-minute fitness information online. You also can get plenty of hogwash.

The World Wide Web features hundreds, if not thousands, of fitness-related sites. If you're not too tired from typing in `http://www.webrunner.com/webrun/running/genred.html`, you can learn a lot of interesting things about running, including marathon training tips, 10k races in your area, and how to find the right shoes for your feet. On the Web, you find FAQs (Frequently Asked Questions), mailing lists, product directories, and links to other Web sites. If you're a woman who wants to learn about lifting weights, by all means, click to Weight Training for Women, but skip Very Fit Ladies Indeed — there's that porn we were talking about.

We're not going to provide a long list of Web sites because they tend to come and go quickly. Our best advice is to stick with information put out by reputable sources, like the American Heart Association or the National Institutes of Health. Don't bother with "Bob's Exercise Home Page." And recognize that many Web sites are simply product advertisements. Many fitness magazines, including *Self* and *Men's Health,* review fitness-related sites.

You also can join Internet newsgroups such as `misc.fitness` and swap advice with fellow fitness enthusiasts on just about any topic, whether you're looking for a good gym in Hoboken, New Jersey, wondering whether wearing a jock strap while weight lifting can prevent you from getting a hernia, or not sure whether the military press exercise can give you hemorrhoids (three topics we don't cover in this book).

Chapter 4
Nutrition Basics

● ●

In This Chapter

▶ The skinny on fat

▶ Counting calories

▶ Knowing your carbohydrates

▶ Protein myths

▶ The lowdown on fiber

▶ Why you need those eight glasses of water

▶ Vitamins and minerals

▶ The Food Guide Pyramid

● ●

*W*e recently came across a fitness book that said, "A great exercise program can make up for lack of a great diet." Unfortunately, that just isn't so. As you get going on your workout program, keep in mind that no amount of exercise can compensate for lousy eating habits.

But wait — if you scarf an extra donut at the office, can't you just burn off the calories on the treadmill? Sure, except that it takes an entire hour of brisk walking to burn off that single honey-dipped cruller. On a daily basis, exercise isn't a realistic way to make up for overeating. Besides, weight control isn't the only reason you should watch what you eat. If you make consistently poor choices, you deprive your body of nutrients that fight cancer and heart disease, prevent your bones from becoming brittle, and keep you from falling asleep while reading this book. Not that this book isn't a real page turner, of course.

We know several athletes who exercise four hours a day but live on junk food or virtually no food at all. They may be *fit* — maybe they can run marathons, do backflips, or bench press 400 pounds — but they are not *healthy*. And surely they would perform better if they cleaned up their diet. When you're short on nutrients, you can't live up to your potential in the gym, at the office, or at the park with your kids.

This chapter covers nutrition basics: how to trim fat from your diet, how to boost your fiber intake, how to choose a vitamin supplement, and how to cut calories without feeling like a hunger striker. We make sense of terms such as *saturated fat* and *cholesterol* and explain how you can get fat on fat-free foods. And we answer the question that inquiring minds want to know: What ever happened to the Basic Four Food Groups?

Throughout this chapter, we give you formulas for figuring out how much of various nutrients you need. But don't give these numbers too much authority: Use them as a general guide, listen to your body, and experiment with what works for you.

The Skinny on Fat

Here's a fact that's not going to stop any presses: Americans eat too much fat. Even though we know better, we're still wolfing down potato chips and drowning our tuna in mayo. McDonald's sold so few McLean burgers that the Golden Arches yanked the low-fat burger from the menu. Of course, maybe that was because the McLean tasted like paper-mache. Americans seem to want the real deal: grease. Health experts implore us to get less than 30 percent of our total calories from fat, but $2/3$ of Americans exceed that limit. Many believe that 20 percent is a better goal for fat consumption.

We're not opposed to fat. In fact, we *love* fat. We especially love Ben & Jerry's Peanut Butter Cup ice cream, which has 104 grams of fat in one pint and may very well be the most compelling evidence yet of a benevolent deity. Besides, we all need *some* fat in our diet. Fat is essential for absorbing certain vitamins, providing fuel, keeping your immune system healthy, and keeping your skin moist. But if we consume mass quantities of Peanut Butter Cup ice cream on a daily basis, we'll join the ranks of the 58 million obese Americans who are at increased risk for heart disease, cancer, high cholesterol, and premature death. Fortunately, cutting fat from your diet isn't as tough as it might seem.

Three strategies to trim the fat

Fat is one of the four nutrients your body can convert to fuel—the others are carbohydrates, protein, and alcohol. Fat is also the one that packs the largest caloric punch: Each gram of fat holds nine calories worth of potential energy (or potential spare tire material). A gram of carbohydrate or protein contains just four calories, and alcohol contains seven.

Trimming the fat means more than simply slicing the white edges off of your steak or driving past Burger King on the highway. In the next section, we cover several ways to eliminate excess fat that you might not realize has been sneaking into your diet.

Find out how much fat you eat

Are you getting 50 percent of your calories from fat? Are you getting 20 percent? Do you have any *idea?* To get a ballpark figure, jot down everything that you eat for three days — every french fry, every Hershey's kiss, every slice of meatloaf. Also, take careful note of your serving size. Don't just write "peach yogurt." Write "8 oz. peach yogurt." Save this food diary; you need it for another exercise later in this chapter. Then buy one of those $10 paperback books that list the number of fat grams and calories in nearly every food that you can think of, from brussels sprouts to Japanese fish paste cake, whatever that is. We recommend books that include saturated fat numbers, too. Among our favorites are *The Calorie Factor: The Dieter's Companion* by Margo Feiden (Simon & Schuster), which even lists the calorie content of licking a postage stamp (.07 of a calorie), and the *Barbara Kraus Calorie Guide* (Signet). We also recommend computerized and CD-ROM nutritional analyzers available at software stores.

Next to every food you eat, write down the number of calories and fat grams, and calculate your daily total for each. Then use the following formula to figure out what percent of your calories came from fat. Here's how you'd do the math if you ate 2,400 calories, including 102 fat grams.

Step 1: **Determine how many *fat calories* you ate — in other words, how many calories were supplied by the grams of fat that you ate.**

Determine your fat calories by multiplying the number of fat grams (in this case 102) by 9 because each fat gram has 9 calories.

$102 \times 9 = 918$

So you ate 918 calories of fat.

Step 2: **Calculate what *percentage* of your total daily calories came from fat.**

To find this number, divide the number of fat calories (in this case 918) by the number of total calories (in this case 2,400).

$918/2400 = .38.$

This means 38 percent of your total calories were from fat.

Do these calculations for three consecutive days, to make sure that the first day wasn't an aberration. If you get similar results, you need work in the fat department.

Look at where you get your fat

Now you need to figure out which foods are supplying your fat. The answers are not always obvious. For instance, which has more fat:

- One ounce of Nature Valley Honey Nut Granola Bites or an ounce of ChipsAhoy! chocolate chip cookies?

- A Taco Bell Taco Salad or a McDonald's Quarter Pounder with Cheese?

The four food groups: where are they now?

Back in the days of Wonder Bread and Bosco, you and your fellow fourth-graders probably were treated to an educational film about the Basic Four Food Groups: Meat, Dairy, Fruits & Vegetables, and Cereals & Grains (in case you forgot). The idea was that if you got enough servings from each group, you'd cover all of your nutritional bases. You got to test this theory first-hand when the school cafeteria worker — who both fascinated and repelled you — slapped an approximate representative of each food group on your plate.

Well, the U.S. government's definition of a balanced diet has changed since then. Turns out, you can follow the Four Food Groups plan and still come up woefully short on some nutrients and overdo it on others. The plan isn't specific enough, and it doesn't take into consideration how foods are prepared — ketchup and broccoli both count as vegetables.

In 1992, the federal government exiled the Four Food Groups and unveiled the Food Guide Pyramid. Although the new plan looks like a complete departure from the four basics, it's simply a more detailed look at the same picture. (See the Pyramid on the next page.)

You're supposed to get the lion's share of your calories from the foods at the bottom of the pyramid: grains, cereals, rice, pasta, fruits, and vegetables. Meat, poultry, fish, eggs, and dairy products fall in the center, and fats, oils, and sweets are at the very top, under the heading of "use sparingly." The pyramid isn't perfect; for instance, it doesn't distinguish between the saturated fats found in meat and dairy products and the healthier unsaturated fats found in vegetable and nut oils. Harvard University recently unveiled a Mediterranean Diet Pyramid that derives most of its fat from olive oil, whereas the U.S. government's pyramid has more saturated fat sources such as meat and cheese. Still, the government's pyramid is a big improvement over the Four Food Groups.

To make sure that you don't go overboard on calories, pay attention to what counts as a serving. For instance, according to the pyramid, a serving of pasta is a half cup. This, we suspect, is not how the Italian restaurant in your neighborhood defines a serving. The federal government's idea of a meat serving — 3 ounces — is about the size of a deck of cards. Here's a rundown of serving sizes as defined by the government.

- Fats, oils, and sweets: Use sparingly. This means as little as possible — or, according to most health organizations, less than 30 percent of your total calories.

- Meat, poultry, fish, dry beans, eggs, and nuts: One serving equals 2–3 ounces of lean cooked meat, fish, or poultry; 1 egg; $1/2$ cup cooked beans; or 2 tablespoons seeds and nuts.

- Milk, yogurt, and cheese: One serving equals one cup (or $1^1/2$ ounces) of milk or yogurt — enough to fill your cereal bowl in the morning — or about a slice and a half of pre-cut cheese. Choose the low-fat varieties most of the time.

- Fruits: One serving equals one medium apple, banana, or orange; $1/2$ cup of chopped fruit or berries; or $3/4$ cup of fruit juice. Fresh fruits are preferable to canned or juiced.

- Vegetables: One serving equals 1 cup of raw, leafy veggies; $1/2$ cup of other vegetables, chopped; or $1/2$ cup of cooked cereal, rice, or pasta.

(continued)

(continued)

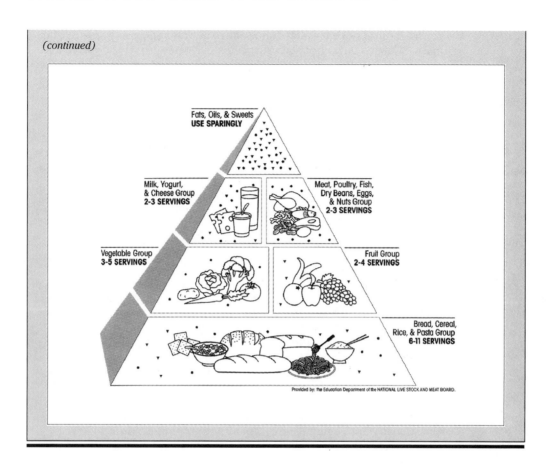

Fats, Oils, & Sweets
USE SPARINGLY

Milk, Yogurt,
& Cheese Group
2-3 SERVINGS

Meat, Poultry, Fish,
Dry Beans, Eggs,
& Nuts Group
2-3 SERVINGS

Vegetable Group
3-5 SERVINGS

Fruit Group
2-4 SERVINGS

Bread, Cereal,
Rice, & Pasta Group
6-11 SERVINGS

Provided by: the Education Department of the NATIONAL LIVE STOCK AND MEAT BOARD.

Granola and salad sound a lot leaner than cookies and burgers, but in these cases, they have even *more* fat. To ferret out your hidden fat, scrutinize your three-day diary. Start reading food labels on packages you buy and refer to your fat-gram book when you eat out or buy nonpackaged foods. Read labels carefully. Low-fat 2% milk doesn't get 2 percent of its calories from fat — it gets 38 percent. The "2%" refers to the amount of weight that comes from fat. Similarly, ground lean turkey that's labeled "7% fat" is really 39 percent fat.

Make simple substitutions

Cutting your fat calories from 40 percent to 30 percent or 20 percent sounds like a punishment that should be reserved for Third World dictators and evil dentists. But you don't have to give up your favorite foods or eat bird-sized portions. A few simple substitutions can drastically slash your fat intake.

Switch from tuna packed in oil to tuna packed in water and you'll save 5 $^{1}/_{2}$ fat grams. Eat Haagen Dazs chocolate sorbet instead of ice cream and you'll save 17 fat grams. When you make oatmeal raisin cookies, replace whole eggs with egg whites, and cut back on the oil by combining fat-free cream cheese and molasses; you'll save 3 grams of fat per cookie.

For innovative substitution ideas, invest in a few low-fat cookbooks and subscribe to magazines such as *Cooking Light* and *Eating Well,* which are filled with low-fat recipes. Many health and fitness magazines, including *Health* and *Men's Fitness,* also feature low-fat recipes. We especially like *Shape's* monthly "Recipe Makeover" column, which shows you step-by-step how to turn, say, a 43 percent fat creamy chicken casserole into a tasty 13 percent fat version. For ideas on how to trim the fat from your favorite foods, consult a registered dietitian.

But don't get obsessive about this fat-trimming business. Some dishes are sacred, like Freihoffer's Chocolate Chip Cookies and Grandma Ruth's pecan pie. You needn't apply the 30 percent rule to every food you eat; the guideline applies to your eating habits as a whole. You still have room for an occassional breakfast of bacon (78 percent fat) and eggs (67 percent fat). There are no "bad" foods that you must swear off for good.

Reduce the fat in your diet gradually — otherwise, you *will* feel deprived. Start with a few foods at a time, or focus on reducing the amount of fat you eat at lunch. Using the gradual approach, you can actually train your body to *like* low-fat foods.

Consider what happened to Kathy Schneider and her co-workers at Bayer Corporation in West Virginia. The company held a competition in which employees were divided into teams of 10. Over the next 10 weeks, the teams competed against each other, scoring points for exercise and weight loss. The members of Kathy's team decided that if they won the contest, they'd celebrate by pigging out at Red Lobster. "We thought we'd go for deep fried shrimp with lots of garlic butter," Kathy told us.

Well, after 10 weeks of sticking to fruits, vegetables, and low-fat chicken and fish, Kathy's team won the contest. But when the members got to Red Lobster for their victory dinner, nobody ordered the fried foods they'd been talking about for weeks. "We all ended up getting salads and grilled shrimp," Kathy says. "I used to love steak and deep fried food. But now I can't even stomach it."

What the heck is cholesterol?

Fat and cholesterol are frequently mistaken for one another, so let's clear up the confusion. Unlike fat, cholesterol has *no* calories. Cholesterol is a fatty substance found *only* in animal products, including beef, chicken, fish, cheese, eggs, and milk. Eating foods high in cholesterol will raise the level of cholesterol in

your blood. However, eating certain types of fat will raise your blood cholesterol even more. (A healthy diet and regular aerobic exercise can lower your
blood cholesterol level.)

Once inside your body, cholesterol combines with other substances to form
lipoproteins. There are two types of lipoproteins: LDLs (low-density lipoproteins, nicknamed the *bad cholesterol*) and HDLs (high-density lipoproteins, the
good cholesterol). If you have too many LDLs, they stick to the walls of your
arteries, gradually obstructing your blood flow. HDLs, meanwhile, act as
vacuum cleaners within your bloodstream, removing the bad lipoproteins from
your body. We picture HDLs as scrubbing bubbles, like the ones in the bathroom cleaner commercials.

The higher your HDL level, the lower your risk of developing coronary heart
disease. When your doctor checks your blood cholesterol levels, don't just ask
about the total cholesterol level (which should be less than 200 mg per 100 ml).
Ask to see your LDL/HDL breakdown. Your ratio of total cholesterol to HDL
should be 5:1 or less. To do the math, divide your total cholesterol number by
your HDL number. If your total cholesterol is 175 and your HDL is 55, your ratio
is 3:1. That's good.

All fats are not created equal

Any fat you eat — whether it comes from olive oil, filet mignon, or avocados —
has 9 calories per gram. But some types of fat are more hazardous to your
health than others because of their effect on blood cholesterol levels. Keep in
mind that most foods contain mixtures of different types of fat, with one type
predominating. This section discusses the different varieties of fat.

Saturated fat

Saturated fat is the really bad stuff. It's found primarily in meats, such as beef,
pork, and ham, and in dairy products, such as whole milk, cream, ice cream, and
cheese. Excess saturated fat raises your total cholesterol level and increases
your risk of developing heart disease. Simply keeping your fat intake to less
than 30 percent is not enough for good health; it's even more important, experts
say, to keep saturated fat intake at less than 10 percent of your total calories.

Become aware of your saturated fat intake by reading food labels and consulting a fat-gram book that includes saturated fat grams. To figure out the percentage of your calories that come from saturated fat, first add up your total
calories and the number of saturated fat grams you ate. Then use the following
formula, which is similar to the fat percentage formula we describe earlier in
this chapter.

Let's say you ate a Quarter Pounder and medium french fries at McDonald's for lunch. The Quarter Pounder has 414 calories and 8 grams of saturated fat. The fries have 312 calories and 7 grams of saturated fat, so you ate a total of 726 calories and 15 saturated fat grams. Here's how to figure out what percentage of those calories came from saturated fat.

Step 1: **Determine how many *saturated fat calories* you ate by multiplying the number of saturated fat grams (in this case 15) by 9 (the number of calories per saturated fat gram).**

$15 \times 9 = 135$

So you ate 135 calories of saturated fat.

Step 2: **To calculate what *percentage* of your calories came from saturated fat, divide the number of saturated fat calories (in this case 135) by the number of total calories (in this case 726).**

$135/726 = .19$

This means 19 percent of your total calories were from saturated fat. The Quarter Pounder and fries are — surprise — not a good choice.

Unsaturated fats

Unsaturated fats fall into two categories: mono and poly. Olive and canola oils are predominantly monounsaturated; corn, soybean, safflower, and sunflower oils are mainly polyunsaturated. Which type is healthiest for your heart? A debate continues to rage among nutrition experts.

Monounsaturated fats get so much good press that olive oil comes off sounding like a health food. Proponents point to research suggesting that monounsaturated fats can reduce LDL (the bad stuff) without affecting HDLs, whereas polyunsaturated fats may reduce your supply of those helpful HDLs. However, other research suggests that there is no difference in the ways that monounsaturated fats and polyunsaturated fats affect cholesterol levels.

Experts do agree on two points: First, unsaturated fats, whether polys or monos, are better choices than saturated fats. Second, all fats should be used sparingly.

Trans Fatty Acids (TFAs)

These fats are created when polyunsaturated oils are chemically altered through *hydrogenation,* a process used to turn liquid vegetable oils into solids like margarine and shortening. Hydrogenation keeps baked goods fresh longer, but research suggests that TFAs act like saturated fats, raising LDL levels and increasing heart disease risk. Common sources of TFAs include fried foods, cookies, and crackers. Labels don't reveal how much fat comes from trans fatty acids, so watch out for foods that contain "hydrogenated vegetable oil."

Fake fats: a good idea?

Olestra is coming to a supermarket near you. In a move that has enraged a number of nutrition experts, the U.S. Food and Drug Administration has given the OK to olestra, the first fake fat approved for human consumption.

What's the big deal? Don't we already have tons of fat-free products on the market? Yes, but those products are made with fat *substitutes,* developed from substances like proteins and carbohydrates. Fat substitutes can't withstand high cooking temperatures, so they can't be used to make fried snack foods like chips and cheese puffs. Manufacturers have been left to use alternative processes such as baking, which is why most low-fat snack foods taste like Styrofoam.

Olestra is different because it's bona fide fat, made from a combination of vegetable oil and sugar. It looks like fat, cooks like fat, and tastes like fat. However, it doesn't cost you 9 calories a gram. Olestra molecules are too large to be digested by your body, so they pass right through you. An ounce of olestra potato chips has no fat and just 70 calories, compared to 10 grams of fat and 150 calories for a one-ounce bag of regular potato chips.

So why are many health experts up in arms over the FDA's decision? Because, when olestra molecules pass through your body, they take certain nutrients right along with them. Some of these nutrients are thought to protect against cancer, and some experts worry that people who eat a lot of olestra products will be compromising their health. Procter & Gamble, the company that markets olestra products under the name Olean, maintains that if you eat olestra products in moderation, your nutrient levels will remain normal.

Another concern about olestra is that in some people, the substances cause abdominal cramps and what the FDA politely refers to as *loose stools*. P & G, which spent $200 million developing olestra, counters that the side-effects of olestra aren't significant. After examining some 270 studies, the FDA agreed.

We'll stay tuned to see how this drama plays out. In the meantime, don't consider olestra (or the fat substitutes) the answer to any weight problems you might have. Even if you're willing to find out what it's like to have loose stools (we're not all that interested), go easy on processed snack foods. Instead, work on developing a taste for foods that are *naturally* low in fat.

Watch Your Calories

In 1994, Snackwell's Devil's Food Cookie Cake supplanted the Oreo as America's best selling cookie. This was pretty ironic because, as a nation, we're the fattest we've ever been. We've somehow convinced ourselves that *fat*-free means *calorie*-free and that we can gorge on fat-free foods without any consequences. In reality, when you eat more calories than you burn off, your body converts these extra calories to fat — whether they came from a high-fat cookie, a low-fat cookie, or an orange. Many fat-free foods are plenty high in calories because they make up for the lost fat by adding sugar. One Reduced Fat ChipsAhoy! cookie has 50 calories, while a regular ChipsAhoy! has 53. Not exactly major savings.

What's more, because the low-fat versions tend to offer less than complete satisfaction, you often eat much more of them than you would the real thing. Psychology plays a role, too: Studies show that when people are *told* that they are eating low-fat foods, they tend to eat more than when they aren't told anything about their food.

To estimate your daily calorie budget (which depends a lot on your activity level), use the formula in Chapter 27. Don't drop your calorie intake too low, especially if you are exercising regularly. If you drastically cut calories — particularly if you drop below 1,200 — your body will think it's being starved and compensate by hanging on to the few calories that you *do* eat. Use the following strategies to keep your calories under control. It's not as tough as you think.

- ✔ **Start with small portions.** You don't need to model your dinner plate after the Eiffel Tower. You can always go back for more. Also, buy single-serving packages of snack foods. You're less likely to keep eating if you have to rip open a whole new bag of chips than if you have your hand buried in a bargain-sized package.

- ✔ **Don't deprive yourself.** If you lust after a slice of chocolate cake, go for it; otherwise you'll end up inhaling an entire cake tomorrow. Live by the 90–10 rule. Eat what you should 90 percent of the time and cut yourself some slack the other 10 percent of the time.

- ✔ **Be selective.** Permission to satisfy yourself isn't license to gorge on every dish in sight. Buffets and salad bars require you to be extra-selective. See Chapter 26 for tips on eating out in restaurants.

- ✔ **Eat slowly.** Utter at least one complete sentence between bites. Many people eat so fast that they don't taste anything and then rush back for seconds. Give your body a chance to feel full.

- ✔ **Go easy on the booze.** Alcohol stimulates your appetite and weakens your reserve. This combination can lead to some serious overeating. Rather than drink before a meal, drink *while* you eat.

- ✔ **Stop when you're full.** Quit eating *before* your belt makes a permanent indentation on your stomach. Eat half of what's on your plate and then take a 10-minute break and assess whether you're still hungry. People often eat for reasons other than hunger, such as depression and exhaustion. Make sure that you're eating for the right reasons.

- ✔ **Eat regular meals.** Skipping meals sets you up for losing control and overeating. You're less likely to pig out if you avoid becoming a ravenous monster in the first place. Your meals should include some protein; if you just eat fat and sugar all day long, that's what you'll crave.

- ✔ **Avoid temptation.** Don't sabotage your efforts by keeping a bowl of chocolate-covered espresso beans in your living room. Instead, fill your fridge with crunchy vegetables, fruit, and low-fat cottage cheese or yogurt. Don't keep a jar of caramels on your desk at work. Bring fruit and low-fat crackers to the office.

✔ **Make meals a special time.** Don't eat while you're simultaneously reading *People* magazine, watching "Entertainment Tonight," and chatting online with your antique lover's support group. You might devour an entire box of Mallomars without even realizing it.

✔ **Don't strive for perfection.** If you do overeat, forgive yourself and get back on track. Don't think, "Heck, I've already blown it. A few more peanut butter cookies won't matter." They *will.*

Know Your Carbs

So far we've been talking about what you *shouldn't* eat — too much fat and too many calories. Now let's shift to a nutrient that you need in abundance: carbohydrates, or *carbs,* as athlete-types like to call 'em. Carbohydrates are somewhat of a nutritional bargain. While a single gram of fat has 9 calories, a single gram of carbohydrate has only 4 calories. Carbohydrates are your body's main source of fuel. If necessary, your body can turn to fat and protein for energy, but it prefers to use carbohydrates. However, your body stores very little carbohydrate, so you constantly have to restock. Carbs should make up at least 50 percent of your total calories, most experts believe.

Not all carbs are created equal

As with fat, not all carbohydrates are created equal. Some are nutritious, like whole-wheat bread and sweet potatoes; others, like Pepsi and Twinkies, are nutritional zeros. You've probably heard about complex carbs and simple carbs. *Complex carbohydrates* have sugar molecules strung together in long chemically bonded chains. They're found in beans, pasta, grains, veggies, and the like. Most complex carbs are low in calories, low in fat, and high in fiber. The sugar in complex carbohydrates is absorbed slowly into your bloodstream because it takes time for those chains of molecules to break down. Your blood-sugar level and energy level remain fairly constant, and you feel full for a good while.

Simple carbohydrates, on the other hand, are single or double sugar molecules. Simple carbohydrates, also called simple sugars, are found in table sugar and processed foods, but they also occur naturally, like in fruit. Simple carbs, whether they're found in a papaya or a Pop Tart, are absorbed quickly, causing the amount of sugar in your blood to skyrocket. Soon after, the sugar level in your blood plunges, often to a level below where you started — leaving you feeling tired and hungry. This change in blood sugar is what people call sugar *highs* and *lows.*

Fuel up for your workouts

Don't underestimate the power of food to get you through a workout — and beyond. This goes for novices and athletes alike. A few years back, professional triathlete Brad Kearns, in an attempt to lose weight and win races, went on a wacky diet that had one rule: Eat nothing but fruit until noon. "I'd have a melon, a banana, and some berries, then I'd go ride my bike for 3 hours and swim for an hour and a half," Brad told us. Three months later, he hadn't lost any weight and was struggling to even finish his races. "I was cooked," he says. "I was so starved that, for months after, I was eating peanut butter straight from the jar. It made me realize that your body doesn't like you messing with it. You have to eat."

You also have to drink. We're talking lots and lots of water — before, during, and after your workout. Some people are afraid to drink water during a workout because they fear getting cramps; in reality, dehydration often gives you cramps. What about those high-tech sports drinks with "unique glucose polymers that provide optimal fluid replacement"? Gatorade, Cytomax, and the like are good idea if you exercise for more than an hour — they provide fluid as well as easily-digestible energy — but water is perfectly sufficient for shorter workouts.

Here are eating tips for anyone who exercises.

Before you work out: Most people don't eat enough before a workout. At a gym where one of us works, the staff members witness at least one fainting a month; usually it's someone who shows up for a lunchtime workout without having eaten anything since the English muffin at 6 a.m. Your mom may have told you not to go swimming until at least an hour after you eat, but we're going to tell you the opposite: Eat *within* an hour of your workout. We don't recommend a seven-course meal, nor do we suggest scarfing down a turkey sandwich 10 seconds before you press "Start" on the treadmill. We do recommend a couple hundred calories of (primarily) complex carbohydrates, such as a bagel or a couple pieces of fruit. A little protein may help if you're going for a long workout.

During your workout: During most workouts, you don't need to eat anything unless you feel a major dip in energy. But if you're going for a three-hour bike ride or an afternoon hike, bring along snacks. Energy bars like Powerbars and Cliff Bars are a convenient choice. They easily slip into your pocket or fanny pack, and they don't get crushed like Fig Newtons or smashed like a banana. The good ones are low in fat and stocked with vitamins and minerals. However, real foods tend to taste better and cost less. Besides, some of those energy bars have as much fat as a Milky Way.

After your workout: Some people are under the impression that, if they eat right after exercise, they're somehow negating the benefits of their hard work. Just the opposite is true. If you eat within an hour of your workout, your body is more receptive to replenishing your energy stores. Eat a meal that's high in carbohydrates, but know that carbs alone won't cut it: You need to mix in some protein and even a little fat, to feel satisfied and to get the right balance of vitamins, minerals, and other nutrients.

But there's a difference between the *natural simple sugars* found in fruit and the *refined simple sugars* found in candy. When you eat that papaya, the natural sugar comes packaged with lots of vitamins, minerals, water, and fiber. Also, natural sugars are often mixed with complex carbs. When you eat the Pop Tart, you get zippo that's good for you — although we have to admit, Pop Tarts taste pretty good.

Try to stick to complex carbohydrates and the natural simple sugars. In general, eat foods that are processed as little as possible. In other words, choose an apple over apple juice, and whole-wheat bread over white bread. Be sure to buy bread that is actually labeled *whole wheat;* many wheat and grain breads are mostly refined white bread colored with molasses, despite the brown wrapping that depicts wheat fields waving in the wind and names like "12-grain health nut bread."

Is sugar really that bad for you?

Unlike fat, sugar hasn't been directly implicated in any disease other than tooth decay. However, sugar — in the mass quantities that Americans consume — can contribute to obesity, which in turn can lead to heart disease and cancer. (In 1840, the typical American consumed 4 teaspoons of refined sugar a day; today, we've shot up to 43.) Also, some people are so sensitive to sugar that even one glazed donut can send them on a mood-swing roller coaster. For some people, clinical depression literally vanishes within a week when they eliminate sugar.

Read food labels carefully and learn where you're getting most of your refined sugar. Like fat, sugar is often hidden. A cup of strawberry low-fat yogurt has $8^1/_2$ teaspoons. Even salty snacks like Bugles and Chex snacks have a lot of sugar. Breakfast cereals are classic culprits; Kellogg's Raisin Bran and Frosted Flakes are more than 42 percent sugar. When you read labels, know that sugar goes by other aliases, including corn syrup, honey, maple syrup, maltodextrin, sucrose, and other words that end in "ose." Sugar is sugar; honey and raw sugar are no better than the white stuff. The label for Wishbone low-fat salad dressing, which gets nearly 70 percent of its calories from sugar, lists maltodextrine, high fructose corn syrup, *and* sugar.

Studies show that, on average, Americans get 20 percent of their calories from sugar. Most health organizations suggest that we cut back to 10 percent. Pay attention to the number of sugar grams listed on food labels. The number of sugar grams tells you more than the number of carbohydrate grams, since not all carbohydrates are sugar.

Free radicals: the insecure molecules

Those gray hairs. Those laugh lines. They're the visible signs of aging, an outward indication of the chemical processes going on inside of you. You can thank mischievous little molecules called free radicals for the breakdown of your body.

Free radicals may sound like something out of the Woodstock era, but actually they're insecure oxygen molecules that roam around your body desperately trying to grab a hold of something. Free radicals are found in pollution, ozone, and tobacco smoke, and they're found naturally in your body. When they latch onto molecules that are more stable, they create a situation similar to what happens when you leave your bike out in the rain: In a sense, free radicals cause your body to rust. A free radical free-for-all can cause severe enough damage to weaken your immune system and leave your cells vulnerable to diseases as serious as cancer.

Enter antioxidants, the super heroes of your cell biology. *Antioxidants* destroy free radicals and protect your body's cells from harm. Research suggests that vitamin C, vitamin E, and beta carotene (a form of vitamin A) act together as powerful antioxidants. Beta carotene lost some of its luster when two studies found that smokers who took beta carotene supplements showed an *increased* risk of lung cancer — a result that so far defies explanation. Another study found that people who have never smoked did not benefit from beta carotene supplements. However, these results do not mean that beta carotene has no value. Perhaps it's just the supplement form that is not beneficial. Also, research has overwhelmingly shown that antioxidants work as a team.

In general, antioxidants show promise for preventing cancer, heart disease, and other conditions, but there's little evidence to back up claims that they're molecular fountains of youth.

Sugar substitutes

If refined sugar isn't such a hot idea, what about sugar substitutes like aspartame, also know as NutraSweet? Aspartame is probably safe, at least in moderation, although some people do report headaches and nausea. Still, aspartame has not been shown to aid in weight loss. When people switch to sugar substitutes, they tend to make up for the calories by eating more of other foods. Diet soda has been around for 20 years, and America is fatter than ever.

Protein Myths

Americans tend to treat protein two different ways: On one hand, most people get far more than they need — and from sources like steak and cheese that are loaded with fat, especially saturated fat. On the other hand, some obsessive dieters equate protein with fat, so they eat none at all. We know a high school track coach struggling to get her protein-phobic girls off what she calls the Bagel and Pasta Diet.

Protein is crucial because it's made up of amino acids, which your body uses to build and repair your muscles, red blood cells, enzymes, and other tissues. Your body needs more than 20 different amino acids, 11 of which your body can produce on its own. The remaining 9 must come from food. These 9 amino acids are called *essential amino acids.*

Before you go adjusting your protein intake, find whether you're a out protein overeater or undereater, or whether you're right on target. A good rule of thumb for protein is .4 grams per 1 pound of body weight. For example, a 180-pound person multiplies 180 by .4. He needs about 72 grams of protein a day; a 130-pound person needs about 52. To get an idea of how easy it is to rack up protein, consider that a Philly Cheese steak (36 grams), a side of fries (6 grams), and an 8-ounce glass of chocolate milk (8 grams) provide 50 grams of protein. In general, about 15 to 20 percent of your total calories should come from protein.

Estimating your daily protein intake is tougher than estimating your daily fat and calorie intake because most fat-gram books don't list protein grams (although all food labels and most nutritional software programs do). Use Table 4-1 to fill in the gaps:

Table 4-1	Average Protein Content of Foods	
Source	*Amount*	*Protein Grams*
Cooked legumes (beans, peas)	1 cup	12
Milk, yogurt	1 cup	8 to 10
Meat, fish, poultry, cheese	1 ounce	7
Most starches	1/2 cup	3
Vegetables	1/2 cup	2

It's fine to eat more protein than your body needs, as long as you don't go overboard. If you're way overshooting the mark on protein, cut back by using protein foods as a side-dish rather than as your main course. Sprinkle meat on your spaghetti or top your salad with strips of grilled chicken rather than plan your entire meal around hamburgers or fried chicken. If you find that you're not getting enough protein because you fear the fat, focus on the plant sources, such as dried peas and beans, lentils, soybeans, and black beans. Also, turn to dairy foods like fat-free cottage cheese and fat-free plain yogurt. If you're a vegetarian, even a vegan, you have plenty of protein choices.

Protein powder and pill manufacturers would have you believe that protein has magical powers. One protein powder advertisement says that drinking protein shakes might be the answer "whether you need to shed some flab or sculpt some amazing abs." This ad is misleading: Extra protein doesn't help you lose fat or build muscle. Besides, most people already consume two to three times as much protein as they need.

Protein supplements are a huge waste of money. One-half cup of cottage cheese has the same amount of protein as 14 protein wafers we saw in one health food store; the serving of cottage cheese costs 35 cents; the 14 wafers cost $2.30. And if you consume too much protein, your body will break it down to form fat. Excess protein also can damage your kidneys and liver.

Load Up on Fiber

Up until the '80s, when people mentioned fiber, they were usually talking about rugs or clothing. What we call fiber today, we used to call roughage. Whatever you call it, we're referring to a whole group of compounds that your body does not digest. Fiber comes only from plant foods — not animal products — and most of us don't get nearly enough of it. Experts recommend at least 25 to 30 grams per day, but the typical American gets 10 to 15 grams.

By helping to keep waste moving through your intestines, fiber keeps you regular and prevents hemorrhoids. Research suggests high-fiber foods also can prevent heart disease and colon cancer. Plus, they're bulky *and* low in fat, so you can feel full without overeating. People who eat a lot of fiber tend to eat fewer calories than people who skimp on fiber.

Wheat bran, oat bran, barley, and lentils have lots of fiber, but fiber isn't just brown stuff. It comes in many colors and textures. Apples, blueberries, and apricots are good sources, whereas some of those crunchy, brown foods are deceiving. You get only $1/2$ a gram of fiber from seven Nabisco Harvest Crisps 5-Grain crackers; a Snickers candy bar has twice that amount of fiber, and a peach has four times the fiber. So read labels carefully. Some breads have 4 grams of fiber per slice; other breads have less than 1 gram of fiber per slice.

The best way to get your fiber is through unprocessed high-fiber foods, which are low in fat and packed with vitamins and minerals. Forget fiber pills. Researchers think that fiber alone doesn't lower the risk of heart disease and cancer but rather the interaction of fiber with other components of these foods, like vitamin C or E. In order for a package to say "good source" of fiber, government regulations require the food to have at least $2^1/2$ grams of fiber per serving. "High fiber" foods need 5 grams of fiber or more to qualify. Fi-Bar granola bars can't make either claim; each bar has only 2 grams of fiber.

Table 4-2 lists the fiber content of some healthy foods.

Table 4-2	Where to Find Fiber	
Fiber Sources	*Portion*	*Grams of Fiber*
Pinto beans, cooked	3/4 cup	14.2
Kidney beans, cooked	3/4 cup	13.8
Split-pea soup	10 ounces	10.4
Whole-wheat spaghetti	1 cup	5.9
Dried figs	3	5.2
Whole-wheat pita bread	1 pocket	4.4
Pear	1	4.3
Baked potato with skin	1 medium	4.2
Raisins	1/2 cup	3.9
Wheat germ	1/4 cup	3.7
Brown rice	1 cup	3.3

A word of caution: If you don't normally eat a lot of fiber, increase your intake gradually. Give your body time to adjust or you may be indisposed for a good part of the day. Increasing your fiber intake drastically or eating more than 50 grams of fiber a day can cause diarrhea. Aim to eat a *variety* of high-fiber foods. Some types of fiber, such as the fiber found in wheat bran, can help prevent constipation; other types of fiber, such as the fiber found in fruit, oat bran, and cooked dried beans, can lower your cholesterol and risk of cancer. When you increase your fiber intake, be sure to drink a lot of water to help carry the bulk through your intestines.

Drink Water

We can't overstate the importance of guzzling water, particularly if you exercise. Even a tiny water deficit can radically affect how your body performs. More than 75 percent of our body is made up of water — even bone is more than 20 percent water. When you don't drink enough, your blood doesn't flow properly, and your digestive track doesn't run smoothly.

You've probably heard that you need to drink 8 glasses of water a day, 9 to 13 if you're exercising. Here's where that number comes from: You typically lose 10 cups of water per day — 2 cups to sweating and evaporation, 2 cups to breathing, and 6 cups to waste removal. You can replace up to 2 cups through the water in the foods that you eat, but you have to make up the remaining 8 cups by drinking fluids — water being the best choice. You also can meet your daily water quota by drinking juice and skim milk and by eating juicy fruits and veggies. Alcohol and caffeinated drinks, however, tend to have a dehydrating effect.

Don't rely on thirst to tell you when to drink. By the time your mouth feels parched, you're already dehydrated. Prevent dehydration by drinking all day long. Keep a water bottle at your desk, and always carry a bottle when you work out. See Chapter 23 for some innovative products that make drinking water more convenient. You know that you're not drinking enough if your urine is dark and scanty rather than clear and plentiful. However, vitamin supplements can make your urine dark; in this case, volume is a better indicator.

The Lowdown on Vitamins and Minerals

Contrary to what some hucksters might have you believe, vitamins and minerals don't give you energy. They can't because they don't supply calories. However, if you are deficient in certain vitamins or minerals, you may feel lethargic, in which case replenishing these nutrients can get you back up to speed. In addition to performing countless other jobs, vitamins and minerals help convert food into energy; they're the compounds that allow chemical reactions to take place in your body. If fats, carbs, and protein are the bricks from which your body is made, then vitamins and minerals are the cement that holds the structure together. Vitamins, by the way, come from living sources; minerals come from inorganic sources.

Despite the sleazy marketing tactics of many vitamin manufacturers, we believe — for two reasons — that virtually everyone can benefit from taking a daily multivitamin/mineral supplement. First, although you can get most of the vitamins and minerals you need from eating nutritious foods, the fact is, most of us don't eat that elusive *balanced* diet. According to the United States Department of Agriculture, about 90 percent of us fail to get enough magnesium, chromium, vitamin A, B vitamins, vitamin E, zinc, and many other nutrients. The typical woman gets less than two-thirds the calcium she needs to help prevent osteoporosis. In a typical four-day period, nearly half of all women fail to eat a single piece of fresh fruit, and the vast majority fail to eat even one dark green leafy vegetable. This explains why women are so deficient in vitamin C, folic acid, and other vital nutrients.

The second reason we recommend supplements is that, even if you make all the right food choices, it's tough to get optimal amounts of a few particular vitamins and minerals. For instance, research suggests that vitamin E might lower your risk of cancer and heart disease, but only when you consume at least 100 IU (international units, a way of measuring tiny amounts). To get this much vitamin E from your diet, you'd have to eat 25 cups of cooked spinach or drink 1¼ cups of vegetable oil (not recommended, by the way). Unlike with vitamin C, there's no easy way to get vitamin E from food.

However, none of this means that you should rely on supplements for your vitamins and minerals. Scientists are learning that the vitamins or minerals alone may not prevent certain diseases; instead the benefit may come from the way these nutrients mingle with other components in food. Aim to get the vast majority of your vitamins and minerals from food and take the word *supplement* literally. No pill is going to compensate for a diet of Doritos and Budweiser. When you eat healthy foods, you not only get vitamins and minerals, but you also get protein, carbohydrates, fiber, and other nutrients.

Choose a multivitamin (rather than individual pills) with doses that don't go much beyond 100 percent of the U.S. RDA (Recommended Daily Allowance). Don't bother with *super potency megavitamins,* which often contain more than 10 times the U.S. RDA (and cost you bundles). More isn't always better. Your body can absorb only so much of each nutrient; if you go overboard, the rest is just excreted when you go to the bathroom. As one doctor told us, "You'll have very expensive urine." With some vitamins, such as A and D, extra-high doses can be toxic. In general, you get all the nutritional insurance that you need from a single multisupplement; however, because most *multis* don't supply adequate calcium, you may want to take an extra calcium pill. Consult your doctor about other exceptions.

Also, forget those designer vitamins hawked infomercial-style by has-been celebrities and former athletes. Generic drug store brands are identical. Manufacturers have yet to come up with the magical combination of dosages to banish wrinkles or to make you live to 196, although a telemarketer recently called to inform us that every single Olympic athlete today swears by her particular brand of supplements. "Really, every single one?" we asked. Yes, she said. She was quite sure — every single one. Finally, don't be suckered by vitamins called *organic, natural,* and *time-released.* They cost more, but don't offer more benefits.

Vitamins: as easy as A, B₁₂, and C

Human beings knew about the importance of vitamins before we even knew about their existence. Seventeenth century seafarers found they could cure certain diseases by eating different kinds of foods. Oranges, for example, could cure scurvy, a horrible skin disease sailors seemed prone to catching. Then, in the early 1900s, a scientist isolated a substance in unpolished rice that he dubbed a "Vital Amine," which translates to essential protein. Early conclusions were that there was only one vitamin and that it was derived from protein. Oh well, even scientists are entitled to a few mistakes.

Progress being what it is, we now know that there are roughly 20 different vitamins, some that are absorbed into our body fat and organs and others that dissolve in the body's water. Scurvy and other vitamin-deficiency diseases have all but vanished in industrialized countries. However, scientists believe most of us still don't get enough of many vitamins to help prevent conditions such as cancer and heart disease. Here's a rundown of the major vitamins and minerals your body needs.

- **Vitamin A**

  What it does: Helps you see better in the dark; gives you shiny hair, clear skin, and cavity-resistant teeth.

  Best sources: Liver, eggs, dairy products, dark green vegetables, apricots, peaches, cantaloupes, carrots, squash.

- **Vitamin B₁ (Thiamin)**

  What it does: Although it doesn't supply energy, it helps you burn carbohydrates for fuel.

  Best sources: Lean meat, green peas, legumes, oranges, asparagus, whole grains, enriched and fortified grains, avocados.

- **Vitamin B₂ (Riboflavin)**

  What it does: Helps you unlock the energy found in carbohydrates, and helps you manufacture red blood cells.

  Best sources: Organ meats, dairy, oysters, lean meats, chicken, dark green vegetables, sardines, eggs, tuna, whole grains, legumes.

- **Vitamin B₃ (Niacin)**

  What it does: Helps keeps skin, nerves, and digestive tract healthy. Another key to unlocking the energy in carbohydrates. May also help lower total cholesterol while raising levels of HDL (the good cholesterol).

  Best sources: Lean meats, fish, poultry, legumes, whole grains, eggs.

✔ **Vitamin B₆ (Pyroxdine)**

What it does: Helps fight infections; helps you produce amino acids, the building blocks of protein.

Best sources: Lean meat, liver, fish, nuts, legumes, whole grains, poultry, bananas.

✔ **Vitamin B₁₂ (Cobalamin)**

What it does: Helps reduce risk of heart disease, some cancers, and birth defects like spina bifida.

Best sources: Organ meats, lean meat, egg yolks, dairy, fish, shellfish.

✔ **Folic Acid (Folacin)**

What it does: Helps form enzymes and hemoglobin.

Best sources: Meat, dark green and leafy vegetables, asparagus, lima beans, whole grains, nuts, legumes.

✔ **Vitamin C (Citric Acid)**

What it does: Helps you resist infections, although there's still no proof it cures the common cold. Helps cuts heal faster. Vitamin C is also a powerful antioxidant (see the sidebar in this chapter).

Best sources: Strawberries, citrus fruits, cauliflower, cabbage, tomatoes, asparagus, dark green vegetables.

✔ **Vitamin D**

What it does: Helps you absorb calcium for strong bones and teeth. May help prevent colon cancer.

Best sources: Milk, egg yolks, fortified breakfast cereals, sunlight.

✔ **Vitamin E**

What it does: Helps keep your body's tissues healthy and acts as an antioxidant.

Best sources: Plant oils, wheat germ, green leafy vegetables, nuts, whole grains, liver, egg yolks, legumes.

Precious minerals

Minerals do several jobs, from helping produce energy to regulating your blood pressure. Sometimes two minerals act together. Sodium and potassium perform a delicate dance with each other to regulate the balance of fluids in your body.

On the other hand, one mineral may interfere with the absorption of another, as iron supplements have been shown to prevent the body from absorbing calcium. You'll be fine if you make sure to eat a variety of foods packed with vitamins and minerals.

Here's the scoop on 10 important minerals. You need 24 overall:

- **Calcium**

  What it does: Keeps your bones healthy. Lack of calcium leads to osteoporosis, the brittle bone disease.

  Best sources: Dairy products, leafy green vegetables, broccoli, dried fruit.

- **Chromium**

  What it does: Helps break down carbohydrates so your body can use them for energy.

  Best sources: Brewer's yeast, meat, clams, whole grains, cheese, nuts.

- **Copper**

  What it does: Boosts your immune system. Too little of this mineral can lead to elevated cholesterol levels.

  Best sources: Organ meats, shellfish, whole grains, nuts, legumes, lean meat, fish, fruits, vegetables.

- **Iodine**

  What it does: Helps regulate metabolism. (See Chapter 27 for a discussion on metabolism.)

  Best sources: Iodized salt, seafood, seaweed, dairy, meats.

- **Iron**

  What it does: Keeps your blood healthy and bolsters your immune system.

  Best sources: Organ meats, red meat, fish, shellfish, poultry, enriched cereals, egg yolks, leafy green vegetables, dried fruits.

- **Magnesium**

  What it does: Helps protect against heart disease and kidney stones.

  Best sources: Whole grains, nuts, legumes, dark green vegetables, seafood, chocolate.

- **Phosphorus**

  What it does: Helps build strong bones and teeth, transmits nerve impulses. However, too much phosphorous may contribute to bone loss. Limit soft drinks and processed foods that contain large amounts of phosphorous.

  Best sources: Dairy, fish, meat, poultry, egg yolks, nuts, legumes, whole grains.

✔ **Potassium**

What it does: Helps keep your blood pressure low.

Best sources: Lean meat, fresh fruits and vegetables, dairy, nuts, legumes.

✔ **Selenium**

What it does: Acts as an antioxidant.

Best sources: Organ meats, seafood, lean meats, whole grains, dairy.

✔ **Sodium**

What it does: Helps keep your body's fluids in balance. However, most of us get too much of a good thing by overeating salted and processed foods.

Best sources: Salt, soy sauce, soups, sauces, cured meats.

✔ **Zinc**

What it does: Helps maintain your sense of taste. No, not the sense of taste that makes you realize stripes clash with flower prints — the sense of taste that makes you appreciate fudge brownies.

Best sources: Oysters, lobster, crab, extra-lean beef, dark turkey meat.

Part II

Working Your Heart

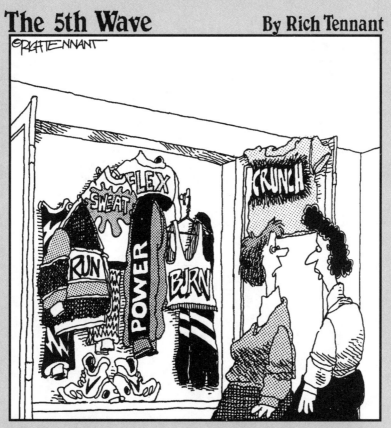

The 5th Wave   By Rich Tennant

"I'm not sure I can live up to my workout clothes."

In this part . . .

We explain what the heck "aerobic" means and tell you everything you need to know about this type of exercise. In Chapter 5 we cover how often you need to exercise and how hard you need to push yourself. Chapter 6 explains what it takes to lose fat. We also tell you which activities burn the most calories. In Chapter 7 we cover the three most neglected components of exercise: warming up, cooling down, and stretching. In Chapter 8 we explain how to use indoor aerobic equipment such as stairclimbers and treadmills and introduce high-tech machines coming soon to health clubs near you. Chapter 9 covers tips and equipment for your major outdoor aerobic activities: walking, running, cycling, Rollerblading, and swimming.

Chapter 5

The Truth About "No Pain, No Gain"

- -

In This Chapter
▶ How hard to push yourself

▶ Finding your target heart rate zone

▶ Measuring your progress

▶ What does *aerobic* mean, anyway?

▶ The best pace for burning fat

- -

If we could eliminate two phrases from the English language, they would be "no pain, no gain" and "feel the burn." We'd also like to eliminate "It's the economy, stupid," but one thing at a time. The truth is, exercise does not need to hurt to be good for you. In fact, if it does hurt, you're probably doing something wrong. Even Jane Fonda, who popularized those annoying adages, has mellowed in recent years.

However, this doesn't mean you can benefit much from walking around the track at the same pace you stroll down the aisles at the grocery store. They don't call it *working out* for nothing. Your heart is like any other muscle: The more you challenge it, the stronger it gets. In this chapter, we explain just how hard you need to push yourself, whether you're training to run a fast marathon or training to chase the ice cream truck down the street. We tell you what the heck people are doing when they poke their fingers into their neck in the middle of an aerobics class. And we explain the concept of your *target heart rate zone*, which — in case you were wondering — has nothing to do with what happens to your heart when there's a sale at Target.

Finding the Right Pace

If you don't push yourself hard enough, you'll miss out on many of the benefits of exercise — such as a reduced risk of heart disease, diabetes, and high blood pressure — and you won't burn a significant number of calories. On the other hand, exercising too hard can lead to injury and inhibit your progress; plus, you may get so burned out that you want to set fire to your treadmill.

To get fit and stay healthy, you need to find the middle ground: a moderate, or aerobic, pace. (For a more scientific definition of aerobic, see the sidebar, "What does *aerobic* mean, anyway?" later in this chapter.) You can find the middle ground in a number of different ways. Some methods of gauging your intensity are extremely simple, and some require a foray into arithmetic. This section looks at three popular ways to gauge your intensity.

The talk test

The simplest way to monitor how hard you're working is to talk. You should be able to carry on a conversation while you're exercising. If you're so out of breath that you can't even string together the words "Dear God, help me," you need to slow down. On the other hand, if you're able to sing "Achy Breaky Heart" at the top of your lungs, that's a pretty big clue you need to pick up the pace. Basically, you should feel like you're working, but not so hard that you feel like your lungs are about to burst.

You can use the talk test even if you're exercising alone. Simply ask yourself out loud from time to time, "How's it hanging?" Or say, "Keep it up. You're doing great." You may get some weird stares, but at least you know you're humming along at the right pace.

Rating of perceived exertion

If you're the type of person who needs more precision in life than the talk test offers, you might like the so-called *RPE* (short for *rating of perceived exertion*) method of gauging intensity. This method uses a numerical scale, typically from 1 to 10, that corresponds to how hard you feel you're working — the rate at which you *perceive* that you are exerting yourself.

An activity rated "1" on an RPE scale would be something that you feel you could do forever, like sit in bed and watch *Chariots of Fire*. A 10 represents all-out effort, like the last few feet of an uphill sprint, about 20 seconds before your legs buckle. Your workout intensity should fall somewhere between 5 and 8. To decide on a number, pay attention to how hard you're breathing, how fast your heart is beating, how much you're sweating, and how tired your legs feel — anything that contributes to the effort of sustaining the exercise.

The purpose of putting a numerical value on exercise is not to make your life more complicated but rather to help you maintain a proper workout intensity. For instance, let's say that you run two miles around your neighborhood and it feels like an 8. If after a few weeks running those two miles feels like a 4, you know it's time to pick up the pace. Initially, you may want to have an RPE chart in front of you. Many gyms post these charts on the walls, and you can easily create one at home. After a few workouts you can use a mental RPE chart. Table 5-1 shows a sample RPE chart.

Table 5-1	RPE Chart	
Numerical Rating	*Subjective Rating*	*Sample Activities*
0	Nothing at All	Sitting still, reading
1	Very Light	
2	Light	Standing in line, taking a leisurely stroll
3		
4	Light/Moderate	
5	Moderate	Walking at a moderate pace, gardening
6		
7	Hard	Jogging briskly, cycling over rolling hills
8	Very Hard	
9		
10	Extremely hard	Sprinting up a steep hill

Measuring your heart rate

The talk test and the RPE chart are both valid ways to make sure that you're exercising at the right pace. But there's a more precise way: Measuring your *heart rate,* the number of times your heart beats per minute. (Your heart rate is also called your pulse.) You can determine this number either by counting the beats at your wrist or neck or by wearing a gadget called a heart rate monitor. We explain these methods in detail later in this chapter.

If you're the type of person who likes to balance your checkbook, you'll love measuring your heart rate. Actually, if you hate balancing your checkbook, you still might like keeping track of your pulse. Your heart rate can tell you so much about your body — how fit you are, how much you've improved, and whether you've recovered from yesterday's workout.

What does *aerobic* mean, anyway?

At some point, you're going to run into the terms aerobic and anaerobic. So here's what those terms mean.

Aerobic exercise is any repetitive activity that you do long enough and hard enough to challenge your heart and lungs. To get this effect, you generally need to use your big muscles, including your butt, legs, back, and chest. Walking, bicycling, swimming, and stair climbing count as aerobic exercise. If you hopped up and down on one foot long enough and hard enough, we suppose that'd be aerobic, too, though why you'd want to do that is beyond us.

Movements that use your smaller muscles, like your wrists, don't cut it. Channel surfing with your remote control can certainly be repetitive, sustained, and intense — particularly when performed by certain husbands and boyfriends we know — but it's not aerobic. Throughout this book we use the terms *cardiovascular* and *aerobic* interchangeably.

The word aerobic was coined in the late 1960s by fitness guru Dr. Kenneth Cooper, and it literally means *with air*. When you exercise, your body needs an extra supply of oxygen, which, of course, your lungs extract from the air. Think of oxygen as the gas in your car: When you're idling at a stoplight, you don't need as much fuel as when you're zooming across Montana on I90. During your aerobic workouts, your body continuously delivers oxygen to your muscles.

However, if you push yourself hard enough, eventually you'll reach the breaking point: Your lungs can no longer suck in enough oxygen to keep up with your muscles' demand for it. But you won't collapse, at least right away. Instead, you'll begin to rely on your body's limited capacity to keep going without oxygen. During this time, you are exercising *anaerobically*, or *without air*.

Anaerobic exercise refers to high-intensity exercise like all-out sprinting or very heavy weight lifting. After about 90 seconds, you begin gasping for air and you feel a burning sensation in your legs. That's when your body forces you to stop.

The point at which your extra oxygen supply runs out and you slip into the reserve mode is referred to as your *anaerobic threshold*. When you're in poor physical shape, your body isn't very efficient at taking in oxygen, and you hit your anaerobic threshold while exercising at relatively low levels of exercise. As you become more fit, you're able to go farther, faster, yet still supply oxygen to your muscles. If a couch potato tries to run an 8-minute mile pace, he's going to go anaerobic pretty darned fast; an elite runner can run an entire marathon at about a 5-minute pace and still stay primarily aerobic.

But how do you know what heart rate to aim for? There's no single magic number. Rather, there's a whole range of acceptable numbers, commonly called your *target heart rate zone*. This range is the middle ground between slacking off and knocking yourself out. Typically, your target zone (as it's called for short) is between 50 percent and 85 percent of your *maximum heart rate*, the maximum number of times your heart can beat in a minute.

At the low end of your zone, you're barely breaking a sweat; at the high end, you're dripping like a Kentucky Derby winner. Beginners should stick to the lower end so that they can move along comfortably for longer periods of time and with less chance of injury. As you get more fit, you may want to do some of your training in the middle and upper end of your zone.

So how do you know what your maximum heart rate is? Well, we don't recommend running as hard as you can until you keel over and then counting your heart beats for one minute. A safer and more accurate way is to have your max measured by a professional such as a physician or exercise specialist. (See Chapter 1 for details on exercise testing.) You can also use a number of mathematical formulas to estimate your max.

The most time-honored method for determining maximum heart rate is for men to subtract their age from 220 and for women to subtract their age from 226. Keep in mind that this formula gives you only an *estimate.* Your true max might be as much as 15 beats higher or lower. Also, this formula is generally used for activities during which your feet hit the ground. (To estimate your max for bicycling, subtract about 5 beats from the final result; for swimming, subtract about 10 beats.)

Using that easy formula to find your max, find your target heart rate zone by calculating 50 percent and 85 percent of your maximum. Here's the math for a 40-year-old man:

> $220 - 40 = 180$
>
> This is your estimated maximum heart rate.
>
> ---
>
> $180 \times .50 = 90$
>
> This is the low end of your target zone. If your heart beats less than 90 times per minute, you know that you're not pushing hard enough.
>
> ---
>
> $180 \times .85 = 153$
>
> This is the high end of your target zone. If your heart beats faster than 153 beats per minute, you need to slow down.

Okay, so now you know how to figure out your target heart rate zone. But how do you know if you're *in* the zone? In other words, how do you know how fast your heart is beating at any given moment? As we mentioned earlier, you can check your heart rate in two ways: taking your pulse manually or using a heart rate monitor.

Another way to find your target zone

One of the problems with the formula for finding your target heart rate presented earlier in this chapter is that it takes into consideration only your age. This is a valid consideration, because your heart rate tends to decline as you get older. However, the following formula, called the Karvonen method, is somewhat more accurate because it also factors in your *resting heart rate,* the number of times your heart beats when you're sitting still. Typically, as you become more fit, your heart rate drops.

The Karvonen method requires a bit more math, but don't let that intimidate you. Grab your calculator and follow these step-by-step instructions. Let's use the example of a 40-year-old man who has a resting heart rate of 60 beats per minute. Let's say this guy wants to work at between 50 percent and 85 percent of his maximum heart rate.

Step One: Subtract your age from 220.

$$220 - 40 = 180$$

This is your estimated maximum.

Step Two: Subtract your resting heart rate from your estimated maximum.

$$180 - 60 = 120$$

Step Three: Multiply the number you arrived at in Step Two by 50 percent. Then add your resting heart rate back in.

$$120 \times .50 = 60$$

$$60 + 60 = 120$$

120 is the low end of your target zone.

Step Four: Multiply the Step Two result by 85 percent. Then add your resting heart rate back in.

$$120 \times .85 = 102$$

$$102 + 60 = 162$$

162 is the high end of your target zone.

Okay, now that you feel like you've earned your Ph.D. in integral calculus, let's compare the results of this formula with those of the traditional formula. Using the age-related formula, this 40-year-old's target zone is 90 to 153 beats. But when you factor in his resting heart rate, this allows him to work up to 162 beats per minute. And he knows that if he drops below 108 beats, he probably needs to pick up the pace.

Taking your pulse

Watch any quality aerobics video or take any decent class at the gym, and you hear the instructor yell out, "Okay, everybody, time for a heart rate check." On this cue, the participants place their fingers on their neck or on their wrist. Taking your pulse manually can be wildly inaccurate, so concentrate when you do it.

To use the neck method, place your index and middle fingers (not your thumb) in the groove on either side of your throat pipe. When you feel a beat, you've found your carotid artery. The neck method isn't our favorite because your heart rate is harder to find on your neck and because some experts feel that the act of pressing against this artery may actually slow your heart rate down. We prefer the wrist method, which we explain in Chapter 1.

Whichever method you choose, you don't need to keep your fingers on your neck or wrist for an entire minute while you count the beats. Feel the steady pounding of blood flowing through your arteries. Once you are fairly comfortable with the rhythm, count how many beats you feel in 15 seconds. Then multiply this number by four — voilà, your heart rate.

If you flunked Mr. Dyshuck's fifth grade math class and multiplying by four proves to be out of your range of talents, that's okay. Just take your pulse for 6 seconds and add a zero onto the number of beats you count; this, in effect, is multiplying by 10. For example: You take your pulse for 6 seconds and count 14 beats. Add a zero and you get 140 — that's approximately how many times per minute your heart is beating. Just know that this short-cut method can be extremely inaccurate. If you miss a single beat, you miscalculate your heart rate by 10 beats per minute. We mention this method only because it's commonly used in health clubs.

During your workout, take your pulse about every 15 minutes and be sure to concentrate. Otherwise, you might end up counting the number of steps you take on the stairclimber rather than the number of pulses in your wrist. You might want to slow down or even stop while you take your pulse. True, this is disruptive to your workout, but not nearly as disruptive as getting launched off the treadmill.

Using a heart rate monitor

You can eliminate this inaccuracy and inconvenience by wearing a heart rate monitor (see Figure 5-1). With a monitor, you don't need to stop exercising or take the time to count anything. At any given moment you can find out your heart rate by glancing at your wrist. A good monitor can cost less than $100. The really fancy ones cost up to $400. They offer features such as a clock, a timer, and an alarm that you can set to beep when you wander out of your target zone.

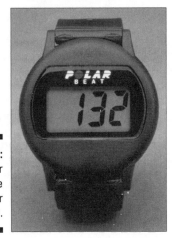

Figure 5-1:
The Polar heart rate monitor wristwatch.

The most accurate type of monitor is the chest-strap variety, which operates on the same principle as a *medical electrocardiogram* (ECG). You hook an inch-wide strap around your chest. This strap acts as an electrode using radio signals to measure the electrical activity of your heart. This information is then translated into a number, which is transmitted to a wrist receiver that looks like a watch with a large face. All you have to do is look at your wrist, and you instantly know how many times your heart is beating that moment, whether it's 92 or 164.

Some companies, such as Body Wrappers, make a special sports bra with loops for the chest strap. The bra works with any brand of monitor.

Chest monitors are very accurate, but they are subject to interference from electromagnetic waves like those given off by some treadmills and climbers. Exercising next to someone else who's wearing a monitor may also scramble signals, a sort of electronic equivalent of getting your braces locked with someone else's when you're kissing. You typically need at least 4 feet between users for monitors to function properly, although at least one brand, Polar, has a model with a special device to eliminate interference. (This is the $400 model.)

Less accurate than chest monitors are photo-optic models. These clip onto your earlobe or fingertip and shine a beam of infrared light through your skin to measure the amount of blood pumped into your blood vessels. Your heart rate shows up on a hand-held or clip-on digital screen or special wrist watch. Those models cost only about $30, but any movement of your wrist, hand, or fingers can cause highly erratic or false readings. Daylight, poor circulation, and high-intensity exercise may also skew the results.

Why Monitor Your Heart Rate?

Keeping track of your heart rate, by whatever method, sounds like an incredibly advanced thing to do — something way beyond the needs of a beginner. But novices actually have the most to learn from heart-rate monitoring.

When you're just starting to work out, you may not have a good sense of how hard to push yourself. And with all that "no pain, no gain" propaganda, you might be working harder than you really need to. Actually, this happens to advanced exercisers and athletes all the time. Left to their own devices, they try to out-do themselves every day. The smart ones use a heart rate monitor to remind them to slow down. However, for most of us the problem is getting into a higher gear.

Knowing how hard you're working during a workout is far more helpful than simply knowing how fast you're going. For instance, running 9-minute miles on a hot, humid afternoon takes a lot more effort than running at the same pace on a cool, overcast morning. If you rely only on your stopwatch, you might push yourself to run 9-minute miles in the heat, when that pace might put excess stress on your body. If you pace yourself according to your heart rate instead, you know when you need to back off.

MYTH BUSTER

Will going slow help you burn fat?

You may have heard about the "fat-burning zone." Experts used to think that if you slowed down your pace, you'd magically lose more fat. Well, it turns out that this concept is no more real than the Twilight Zone.

It is true that during low-intensity aerobic exercise, your body uses fat as its primary fuel source. As you get closer to your breaking point, your body starts using a smaller percentage of fat and a larger percentage of carbohydrates, another fuel source. However, picking up the pace allows you to burn more total calories, as well as more fat calories.

Here's how: If you go in-line skating for 30 minutes at a leisurely roll, you might burn about 100 calories — about 80 percent of them from fat (so

that's 80 fat calories). But if you spend the same amount of time skating with a vengeance over a hilly course, you might burn 300 calories — 30 percent of them from fat (that's 90 fat calories). So at the fast pace, you burn more than *double* the calories and 10 more fat calories.

However, going faster and harder is not always better. If you're just starting out, you probably can't sustain a faster pace long enough to make it worth your while. If you go slower, you may be able to exercise a lot longer, so you'll end up burning more calories and fat that way. If you're prone to injury, you're also better off slowing things down. Or if you just prefer a slow pace, that's great. Whatever gets you through.

The same goes for when you're tired. If you've had a particularly hard week at work, your body might not be up to your usual workout. Without checking your heart rate, you might force yourself to do Level 4 on the stairclimber, when, in fact, your body isn't up to the task. If you monitor your pulse, you might find that in order to keep up with Level 4, you have to exceed the high end of your training zone — a signal to drop down a notch or two.

If you keep track of your heart rate over a long period of time, you'll discover some interesting things about your progress. When you're a beginner, your heart has to work a lot harder to keep up with your body's demands for blood and oxygen. If you work out on a regular basis, your aerobic system gradually becomes more efficient. Let's say that when you started, Level 1 on the exercise bike used to get your heart up to about 140 beats per minute; now, two months later, your heart rate is 125 beats per minute. This drop means that you need to step up the difficulty of your workout. You can see why it's helpful to keep good records of your workouts.

To find out how much your fitness level is improving, watch how fast your heart rate drops after a workout. Measure your heart rate immediately upon finishing your exercise session and then one minute later. The better shape you're in, the faster your heart rate drops. Ideally, your heart rate should plunge at least 20 beats in the first minute. People in really good shape drop 40 beats or more. Keep track of this measure. You'll see a gradual improvement over a period of weeks and months.

Taking prescription or over-the-counter medication may affect the way your heart and blood pressure respond to exercise. Check with your doctor about this.

As we mention in Chapter 1, it's also a good idea to monitor your *resting* heart rate. Your *resting heart rate* is the number of times your heart beats per minute when you're just sitting around. When you start exercising, your resting heart rate might be as high as 90. But after a few months of exercising, your resting heart rate may drop 10 or 20 beats. Top athletes in endurance sports have resting heart rates as low as 30 beats per minute. However, don't compare your heart rate to anyone else's. Your resting heart rate is partly determined by heredity.

Your resting heart rate also can tell you a lot about your recovery from day to day. Keep your monitor by your bed and strap it on first thing in the morning, on a daily basis. Or, take your pulse manually. If your heart rate is 10 beats higher than usual, you probably haven't recovered from yesterday's workout.

Chapter 6

Losing Fat and Getting Fit

- -

In This Chapter

▶ How exercise can help you lose weight

▶ Which activities burn the most calories

▶ How to live longer

▶ How to build stamina

▶ Signs of overtraining

- -

*W*e're not out to cure insomnia, so we won't sermonize about the importance of exercise for preventing heart disease. You already know that you should exercise because it's good for you — a reason that never seems to rate too high on the motivation list. So in this chapter, we focus on the benefits of aerobic exercise that might be more likely to get your butt moving: losing fat and building stamina. We tell you how much exercise it takes to lose weight and how much it takes to build endurance. We explain how you can cut back on your workouts during a serious time crunch without losing your fitness, and we offer a whole bunch of tips to help you get to the next fitness level.

How to Lose Weight — And Keep It Off

You *can* lose weight without exercising. People do it all the time by simply eating less. But — and this is no small concern — you *cannot* expect to keep the weight off if you don't work out. Studies show that among people who are successful at maintaining weight loss, more than 90 percent exercise. On the other hand, at least 90 percent of those who *don't* exercise gain back all of their weight, if not more, within a few years.

What's more, you probably will lose the weight faster if you make a serious commitment to aerobic exercise. It's simply the best way to burn extra calories. Here's how weight loss works: A pound of body fat contains about 3,500 calories. In order to lose a pound in one week, you need to create a 3,500 calorie deficit. You can accomplish this by cutting 3,500 calories from your diet, by burning 3,500 extra calories through exercise, or by a combination of both.

If your goal is permanent weight loss, the best strategy is to meet in the middle. For instance, over the course of a week, you might eat 250 calories less than usual each day by cutting back from two scoops of chocolate ice cream to one; meanwhile, you could burn an extra 250 calories a day by taking a one-hour walk or a half-hour jog. For details on what exactly a calorie is and what *burning* a calorie means, see Chapter 27.

Losing weight is not as easy as it sounds on TV diet commercials. It takes a lot more commitment than just eating that delicious shake for breakfast. And it takes time. Exercising 20 minutes three times a week certainly can improve your health, as we explain later in this chapter, but it's not enough to make a significant dent in your weight-loss efforts. If you want to lose fat, build up to at least 45 minutes of aerobic exercise 5 days a week. Keep in mind that genetics play a large role in weight loss. It's easier for some people to lose weight than it is for others.

No matter how dedicated you become to exercise or calorie cutting, don't try to lose more than a half pound or a pound each week and don't eat fewer than 1,200 calories per day (preferably more). On a super-low-calorie diet, you deprive your body of the nutrients it needs, and you have a tougher time keeping the weight off.

We know one guy who limited himself to 800 calories per day while exercising like a fiend. One day he was riding the stationary bike and fainted mid-pedal. Don't get so enthusiastic about weight loss that you starve yourself while going on a workout binge. Your body *will* rebel.

Which Activities Burn the Most Calories

Maximize your workout and burn over 1,000 calories per hour! That's a claim you're likely to see in advertisements for treadmills, stairclimbers, and cross-country ski machines. And it's true. You can burn 1,000 calories per hour doing those activities — *if* you crank up the machine to the highest level and *if* you happen to have bionic legs. If you're a beginner, you'll last about 30 seconds at that pace, at which point you will have burned 8.3 calories, and the paramedics will be scooping you off the floor and hauling your wilted body away on a stretcher.

There's a better approach to calorie burning: Choose an activity that you can sustain for a good while, say, at least 10 or 15 minutes. Sure, running burns more calories than walking, but if running wipes you out after a half mile or bothers your knees, you're better off walking.

The following chart gives calorie *estimates* for a number of popular aerobic activities. The number of calories you actually burn depends on the intensity of your workout, your weight, your muscle mass, and your metabolism. In general, a beginner is capable of burning 4 or 5 calories per minute of exercise, while a very fit person can burn 10 to 12 calories per minute.

Table 6-1 includes a few stop-and-go sports such as tennis and basketball. Activities like these are not aerobic in the truest sense, but they can still give you a great workout and contribute to good health and weight loss. The numbers in this chart apply to a 150-pound person.

Table 6-1	Calories Burned During Popular Activities			
Activity	*15 min.*	*30 min.*	*45 min.*	*60 min.*
Aerobic dance	171	342	513	684
Basketball	141	282	432	564
Bicycling				
12 mph	142	283	425	566
15 mph	177	354	531	708
18 mph	213	425	638	850
Circuit weight training	189	378	576	756
Cross-country skiing	146	291	437	583
Downhill skiing	105	210	315	420
Golf (carrying clubs)	87	174	261	348
In-line skating	150	300	450	600
Jumping rope				
60-80 skips/min.	143	286	429	572
Karate, tae kwon do	192	834	576	768
Kayaking	75	150	225	300
Racquetball	114	228	342	456
Rowing machine	104	208	310	415
Running				
10-minute mile	183	365	548	731
8-minute mile	223	446	670	893
Ski machine	141	282	423	564
Slide	152	304	456	608
Swimming				
freestyle, 35 yds/min.	124	248	371	497
freestyle, 50 yds/min.	131	261	392	523

(continued)

Activity	15 min.	30 min.	45 min.	60 min.
Table 6-1 *(continued)*				
Tennis				
singles	116	232	348	464
doubles	43	85	128	170
Walking				
20-minute mile, flat	60	120	180	240
20-minute mile, hills	81	162	243	324
15-minute mile, flat	73	146	219	292
15-minute mile, hills	102	206	279	412
VersaClimber (see Chapter 8 for a description)				
100 ft./min.	188	375	563	750
Water aerobics	70	140	210	280

How Fit Do You Want to Be?

When you start an exercise program, consider not only whether you want to lose weight, but also how fit you want to be. (Even if you're thin, it doesn't mean that you are fit. Many skinny people can't last 10 minutes on a stairclimber. And many hefty folks can run marathons.) Contrary to popular opinion, exercise is not an all-or-nothing proposition. Many people think that you're either fit or you're not, either you're an Ironman triathlete or you're a total slob. But fitness has many definitions. You can be fit to live a long life, fit to go hiking with your kids, fit to run the Mount Everest Marathon (there really is such a thing) — or anywhere in between. In the next section, we discuss how much aerobic exercise you need to do to achieve your goals.

Fit to live longer

If your goal is to feel better and live longer, a little aerobic exercise goes a remarkably long way. Research shows that the people who gain the most from aerobic exercise are those who go from being completely slothful to only marginally slothful — not the ones who go from being fit to super fit. The people in the bottom 20 percent of the population, fitness-wise, are 65 percent more likely to die from heart attack, stroke, diabetes, or cancer than the highly fit people in the top 20 percent. However, when those couch potatoes move up just one notch on the fitness scale, by simply adding a daily 30-minute walk, they're only 10 percent more likely to die from these causes than super-fit people.

More good news: If your goal is to improve your health, you do *not* need to do all your exercise in big chunks. Nowhere is it written — in the U.S. Constitution, the Talmud, or the California Penal Code — that in order to benefit from aerobic exercise, you need to do it for 30 consecutive minutes. Studies show that doing three 10-minute bouts of aerobic exercise has nearly the same health benefits as doing one half-hour session.

What's the minimum amount of exercise that can make a difference in your health? The latest research suggests that you can lower your risk of heart disease just by walking for 20 minutes three times a week.

Fit for endurance

Some people can go dancing Friday night, run a marathon on Saturday morning, and then go mountain climbing on Sunday afternoon. They have enough stamina for an entire French village. To be one of those people takes a bit of commitment. But virtually anyone can build up that kind of endurance.

Bernie Kalkbrenner, a funeral director we know from Duluth, Minnesota, smoked 2½ packs of cigarettes a day for 25 years. One day, Bernie realized that if he didn't get his act together, he was going to become one of his own customers. So he quit smoking and took up bicycling. At age 51 he pedaled 3,230 miles across the United States in less than seven weeks. "I've never felt this good in my life," Bernie said upon finishing. "To be able to pedal my butt up a hill without any shortness of breath — that's exhilarating."

Treat getting into good cardiovascular shape like a really important ongoing project. You might struggle through the first session, maybe even the first 5 to 10. But if you stick with it three times a week for at least six weeks, you'll start to notice dramatic changes. At that point, you'll recover much more quickly from your workouts. Instead of going home and crashing on the couch, you might feel ready to go bowling or out for a walk. You'll feel stronger and have more stamina, your moods will improve, your blood pressure will drop, and so will your total cholesterol level. If you watch what you eat, you probably will lose some fat, too. You might reach some of these goals more quickly than other folks. It's a matter of where you start from, how hard you work, and your genetics.

Almost every athletic goal requires a good deal of motivation and time. But once you get going, you will find that this time commitment isn't a burden; exercise just becomes a regular part of your life — like tying your shoes, only a lot more fun. As you get in better shape, you'll actually look forward to exercising. Your workouts will give you a sense of pride and accomplishment. You may even get that rush of euphoria, known as the *runner's high.*

Realize, though, that the fitness lifestyle is not for everyone. You don't need to train for a cross-country bike ride to improve the way you function or feel. You shouldn't feel guilty if your commitment is simply a 20-minute walk three days a week; you should feel proud of yourself for sticking with it. And if you do become one of those people who rises every day at 5 a.m. for a 10-mile run, don't go around feeling morally superior to everyone else.

What Happens if You Stop Exercising?

Aerobic conditioning is a use-it-or-lose-it proposition. A couple of days of inactivity won't set you back, but if you continue to slack off, your improvements will fade in a matter of weeks. Research indicates that most of the benefits from aerobic training are lost within two weeks to three months. You seem to lose your conditioning in this short period of time no matter how long or how hard you've worked out in the past.

But there's good news, too. You can preserve your hard-earned fitness even if you go through a period when you don't exercise as much as usual. Let's say that you're a CPA. You get into a really good routine of jogging on the treadmill four days a week for a half hour, and you keep up the routine for four straight months. Then, suddenly, tax time arrives, and for two months you're buried in 1099s, IRS long forms, and 401k plans. Well, instead of abandoning exercise altogether, which would practically guarantee that you lose all your conditioning, you can cut back and still maintain your fitness for up to 12 weeks.

Instead of running a half an hour four days a week, you could get by with a half hour twice a week or 15 minutes four times a week. The only requirement is that you keep up your usual pace. When you get back to your regular routine after tax time, you may find that you've lost no fitness at all — or maybe just a tiny bit. Use the same approach if you get injured. If you're a walker and you sprain your ankle, don't simply give up exercise while you wait for your ankle to heal. Preserve your fitness by swimming with a pull buoy between your legs or by using the arm handles on a *dual action* stationary bike.

Strategies to Boost Your Fitness

As you get in better shape, you may want to challenge your body by exercising longer, more often, and harder. But don't do all of these things at once, and don't increase the length of your workouts by more than 10 percent a week. Otherwise, you really increase your chances of getting injured. In other words, it's not a great idea to do three 20-minute workouts one week and then jump to three 45-minute workouts the next. It's more sensible to increase the time of just *one* of your workouts to 25 minutes and keep the others at 20.

One of the best ways to improve your fitness is to experiment with your intensity. There are plenty of games you can play to challenge your body. This section discusses four training techniques that you can try after about a month or two of training at 50 to 60 percent of your maximum heart rate or 5 or 6 on the RPE scale. (For more information about your heart rate and the RPE scale, see Chapter 5.)

The less conditioning you start with, the more cautious you should be. Give your body time to adjust to this exercise business. And remember: The great thing about being totally out of shape is that you have nowhere to go but up.

Interval training

With interval training, you alternate short, fairly intense spurts of exercise with periods of relatively easy exercise. For example, say you're out bicycling. After warming up for 15 minutes or so, you might cycle all out for 30 seconds and follow this with a few minutes of easy pedaling until your heart rate slows down a little, to about 120 or fewer beats per minute. Then you do another tough 30-second interval, and so on. In essence, you're switching between the low and high ends of your target zone.

When you first try interval training, keep the high intensity periods short — 15 to 30 seconds. Follow these periods with at least three times as much active rest. *Active rest* means that you keep moving between intervals rather than stopping dead. So if you do that 30-second bike sprint, pedal slowly for about 90 seconds. You might need even more recovery than that, especially if you're a beginner. As you become more accustomed to higher levels, you can increase the length of the high-intensity intervals as you decrease the length of the low-intensity intervals. Eventually, you can aim for a 1:1 hard/easy ratio. You can measure intervals in terms of time or distance.

Fartlek

This charming word means *speed play* in Swedish. Fartlek is basically interval training without an exact measure of time or distance. You just do your intervals whenever you feel like it. You might try sprinting to every other telephone pole. Or set your sights on that horse standing in the field down the road and pick up your pace until you reach him.

Uphill battles

You can add hills to walking, biking, running, or skating workouts. You've got to work harder when you come to a hill, but ultimately you're rewarded with extra strength and stamina. As a bonus, going uphill can burn twice as many calories as exercising on flat land. One fun drill is to do *hill repeats.* Find a long, fairly steep hill and then sprint up it and jog down it, repeating this sequence four to eight times.

Here's a trick to make hill workouts seem easier: Pick a landmark that's partway up the hill, such as a bush or mailbox. Pretend that you have a rope in your hands and cast it over your landmark. Now pull yourself up the hill with your imaginary rope. When you reach your landmark, cast your rope on something farther up the hill and keep doing this until you reach the top.

Tempo workouts

Tempo workouts help you learn to move faster. During a tempo drill, you move at a pace that you consider challenging but not brutal, keeping that pace for 4 to 10 minutes. Do that a couple of times each workout. In between, exercise at your normal pace. If you're new to tempo training, begin with short tempos and gradually increase their length. Anyone training for a local road race or a bike-a-thon will find tempo work helpful.

Give It a Rest

For most of us, exercising too much is about as big a problem as saving too much money. However, some beginners — in their zeal to make up for 20 years of neglecting their bodies — vow to exercise every day for the *next* 20 years. This is not a good idea. If you're trying to get fit, your workouts are only part of the equation; *rest* is just as important.

Aim for a balance between hard days and easy days. If you do an intense interval day on Monday, do an easy workout Tuesday. If you do two tough days in a row, your legs will feel like someone inserted lead pipes in them while you were sleeping. Everyone should rest at least one day a week. (Just don't let that one day off slip into three years.) And when we say take a rest day, we mean *no* exercise. Nada. Zippo. An easy day does not count as a rest day. In addition to taking a day or two off each week, you might also want to take an easy week every month or two. So if you usually jog 15 miles a week, cut back to 7 just for the week. Drastic cutbacks can help remotivate you and give your body a vacation it might need.

Three more reasons to break a sweat

You know that aerobic exercise can help you lose weight, prevent heart disease, and lower your blood pressure. But did you realize that regular workouts may keep you from catching a cold or getting depressed?

Scientists are continually discovering new benefits of cardiovascular workouts. Here are three benefits that don't get much attention.

✔ A strengthened immune system

Some research suggests that moderate aerobic exercise can help ward off colds and other infections. For example, one study found that women who walked 45 minutes a day 5 days a week reported cold symptoms on only 5 days over a 4-month period. A comparison group of inactive women averaged 11 days of sickness during the same time period.

These findings, however, apply only to *moderate* exercise. Repeated high-intensity or extra long workouts can actually have the opposite effect, suppressing your immune system and making you *more* susceptible to infection. Studies have shown that runners who log more than 70 miles a week get more colds than the average person.

✔ Less stress and depression

More than 150 studies confirm that exercise can combat stress. Exercise decreases muscle tension while increasing your heart rate. This combination makes you both relaxed *and* alert, so you can deal better with your problems. It feels a lot better to take out your frustrations on the leg press machine than on your spouse or coworkers. Some studies suggest that exercise can even reduce clinical depression.

✔ A reduced risk of osteoporosis

In Chapter 8, we explain that lifting weights can help prevent osteoporosis. But aerobic exercise that you do on land — such as walking, jogging, and aerobic dance — also can help prevent this bone disease.

These activities place stress — or *impact*— on your bones, and this impact keeps them strong. The concept of impact has gotten an evil reputation in recent years because of all the injuries from the sadistic high-impact aerobics craze in the 1980s. But as long as you don't go overboard, impact is actually a good thing. Keep in mind that aerobic activities like cycling and swimming don't offer much help to your bones, although they have countless other benefits.

There's no magic formula to determine exactly how much rest is best for your goals and fitness level. But here's a good rule: If you're doing everything right, you should be able to wake up in the morning and say, "I know my workout's going to be really good," rather than, "How the heck am I gonna drag my butt to the gym?"

Exercisers of all levels are susceptible to overtraining. For an elite athlete, overtraining might be running 80 miles in a week; for a beginner, running 8 miles might be too much. Here are some signs that you've overdone it:

- Your resting heart rate sounds like Aerosmith's "Dude Looks Like A Lady." In other words, if your heart rate is way above what it normally is — say, about 10 beats — take it very easy or take a day or two off. (For details about your resting heart rate, see Chapter 1.)

- You feel chronically sore or weak. If you lift a ketchup bottle and it feels like a 10-pound dumbbell, stay home.

- You get chronic colds and infections.

- You're not sleeping well.

- You're irritable, anxious, or depressed. It's not a good sign if you lock your keys inside your car and smash the window to retrieve them instead of calling the auto club.

- You can't concentrate, or you feel disoriented. If you make a left-hand turn signal while you're on a stationary bike, it's time for a rest.

Chapter 7
Warming Up, Cooling Down, and Stretching

*W*arming up, cooling down, and stretching — they're not exactly sex, drugs, and rock 'n roll. In fact, these three workout essentials are more like flossing your teeth: They're considered a chore and neglected by most people. But if you nudge yourself to do these things regularly, you'll start to appreciate their value. Eventually, you'll even feel weird if you skip a day. This chapter explains how to prepare your body for a workout and what to do after you finish. We also dispel some major myths about stretching.

Warming Up

Before any type of workout — whether it's jogging, playing basketball, or lifting weight — you've got to do a *warm-up,* which simply means 5 to 15 minutes of easy aerobic exercise. (See Chapter 5 for a definition of *aerobic.*) It's best to choose a warm-up activity that emphasizes the same muscles you plan to use during your workout. For instance, joggers might start out with a brisk walk. Before an upper-body weight-lifting routine, you could walk on the treadmill with an exaggerated arm swing and then step off and do some gentle arm circles (no need to imitate a propeller). Be aware that stretching is not a good warm-up activity; as we explain later, you should stretch *after* you've warmed up.

The longer and harder you plan to work out, the longer you need to warm up. People who are out of shape need to warm up the longest. Their bodies aren't as efficient, and their muscles aren't used to working hard. If you are a beginner, *any* exercise is high-intensity exercise. As you get more fit, your body *remembers* what it's supposed to do and warms up more quickly.

Many people skip their warm-up because they're in a hurry. Cranking up the Life Cycle — or hitting the weight room right away — seems like a more efficient use of time. Bad idea. Skimp on your warm-up, and you're a lot more likely to get injured. Besides, when you ease into your workout, you enjoy it a lot more.

What exactly does warming up do for you? Well, for one thing, a warm-up warms you up — literally. It increases the temperature in your muscles and in the tissues that connect muscle to bone, and bone to bone. Warmer muscles and joints are more pliable and therefore less likely to tear. Warming up also helps redirect your blood flow from places such as your stomach and spleen to the muscles that you're using to exercise. This blood flow gives you more stamina by providing your muscles with more nutrients and oxygen. In other words, you tire more quickly if you don't warm up.

Finally, warming up allows your heart rate to increase at a safe, gradual pace. If you don't warm up, your heart rate will shoot up too quickly, and you'll feel like you're walking through a knee-high snowdrift.

Cooling Down

After you're done with your workout, don't stop suddenly and make a dash for the shower or plop on the couch. Ease out of your workout just as you eased into it, by walking, jogging, or cycling lightly. If you've been using a stairclimber at Level 5 for 20 minutes, you could cool down by dropping to level 4 for a couple minutes, then to level 3, and so on. Your *cool-down* should last 5 to 10 minutes — longer if you've done an especially hard workout.

The purpose of the cool-down is the reverse of the warm-up. At this point, your heart is jumping and blood is pumping furiously through your muscles. You want your body to redirect the blood flow back to normal before you rush back to the office. You also want your body temperature to decrease before you hop into a hot or cold shower; otherwise, you risk fainting. Cooling down prevents your blood from pooling in one place, such as your legs. When you stop exercising suddenly, your blood can quickly collect, which can lead to dizziness, nausea, and fainting. If you're really out of shape or at high risk for heart disease, skipping a cool-down can place undue stress on your heart.

Stretching

Contrary to what you learned in high school, stretching is not the first thing that you should do when you walk into the gym or arrive at the park for a jog. Don't stretch your muscles until you have at least warmed up thoroughly; you might even be better off stretching after your cool-down. A post-workout stretch is a great way to relax and ease back into the rest of your day.

By the way, don't stretch *before* you cool down; putting your head below your heart right after a workout can cause fainting and nausea.

Why you need to stretch

Stretching is the key to maintaining your *flexibility* — how far and how easily you can move your joints. As you get older, your *tendons* (the tissues that connect muscle to bone) begin to shorten and tighten, restricting your flexibility. Your movement becomes slower and less fluid. You don't stand up as straight. You walk more stiffly and with a shorter stride. You find it more difficult to step up to a curb or bend down to pick up the trash. Stretching your rear thigh, hips, and calf muscles can enable you to move a lot more easily.

Flexibility is also important for good posture. If your neck muscles are short and tight, your head angles forward. If your shoulders and chest are tight, your shoulders round inward. If your lower back, rear thigh, and hip muscles are tight, the curve of your back becomes exaggerated. A regular stretching routine also can reduce pain and discomfort, particularly in your lower back. In fact, the pain often disappears when you begin doing simple stretches for your lower back and rear thigh muscles.

What's more, flexibility exercises can correct muscle imbalances. For instance, let's say that your front thigh muscles are strong, but your rear thighs are tight and weak. (This is a common scenario.) As a result, you rely on your front thighs more than you should. Chances are, you won't even notice this imbalance, but it will throw off your movement in subtle ways — you might have a short walking stride or bounce too high off the ground. Muscle imbalances can lead to pulled muscles and also contribute to clumsiness, which in itself can lead to injury. Finally, if you're any kind of a jock — even a bowler or a Saturday afternoon softball player — stretching just might help you perform better: The ability to move freely in a wide variety of directions makes you a better athlete.

Experts have done very little research to determine whether stretching prevents injury, but virtually all of the world's top athletes make stretching an important part of their routine. Good flexibility makes their movements more graceful.

The rules of stretching

Watch runners at a park or a bunch of weight lifters at the gym. Chances are, they have the wrong idea about stretching. Maybe they'll grab their heel for 2 seconds to stretch their front thigh or bend over for a moment to touch their toes. This isn't stretching. Here are the basic rules for a useful and safe flexibility workout:

- Always warm up before you stretch. For best results, stretch after every workout.

- Stretch all of your muscles, not just the ones you've used in your workout. You should include at least one stretch for each of the following muscle groups: lower back, upper back, chest, shoulders, rear thighs, front thighs, hip flexors (the muscles above your front thighs), calves, shins, neck, arms, and wrists. Don't be surprised if you're tighter in some places and more flexible in others.

- Hold each stretch for at least 15 seconds. As you become more flexible, gradually increase the time to about a minute.

- Don't bounce. Ease into a stretch and gently hold it for the entire time. Bouncing may actually increase tightness and can cause muscle pulls.

- Don't force yourself into an uncomfortable stretch position. Stretch only to a point of mild tension — *never* to the point of pain.

- Don't hold your breath. Instead, take long, deep breaths. Inhale through your nose and exhale through your mouth.

- Let your mind slow down as you stretch. Stretching is also a good time to mentally replay your workout and think about your goals.

Stretching videos

Videos are a great way to learn about stretching. For Dummies-approved video instructors, see Chapter 21. It's a good idea to watch a stretch tape all the way through before actually doing the exercises. You'll get a sense of the tape so that next time you won't have to strain your neck to follow the screen. You also can learn about stretching from a trainer or from friends who are experienced exercisers.

JARGON ALERT

Stretching your limits

If you have a trainer or go to a gym, you might come across a stretching technique with a name that, in our opinion, wins Jargon of the Year honors: *proprioceptive neuromuscular facilitation.* Or for short, *PNF.* Still, this technique is quite effective and worth knowing about.

PNF simply means that you tighten a muscle right before you stretch it. The act of tightening, or squeezing, exhausts the muscle so that it becomes more receptive to the stretch. PNF is most often used for stretching the rear thigh muscles (hamstrings). You lie on your back with your heel resting on your trainer's shoulder and your leg almost straight. To exhaust your hamstrings, you press your heel into the trainer's shoulder while he pushes his shoulder into your heel. You hold this position for 5 to 10 seconds. Then you relax and hold the stretch for about 15 seconds. You might repeat the whole push/relax scenario three or four times. You can do a PNF hamstring stretch yourself by wrapping a towel around your ankle and holding an end in each hand.

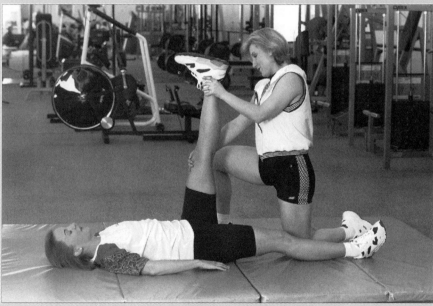

(Photo courtesy of Dan Kron.)

Chapter 8

Using Aerobic Machines

*W*alk into a health club or fitness equipment store and you get the feeling you're not in Kansas anymore. The rows of high-tech, aerobic contraptions bear little resemblance to anything you might encounter in the outside world. These gizmos appear to be part video game, part escalator, part lawn mower. Some gyms have machines that simulate wind surfing, in-line skating, and walking on air, plus fancy versions of the old standbys: treadmills, rowers, bikes, and stairclimbers.

We won't give you a rundown of every crazy invention that finds its way into a gym or an equipment showroom. Many of them will be extinct by the time you read this book. In this chapter, we cover the solid, proven machines that you're most likely to see and, we hope, *use*. We tell you how to take the drudgery out of exercising in place, and we explain how to position your body on each machine so that you burn the most calories and avoid injury. We discuss which equipment is best suited for beginners, and we explain how to hop aboard safely so you don't get ejected from the device like a kernel of popping corn.

About Those Flashing Lights

Indoor aerobic exercise is a lot more fun than it used to be, thanks to the feedback you get from computerized machines. For all your sweat and exhaustion, the screen offers you instant gratification: The number of miles you've walked, steps you've climbed, minutes you've cycled, and calories you've burned. Don't be alarmed by consoles that resemble the control panel of Apollo 13. With help from a gym staff member or equipment manual, even a rookie can understand all the buttons and knobs, flashing red dots, and beeping green arrows.

We love high-tech aerobic machines (see Figure 8-1), but we think that all of this feedback has led to an epidemic of outrageous posture. Many people go to unbelievable lengths to boost the calorie count that flashes on the screen. They crank up the machine to a level higher than they can handle and then compensate by clenching the handrails for dear life or hugging the console like it's a long-lost relative. What they apparently don't realize is that they are *cheating*.

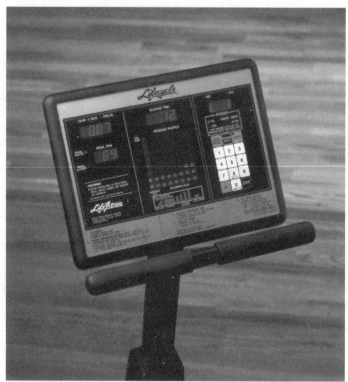

Figure 8-1:
A computerized bike panel.

(Photo courtesy of Color Image.)

When you clutch the rails of a stairclimber, you are transferring your weight from your legs to your arms or the machine. Studies show that cheaters often burn only half the calories that the machine indicates.

Use the computerized feedback to motivate you, but don't be a slave to it, and don't rely on the numbers to validate your efforts. Consider the case of a woman we saw on a stairclimber: Near the end of her 45-minute workout, she looked away from her console to say hello to a friend. When she glanced back at her machine, her workout had ended, and to her absolute horror, she missed the final calorie read-out. She uttered several curse words that we won't repeat — as if not knowing her exact calorie burn negated the entire 45 minutes of effort. She then stormed into the locker room.

Even if you do use perfect form, realize that the calorie figures are simply estimates. The number of calories you actually burn depends on many factors, including your weight, the amount of muscle you have, and your metabolism.

Combating Boredom on Aerobic Machines

It's no coincidence that "treadmill" is listed under "to tedium" in *Roget's Thesaurus;* imitating a laboratory rodent is not among life's thrills. No matter what type of exercise machine you use and no matter how many flashing dots you're rewarded with, boredom is bound to hit you at some point. In this section, we suggest ways to divert your attention so that, before you know it, your 20 or 30 minutes have passed. Eventually, you'll actually begin to enjoy the sensations of sweat and fatigue, and using these machines won't seem like a chore.

But first an important caveat: Tune into your body. If you start to feel faint or your knee hurts, don't try to drown out the pain by cranking up the volume on your stereo headphones. Don't ignore signs that you might be damaging muscles or joints.

Always keep a water bottle and a towel within reach. Many gym machines have water bottle holders, and you can buy them cheaply for your home equipment (see Chapter 18). Water and a towel will help keep you comfortable, and the more comfortable you are, the longer you'll last on the machine.

Vary your workouts

Most machines have a *manual* mode that allows *you* to control how tough the workout is. You push one arrow to speed up the pace, another to slow down the pace. Use the manual mode to design your own workouts, incorporating the training techniques that we describe in Chapter 6.

Also experiment with the various predesigned programs entered in the computer's memory. These programs are great because you don't have to decide what to do next. Most programs have built-in warm-up and cool-down periods. In between, the programs vary your pace. For instance, many machines offer a *random* program; every 10 to 30 seconds, the machine surprises you by changing the tension. Most treadmills offer programs like "A Romp in the Park," which may be a three-mile walk or jog over rolling hills. The treadmill automatically inclines and declines during these workouts.

Read a magazine or do a crossword puzzle

This is a good time to read the fitness magazines we talk about in Chapter 3. Exercise magazines offer lots of encouragement, and tend to contain easy-to-skim lists. When you're drenched in sweat on the stairclimber, it's a lot easier to take in "12 No-Fail Moves for Abs That Impress" than it is to concentrate on an essay about peace-keeping operations in Tajikistan.

Doing a crossword puzzle is also an excellent way to make time fly. Holding a pen and a magazine isn't as cumbersome as it may sound, particularly on a bike or stairclimber. Just don't try this on a day you decide to do go-for-broke sprints on the treadmill. Be sure to choose a puzzle that's not too difficult — you don't need to tax your brain and your body at the same time. Unless you're a whiz with clues such as "a mineral resembling feldspar," pass on The New York Times puzzle. *Dell* crossword magazines are great because they contain puzzles for all levels and include clues like "Mary had a little ___."

Exercise in short spurts

To break up the monotony, alternate 5-minute or 10-minute bouts on a machine with 5 minutes of weight lifting or even 5 minutes on a different machine. As we explain in Chapter 5, it's a myth that you *must* exercise for 20 or 30 consecutive minutes. Breaking up your workout into small chunks isn't a good strategy to use every day if your goal is to build endurance; in that case, you want to do your 20 minutes consecutively. But when you're aiming to burn calories and improve your health, the total time you spend exercising is what really matters.

Think, but not too hard

People tend to have their most creative ideas when they're doing something repetitive that doesn't involve their mind completely. But don't set out to solve the U.S. health-care crisis. Instead, use your time to ponder more solvable dilemmas, like how you can get your boss off your back. You might even keep a tape recorder handy, in case a flash of brilliance comes along.

Watch TV

Tune in to whatever you consider entertaining, whether it's "Truckin' USA" on the Nashville Network or British Parliament debates on C-SPAN. For variety, increase your intensity during the commercials. Many gyms have TVs suspended in front of the aerobic machines, but you might have to negotiate with your fellow gym members to find a show that's agreeable to all.

Listen to music or a book

Rock, rap, pop, or country — go with whatever gets your adrenaline pumping. If the Bee Gees work for you, so be it. A tape that mixes fast and slow songs can add variety to your workout, because your pace tends to be in sync with the music. Or try a book on tape. You might prefer to get wrapped up in a good story or learn how to manage your love life.

Monitor your heart rate

To keep yourself occupied, use a heart rate monitor to create an interval program. For instance, after warming up, you might alternate 5 minutes at the low end of your target zone with 5 minutes at the high end. If all this talk about monitors, intervals, and target zones is complete gibberish to you, read Chapter 5.

Talk to a friend

Some people think that if they're able to speak while exercising, they must not be working hard enough to do their body any good. As we explain in Chapter 5, that's not true. In general, your breathing should be light enough so that you can hold up your end of a conversation.

Exercising in the Great Indoors

Most exercisers have a favorite aerobic machine and one that they probably can't stand. Some people find the treadmill invigorating; others consider it more tedious than peeling potatoes. Some people live to use the Versaclimbers; others consider that machine a form of torture. We suggest you try all the machines at your gym or at an equipment store before you buy one. Here's a look at the most popular cardiovascular machines.

Treadmills

Treadmills are the motorized equivalent of walking or running in place. You simply keep up with a belt that's moving under your feet. Treadmill workouts burn about the same number of calories as walking or running outdoors. The only exception seems to be running uphill. When you incline the treadmill to simulate running uphill, it's somewhat easier than running up real-life hills of the same grade. But walking uphill on a treadmill is virtually the same as walking uphill outdoors.

Who will like it: Treadmills are especially popular in crowded cities, where you need to be part cutting horse, part smog filter to run or walk through the streets. Treadmills are great for beginners because they require little coordination to use. Plus, treadmills can move at a slow enough pace to accommodate even the most out-of-shape exercisers. People with back pain, bad knees, or weak ankles often find treadmills kinder to their joints than concrete or cement. Today's treadmills are springier and more shock-absorbing than ever.

Who will hate it: You need a very strong or very blank mind to do long workouts on a treadmill. Most people find more than a half hour on this machine mind-numbing, even with entertainment. If you crave the wind whipping through your hair and scenery flashing by, reserve the treadmills for emergency aerobic situations only.

Treadmill User Tips

Treadmills are among the easiest aerobic machines to use. Still, treadmill users are not immune to poor posture. And if you're not paying attention, you can stumble. On occasion you see someone slide off the treadmill like a can of beans on a supermarket conveyor belt. Here are some tips to make sure this doesn't happen to you.

✔ **Start slowly.** Most treadmills have safety features that prevent them from starting out at breakneck speeds, but don't take any chances. Always place one foot on either side of the belt as you turn on the machine, and step on the belt only after you determine that it's moving at the slow set-up speed, usually between 1 and 2 miles per hour.

✔ **Don't rely on the handrails.** It's okay to hold on for balance when you learn how to use the machine, but let go as soon as you feel comfortable. You move more naturally if you swing your arms freely. You're working at too high a level if you have to imitate a water skier — in other words, if you hold onto the front rails and lean back. This is a common phenomenon among people who incline the treadmill, and this position is bad news for your elbows and for the machine. Plus, you're not fooling anyone; you're burning far fewer calories than the readout indicates.

✔ **Look straight ahead.** Your feet tend to follow your eyes, so if you focus on what's in front of you, you usually walk straight ahead instead of veering off to the side. When you're in the middle of a workout and someone calls your name, don't turn around to answer. This piece of advice may seem obvious now, but wait until it happens to you.

✔ **Expect to feel disoriented.** The first few times you use a treadmill, you may feel dizzy when you get off. Your body is just wondering why the ground suddenly stopped moving. Don't worry. Most people only experience this vertigo once or twice.

✔ **Never go barefoot.** Always wear a good pair of walking or running shoes for your treadmill workout.

Stationary bicycles

Bikes come in two varieties: upright and recumbent. Upright bikes have been around forever — they simulate a regular bike, only you don't go anywhere (see Figure 8-2). Recumbent bikes, which came onto the scene in the late '80s, have bucket seats so you pedal out in front of you. Neither type is superior; it's a matter of preference. The recumbent does offer more back support and might be more comfortable for people with lower back pain.

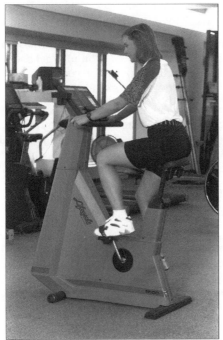

Figure 8-2:
An upright stationary bike.

(Photo courtesy of Dan Kron.)

Who will like it: Bikes are great for toning your thighs (and recumbents are especially good for your butt), and they give your knees a break while offering a terrific aerobic workout. Bikes also suit anyone who wants to read while working out. It's much tougher to hold a book or magazine in place on a stairclimber or treadmill — and it's impossible on a skier or rowing machine.

Who will hate it: Hard-core cyclists complain that most stationary bicycles don't have the same feel as outdoor bikes. They're right: The pedal positions usually are different, and the seats on a stationary bike usually are wider. Also, most indoor bikes force you to sit upright rather than allow you to lean forward, like you do on a regular bike. But these things won't matter to most people. Different bike brands offer very different positioning. You probably will like some bike brands more than others.

Stationary Bike User Tips

Bikes give you less opportunity to use atrocious form than do most other machines. Still, there's room for injury or discomfort. Here are some tips to help you avoid both:

- ✔ **Set the seat height correctly.** With both bikes (recumbent and upright), adjust the seat so that when the pedal is at the lowest position, your leg is almost, but not quite, straight. You shouldn't have to strain or rock your hips to pedal. Your knees shouldn't feel crunched when they're at the top of the pedal stroke. With a recumbent bike, you adjust the seat forward and back, rather than up and down, but the principles are the same.

- ✔ **Before you begin your workout, make sure your handlebars are set correctly.** Otherwise, you'll have to squirm around to get comfortable. Handlebar adjustment is especially important if you're very tall or very short. However, not all bikes allow you to make adjustments.

- ✔ **Get to know the display panel.** Paying attention to the display panel helps you set the proper pace. For instance, notice how many levels the bike has. Some bikes feature 12 levels; others have 40. So if you just hop on and press Level 6, you get two very different workouts. Also, pay attention to your *cadence* — that is, how many *revolutions per minute* (rpm) you're cycling. It's a good idea to vary your cadence. You might want to hum along at 80 rpm for 5 minutes and then do 30-second intervals at 100 rpm using the same tension level.

- ✔ **Don't pedal with just your toes.** Otherwise you may bring on foot and calf cramps. Instead, press from the ball of your foot and through your heel as you pump downward on the pedal, and pull up with the top of your foot on the upstroke. Adjust the pedal straps so that your feet feel snug (but don't let the straps cut off your circulation). Riding a bike with the foot straps is much more comfortable and efficient than pedaling without them.

✔ **Don't hunch over.** Rounding your back is the way to develop back and neck pain. And don't get your upper body into the effort. Unlike some other machines, riding a stationary bike is *not* a total-body workout; don't try to make it one. If you have to rock wildly from side to side, grit your teeth, or clench the handlebars, you need to lighten your load.

✔ **Make sure the bike is sturdy.** At one New York City gym, a guy was pedaling furiously when the frame collapsed and the bike shot forward and out the second story window — with the guy still seated. Ironically, he landed on a bike rack below. This being New York, the doorman said, "Hey buddy, you can't park that thing here." Actually, we made the last part up, but the rest of the story was reported on the news. Although the guy was hospitalized, he walked away more or less unscathed.

Bikes with arm handles

We're not thrilled about the trend of attaching arm handles to treadmills, but we do like the so-called *dual action* bikes, at least the brands that you find in health clubs. On a good bike, it's easy to keep upper and lower body movements coordinated while still getting a smooth ride. Operating one of these bikes looks complicated, but it's not nearly as difficult as, say, rubbing circles on your stomach while patting your head.

We especially like the new recumbent bikes with arm handles, particularly a brand called Cycle Plus. You can adjust the arm and leg tension separately, and the bike offers a variety of hand positions to emphasize different muscles. We're also fond of the upright Schwinn Airdyne; the flywheel fan generates a cool, gentle breeze as you pedal your legs and pump your arms. (See Figure 8-3.)

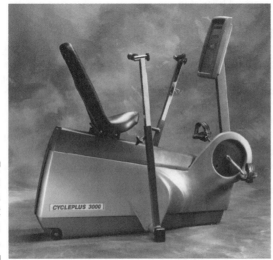

Figure 8-3:
A recumbent bike with arm handles.

Adjust the seat height as you would with a regular bike, and set the arm handles at shoulder height. Coordinating upper and lower body motions can take some getting used to. Start by focusing on your legs and then gradually add in more arm resistance. If you find that exercising your arms and your legs at the same time is too tiring, alternate arm and leg movements until you build more stamina. As long as you keep moving, you're still getting an aerobic workout. (For a definition of *aerobic,* see Chapter 5.) Keep in mind that even if you use a dual-action bike regularly, you still need to do upper-body strength training. The resistance on the bike is too low to build significant strength.

Stairclimbers

The most common type of stairclimber is the pedal stepper, which many exercises refer to as "The StairMaster." In fact, StairMaster is a specific brand, just one of many excellent makes that you find in health clubs and home equipment stores. Stairclimbing on a machine is a big improvement over jogging up and down the bleachers at your local high school football stadium. The machine eliminates most of the wear and tear on your joints.

Who will like it: Women in particular love stairclimbers because these machines do a good job of toning the butt and thighs. People who want to get in shape for skiing, climbing, hiking, and running also love steppers, as they're often called.

This is a good time to clear up the myth that stairclimbing causes you to build big bulky muscles in your legs. The truth is, you're more likely to build bulky muscles doing *any* type of activity if you work very slowly against a lot of tension. And if you have a genetic predisposition toward bulky muscles, you're pretty much going to fight against that no matter what you do. But for most people, this isn't an issue. The fact is, stairclimbing is a terrific way to burn calories and tone your legs.

Who will hate it: Beginners may get frustrated because stairclimbing is no vacation in Maui. If you're a complete novice, you might not last five minutes even on the lowest level. In this case, use other machines until you build up some stamina and strength. Also, stairclimbing bothers some people's knees. If you're one of those people but have your heart set on climbing, you might be able to eliminate the pain with a solid weight-lifting program. Do exercises that strengthen your thighs, both front and back, because those are the muscles that hold your knees together.

Stairclimber User Tips

Proper form is butchered on the stairclimber more than on any other single piece of machinery. We've seen people clutch the railings so tight that their knuckles turn white. Some less-informed exercisers think that it's really cool to be able to climb at the machine's highest level, regardless of their form. But those who know better realize that these people wouldn't be able to keep up if they climbed properly. Here's how to use this machine the right way:

- ✔ **Rest your hands — or better yet, your finger tips — lightly on the bar in front of you or on the side rails.** Do not grip the rails any tighter than you'd grip a paper cup. And never reverse your wrists so that your finger tips are pointing toward the floor and your elbows are turned up to the ceiling. You really should be able to use the stairclimber without holding on to the railing at all, but using the railing for balance (within reason) is okay. If you must hang on in order to keep up with the machine, you're going too fast. Believe us, nobody will think less of you if you drop down a few notches. In fact, you probably will impress people with your stellar posture and noncompetitive attitude. (See Figure 8-4.)

- ✔ **Stand upright with a slight forward lean at the hips.** Don't overcorrect your form by standing upright like a Marine at inspection. A slight — and we mean *slight* — forward lean helps keep your knees from locking and protects your lower back from over-arching.

- ✔ **Take even, moderately deep steps.** Don't take short, quick hopping steps, a technique known as "shaking the machine." This technique is hard on your calf muscles and cuts down on the number of calories you burn.

- ✔ **Keep your entire foot on the pedal.** This helps your buttocks and thighs get a full workout and prevents you from over-burdening your calf muscles.

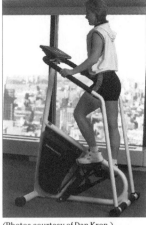 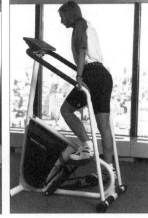 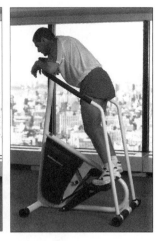

Figure 8-4:
Stairclimber
posture:
good, bad,
and just
as bad.

(Photos courtesy of Dan Kron.)

Rolling Stairclimber

This is the machine that looks like a section of a department-store escalator (only it's hardly a free ride). A set of stairs rotates in a circle so that you climb continuously, like Sisyphus up the mountain, ever upward, but never getting anywhere. You control the speed with a gear shift on the side of the machine and look straight ahead into the console, which tells you how many flights you've climbed. By the way, rolling stair cases have been around a lot longer than steppers. At the turn of the century, federal prisoners were forced to climb on them to provide electrical power to the prison facility.

Who will like it: In many ways, the rolling stairclimber is a better workout than a regular stairclimber. It's harder to cheat, because you're forced to take a fairly deep stride to place your foot onto the next step. (However, you can still cheat by clenching the side rails.) This machines gives you a tremendous butt and thigh workout, and you work up one "helluva" sweat. Start at a very slow speed until you can confidently navigate the height of the step.

Who will hate it: If you're used to the stepper-type climbers, the rolling stair climber takes some getting used to. Also, if you're just getting into shape, this contraption may be a bit much for you. At some health clubs, this workout is referred to as "climbing the stairway from hell." If you have knee or back problems, this form of exercise may not agree with you.

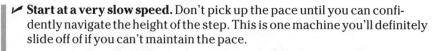

Rolling Stairclimber User Tips

The rolling stairclimber is a good machine to try when you're looking to make stairclimbing even more challenging. We know one woman who used this machine to train for a race up the Empire State Building — 102 flights of stairs. She came in second place.

- ✓ **Start at a very slow speed.** Don't pick up the pace until you can confidently navigate the height of the step. This is one machine you'll definitely slide off of if you can't maintain the pace.

- ✓ **Try climbing every *other* step.** This technique gives you a killer butt workout and a good stretch in your legs. This is not a technique for beginners.

- ✓ **Turn around and climb backwards.** This gives your thighs and calves a great workout. Just be sure you have good balance and a firm (but not *too* firm) grip on the rails.

VersaClimber

In this case, we're using a brand name to refer to a whole class of machines, the ladder-climbing simulator. The VersaClimber is by far the best ladder climber, and the one that you're likely to encounter at gyms (see Figure 8-5). The

VersaClimber is a stick of metal or wood that's about 8-feet high and leans slightly forward. You step on to the foot pedals, grip the handles, and do the vertical equivalent of crawling in place. Some models have hand rails so that you can omit the upper body motion and simply move your legs in an action similar to stair climbing. Other models have detachable seats so that you can do the upper body motion by itself. Many also have a built-in heart rate monitor.

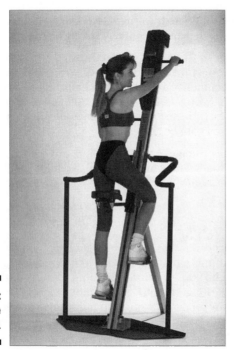

Figure 8-5:
Climbing the
VersaClimber.

Who will like it: The VersaClimber has a reputation for being the exclusive domain of aerobic animals, but actually, it's ideal for beginners, too. You can easily adjust the variables — step height, arm motion, speed, and tension — to customize the workout for any level. People with bad knees who like to climb may have an easier time on this machine than any other type of climber. This total-body trainer is used by many athletes, and in case you care, Madonna has one.

Who will hate it: We have a theory about why the VersaClimber isn't more popular: People don't like to be up high with their butts on display for the rest of the world. Some gyms put their VersaClimber off in a corner where exercisers tend to forget about it. That's a shame because the VersaClimber is a great piece of equipment. Vanity aside, there are some good reasons to avoid it, like if you have a bad back or poor circulation in your feet.

VersaClimber User Tips

Don't be scared off by this admittedly scary-looking contraption. The VersaClimber is not as tough to operate as you think. Here's how to look like a pro:

- ✔ **Always start out with small, quick strokes for 3 to 5 minutes to warm up.** Then experiment with different speeds, stride lengths, and tension levels. If you get tired, you can eliminate the arm movement by holding on to the hand rails or eliminate the leg movements by sitting on the seat, if there is one.

- ✔ **Practice good climbing posture.** Keep your back straight and keep your torso parallel to the machine. Don't round your back or lean back away from the machine. Even if you take long strides, don't stretch out your body so far that your foot hits the floor, your knees and elbows lock, or you're forced to over-arch your back.

- ✔ **Don't get fixated on the mileage.** A vertical mile is not the same as a mile on the treadmill or the road. A mile may still be 5,280 feet (1,609 meters), but we're talking *straight uphill.*

Cross-country skiers

Good cross-country ski machines have two wooden or metal skis that slide along a track of rollers. You clip your toes into a binding so that your feet don't slide around, and you can take long, smooth, gliding movements. Meanwhile, you work your arms by pulling on two cords or moving a set of poles. Your arms and legs work in opposition to one another; as your right arm moves forward, your right leg moves back.

Who will like it: Cross-country skiers love these contraptions because they do such a good job of impersonating the real thing. Even if you wouldn't dream of venturing out when temperatures dip below 50 degrees, you might like this type of workout because it involves virtually all the muscles of your upper and lower body. You can really work up a sweat, and you have a lower risk of injury on this machine than on a treadmill or climber.

Who will hate it: Trying to learn the movement of a ski machine is like trying to perfect the art of walking gracefully on marbles on top of banana peels. Ski simulators are actually harder to get the hang of than the real thing. So if you have zero patience for learning new skills, stick to the bike or treadmill. Consider an alternative, too, if you have weak ankles or lower back pain.

Cross-Country Skier Tips

Be patient while learning this machine. It takes practice to feel like your feet aren't going to slide out from under you.

- ✔ **Set the pad so that it's flush against your hip bones.** If the pad is higher or lower, it may throw you off balance. But don't lean too much of your weight into the hip pad. Otherwise, you probably will fall forward.

- ✔ **Lift your heel at the end of the stride rather than keeping it on the ski the whole time.** The heel lift is what creates the gliding movement. If you don't lift your heel, you will be cross-country shuffling, a much less comfortable activity than cross-country skiing. You might also place too much stress on your ankles and knees.

- ✔ **Get the hang of the leg motion before adding in the arms.** Most machines have a pad or set of handles you can hold onto while you're getting the hang of the lower body movement.

- ✔ **Vary the length of your stride between short, quick steps and long, full strides.** Don't try to ski with fully straightened knees or elbows. This posture is bad for your joints and will cause you to move unnaturally, in a way that resembles Frankenstein running from the villagers.

Rowing machines

Good rowers consist of a flywheel, a fan, and a cable with a handle attached to one end. You pull the handle toward you as you slide the seat backwards. The fan creates air resistance, which makes the movement feel pretty close to skimming across the water.

Who will like it: Anyone looking for a great total-body workout will love rowing. If you're trying to get in shape for a rowing or paddling sport, this is the way to go. Contrary to popular belief, rowing isn't bad for your back. If you row correctly, you initiate the movement from your legs and buttocks, which eliminates excess stress on your back muscles.

Who will hate it: Some people get bored with rowing in a matter of seconds. Others are intimidated because rowing is not as natural as walking, running, or biking. We know one guy who smacked the handle into his forehead over and over again until some kind soul in the gym showed him the proper form.

Rowing User Tips

Experienced rowers make rowing look easy, but when you actually sit down at the machine, it might take more coordination than you think. Here are some tips to fine-tune the motion:

- ✔ **Think legs, legs, legs.** Concentrate on initiating the movement with your buttocks rather than your lower back. Don't fully straighten your knees. Even when you're completely extended, your knees should be a little soft.

- ✔ **Don't round your back.** Hunching over is the way to give yourself back pain. Don't lean all the way back at the end of the stroke, either. You're in proper position when your upper body is leaning backwards about 45 degrees.

- ✔ **Pull the handle in a smooth, continuous stroke.** Don't stop at the most stretched-out and bent positions.

This is not your grandmother's stationary bike

If you build it, they will come. That seems to be the mantra of exercise machine manufacturers. They're always trying to tap into the psyche of the American exerciser to determine what the next big thing will be. We're still waiting for the flying simulator, where you flap your arms up and down like a bird. Here's a look at three new breeds of machines that are starting to pop up in health clubs.

Elliptical Trainer: Elliptical motion trainers have two large, fat foot pedals. Your feet follow a path that's sort of a stretched-out oval. The motion feels like a mix between fast walking, stairclimbing, and cross-country skiing. Precor and Body Glide make the two most popular models.

Reclining Stepper: This machine, the Cross-robics by StairMaster, is the recumbent version of a stairclimber. You recline backward in a position reminiscent of astronauts during take-off and alternately push each leg downward. This may look easier than a regular climber because you're in a reclining position and you have back support, but that thought flies out of your head about one minute into this killer workout.

SkyWalker: This contraption reminds us of a cross-country ski machine in suspended animation. The skis and poles are built into a giant frame and hang a few inches off the ground. The idea is to take all the stress off your joints while providing as good a workout as a ski simulator. This may or may not be true; we do have some concerns about lower back pain over the long haul. But the SkyWalker hasn't been around long enough to gather reliable feedback. Whatever else this machine is, it's a novel idea.

Chapter 9
Exercising Outside

. . . .

. . . .

*F*resh air: What a concept. With all the hoopla these days about space-age, indoor exercise contraptions, it's easy to forget you can get a great workout in the great outdoors. You might even get a better workout — burning more calories per minute — because some outdoor activities involve more muscles than their indoor counterparts. For instance, when you park yourself on a stationary bicycle, your upper body muscles basically get a free ride — you can easily read a magazine while you're pedaling away. But when you take your road or mountain bike out for a spin, your chest, arm, abdominal, and back muscles all get into the act. You use your whole body to power your bike up the hills, fight the wind, and steer your bike around corners. The best part is, while you're burning all of those calories, the time flies by because you're having so much fun.

In this chapter, we cover some of the most popular and invigorating outdoor aerobic activities. We discuss what gear you need and how much it costs, and we offer tips for rookies and klutzes alike on how to have fun and avoid injury.

Walking

Can you really get fit by walking? Absolutely — as long as you walk long enough, hard enough, and often enough. (If you're asking, "How long?" "How hard?" and "How often?" do a U-turn back to Chapter 5.) The beauty of walking is, it's simply a matter of putting one foot in front of the other. Plus, walkers enjoy a relatively low injury rate. Walking burns a lot fewer calories per minute than jogging and in-line skating, but most people last longer on a walk than a run, so it's possible to make up for it.

However, we're not going to sugar-coat this: Some exercisers find walking to be a big, fat bore. We know people who will do anything to avoid walking. We know people who will park in a red zone — at the risk of receiving a $28 parking ticket — simply because they will not walk an extra 100 yards to their office. We know people who spend 20 minutes searching for a good parking space at their *health club* before a one-hour workout on the StairMaster. Okay, we admit it: We *are* those people. (At least one of us is — the one who was raised a half block from a Los Angeles freeway.)

Essential walking gear

Although the rest of the animal kingdom does fine without the benefit of special equipment, human feet don't have adequate padding to meet the demands of walking in the modern world. You need a good pair of walking shoes to avoid foot, ankle, knee, hip, and lower back problems. Expect to spend at least $40 for good walking shoes, which should hold up for 1,000 to 1,500 miles. (Running shoes usually have to be tossed after 300 to 500 miles.) Replace your shoes when the tread begins to wear thin or when the sides start to cave inward or outward.

Walking shoes might sound like a marketing conspiracy hatched by shoe industry executives. After all, it's only *walking* — won't any pair of sneakers suffice? Actually, the concept of a walking shoe is a valid one. Not even running shoes make the grade for a walking workout. Walking shoes need to be more flexible than running shoes because you bend your feet more when you walk, and you push off from your toes with more oomph. Also, because your heels bear most of your weight when you walk, you need a firm, stable *heel counter,* the part of the shoe that wraps around your heel to keep your foot in place.

If you plan to hike or walk over rugged terrain, look for a walking shoe with treaded soles and added heel and ankle support. If you're focusing on speed walking or high mileage, go for a little more cushioning in the *midsole,* the area between the tread and the inside of the shoe. See Chapter 22 for tips on where to shop for athletic shoes.

Walking tips for rookies

Walk as fast as you comfortably can. If you walk very fast — at a 12-minute-mile to 15-minute-mile pace — you can burn twice as many calories as when you walk at a 20-minute-mile pace. You might not be able to move at such super-sonic speeds in the beginning, but as you get fit, you can mix in some fast-paced intervals. (For details about interval training, see Chapter 6.) Keep track of your heart rate to ensure that you're working hard enough to get all the aerobic benefits walking has to offer.

Another way to spice up your walking program is to take a hike. Walking over hilly terrain shapes your butt and thighs and helps you burn extra calories. Plus, communing with nature is a lot more interesting than communing with the white lines on a track, and it's more relaxing than traversing through a cement jungle full of suits and skirts.

Sneak in a walk whenever you can (see Figure 9-1). Leave your car at home and hoof it to the train station. Take a 15-minute walk during your lunch break. Traverse the airport on foot rather than on that automatic walking belt. It all adds up. Sometimes, you actually save time by walking. A few years back, a New York City newspaper timed a walker, a bus, and a subway over some common rush-hour routes. The walker reached his destination faster than mass transit in almost every case, sometimes by more than 10 minutes. Best off all, he didn't have to stand next to a stranger with bad breath.

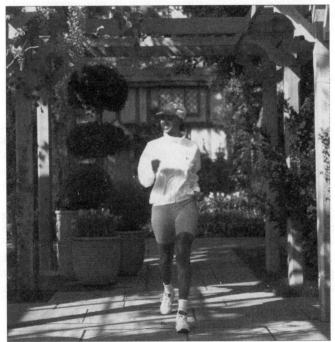

Figure 9-1:
Take a walk
whenever
you can.

(Photo courtesy of Richard Lee.)

Walking the right way

Okay, we lied to you: There actually is more to walking than simply putting one foot in front of the other. To get the most out of fitness walking, you need to pay attention to your form. The biggest mistake walkers make is bending forward, a sure way to develop problems in your lower back, neck, and hips. Your posture should be naturally tall. You needn't force yourself to be ramrod straight, but neither should you slouch, over-arch your back, or lean too far forward from your hips. Relax your shoulders, widen your chest, and pull your abdominals gently inward. Keep your head and chin up and focus straight ahead.

Meanwhile, keep your hands relaxed and cupped gently, and swing your arms so that they brush past your body. On the upswing, your hand should be level with your breast bone; on the downswing, your hand should brush against your hip. Keep your hips loose and relaxed. Your feet should land firmly, heel first. Roll through your heel to your arch, then to the ball of your foot, and then to your toes. Push off from your toes and the ball of your foot.

All this may sound pretty complicated — like we're training you to be a guard at Buckingham Palace. In reality, most people walk with decent form right from the start; they just need some fine-tuning. Run through a mental head-to-toe checklist every so often to see how you're doing.

Running

Like walking, running is a workout that you can take with you anywhere. You don't need a rack on your car or a suitcase full of equipment; you just open the door and go. Plus, as any pathological runner will tell you, nothing is quite as satisfying as getting a good run under your belt. You work up a great sweat, you burn lots of calories, and your muscles feel pleasantly achy after you finish.

But if you learn nothing else from this book, remember this: No single type of exercise is better than all the rest. It's merely a question of what's best for *you*. Running definitely is not for everyone. Runners tend to have frequent, chronic injuries. Many people have joints that simply will not tolerate all that pounding. If you're not built to run, don't argue with your body. You can get in great condition in other ways. Beginners, too, should hold off on running until they've built up stamina and strength.

Cross-Training

To hear some people talk about cross-training, you'd think it was a concept discovered by post-doctoral researchers at some eminent Swedish university. But *cross-training* is just a term that means varying your activities. Instead of running every day, you throw in some cycling, some step aerobics, or some swimming — whatever you want.

Many injuries are the result of repeating the same movement patterns. With cross-training, you never do any one activity long enough to get into trouble. (Unless, like some triathletes, you run, cycle, and swim every day. That's not cross-training; that's *overtraining*.)

Think about mixing high-impact activities like running with low-impact activities like cycling or skating. Also, alternate lower body sports with activities that also use your upper body. For instance, on Monday, you might run hard three miles over a hilly course; on Tuesday, you might go for an easy swim or ride a stationary bicycle with arm handles. Wednesday, you hit the road again — only this time you do a brisk walk. You can see how cross-training is a lot more interesting than doing the same activity over and over again.

Essential running gear

Although you can spend hundreds of dollars on spiffy warm-ups, tights, and tops, the only equipment that's truly essential for running is a good pair of shoes (although women will want a supportive jogging bra, too). Be prepared to spend at least $40 a pair, but know that a hefty price tag does not always correspond to the best shoe. We once asked a podiatrist the difference between a $60 shoe that we were considering and a $100 shoe. His reply? "About $40."

Want us to tell you the best brand of running shoes? We can't. The shoe that's best for you depends on your weight, the shape of your foot, your running style, and any special problems that you may have, such as weak ankles or bad knees. Try on several models at the store, and take each one for a test drive around the mall or at least run a couple of laps around the store. If the salesperson won't allow it, go elsewhere. Your shoes should feel great from the get-go. There's no such thing as "breaking them in." For more tips on buying shoes, see Chapter 22.

Your running shoes should be fairly flexible, especially across the ball of the foot. Hold the shoe at both ends and bend it; it should break right at the ball of the foot. You want cushioning, but not so much that you can't feel your foot hitting the ground. Look for a stable heel counter (we explain what a heel counter is in the "Essential walking gear" section, earlier in this chapter). If your foot slides around a lot, that can mean trouble down the road.

Running tips for rookies

Start by alternating periods of walking with periods of running. Two minutes walking and one minute running is a good place to start. Gradually decrease your walking intervals until you can run continuously for 20 minutes. If you have the inclination, you can build from there.

Even after you phase out walking, vary your pace. Don't always slog along barely lifting your feet off the ground. Experiment with the techniques we describe in Chapter 6. Of course, don't do an all-out sprint every workout, either. Different paces work your heart, lungs, and legs in different ways. Plus, the variety makes running more fun.

To avoid injuries, don't increase your mileage by more than 10 percent a week. So if you run 5 miles a week and want to increase, aim to do 5.5 miles the following week. Jumping from 5 miles to 6 miles doesn't sound like a big deal, but studies show that if you increase your mileage more than 10 percent, you set yourself up for injury. Also, don't run every day. Give your body at least one day per week, although preferably more, to rest and recover. This is a good rule to follow for all athletic activities.

Running the right way

When you're running to catch a bus, you're probably not going to score any points for good form, especially with that cup of coffee in your hand. We'll cut you some slack there. But when you're running for fitness, pay attention to your form so that you can go farther, faster.

Runners have this habit of looking directly at the ground, almost as if they can't bear to see what's coming next. Keeping your head down throws your upper body posture off kilter and can lead to upper back and neck pain. Make sure that you keep your head lifted and your eyes focused straight ahead, even if you're running through a parking lot. (See Figure 9-2.)

An economist we know used to run with his head down, and he actually ran off a bridge. Luckily, a calm stream broke his fall. When he went back later to check out what happened, he realized that he had ran past a whole bunch of flashing lights, cones, and orange signs. Now he runs with his head up.

Keep your shoulders relaxed, your chest open, and your abdominal muscles pulled in tightly. Don't over-arch your back and stick your butt out; that's one of the main reasons runners get back and hip pain.

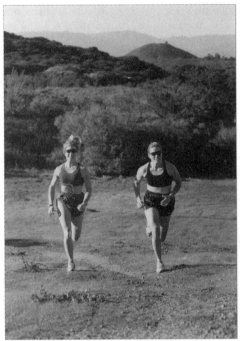

Figure 9-2:
Run with
a buddy.

(Photo courtesy of Tina Gerson.)

Keep your arms close to your body rather than flailing them around. Swing your arms forward and back rather than across your body, and don't clench your fists. Pretend you're holding a butterfly in each hand; you don't want your butterflies to escape, but you don't want to crush them, either. If you're not fond of butterflies, imagine a potato chip. Just don't imagine your boss's neck.

Lift your front knee and extend your back leg. Don't shuffle along like you're wearing cement boots. Let your feet do the work, not your shoes. Land heel first and roll through the entire length of your foot. Push off from the balls of your feet, instead of running flat-footed and pounding off your heels. Otherwise your feet and legs are going to cry uncle long before you cardiovascular system does.

Bicycling: Road and Mountain

Talk to a group of cyclists and, chances are, you're talking to a group of ex-runners. Cycling is the perfect aerobic choice for people who can't take the relentless pounding of running or find the slow pace a real drag. Biking tones your legs and butt, and as a calorie burner, it ranks right up there; even pedaling at 12 mph — not exactly a grueling pace — burns nearly as many calories as jogging and cross-country skiing. (See Chapter 6 for a chart of calorie counts.) And cycling is the best way to cover a lot of ground quickly. Even a novice biker can easily build up to a 20-mile ride. If you have only a half hour to work out, you can go two or three times farther on a bike than you can on foot.

On the other hand, if you have only 30 minutes, you might spend half of it getting your equipment together. The reality is, cycling can be a hassle. You can't just grab your shoes and head out the door. You need your helmet, water bottle, gloves, sunscreen, and glasses, and you need to make sure that your tires are full of air. And even with all of your protective gear, you can never be too cautious. Cycling is a low-impact sport — unless you happen to impact the ground, a car, a tree, a rut, or another cyclist. Accidents send more than half a million bikers to emergency rooms each year.

Essential cycling gear

There's no way around it: Cycling requires lots of gear. You can't just buy a bike and add the rest later. In this section, we cover what's mandatory for road and off-road cycling, also known as mountain biking. We also mention a few extras that we highly recommend.

Buying a bike

If you haven't owned a bike since grammar school, prepare yourself for sticker shock. *Mountain bikes,* the fat-tire bikes with upright handlebars, are somewhat less expensive than comparable *road bikes,* the 10-speed-type bikes with the curved handlebars, which, by the way, now have 14 or 16 speeds. In both categories, you won't find many decent bikes under $400, and you'll see many that cost more than $1,000. Don't take out a second mortgage to buy a fancy bike, but if you have any inkling that you might like this sport, don't skimp, either. You'll just end up buying a more expensive bike later.

Should you buy a mountain bike or a road bike? The answer depends, of course, on where you plan to ride. More than 80 percent of new bikes purchased are mountain bikes. They're more comfortable and more versatile — you can ride on dirt trails, through puddles, and over pot holes in the pavement (see Figure 9-3). But mountain bikes are also clunky and slow. If you plan to cover long distances and stay on the road, you're better off with a road bike. A third option is a hybrid, which is essentially a heavy road bike with upright handlebars and a cushy saddle. Hybrids are good for tooling around town, but they're annoyingly slow for long-distance road riding and very limiting on mountain trails.

You may wonder what distinguishes a $500 bike from a $1,500 steed. Generally, the more expensive the bike, the stronger and lighter its frame. A heavy bike can slow you down, but unless you plan to enter the Tour de France, don't get hung up on a matter of ounces. Cheaper bikes are made from different grades of steel; as you climb the price ladder, you find aluminum, carbon fiber, and titanium (sometimes, but not always, in that order). Which material is better? *Techno-weenies* — that's a nickname for people obsessed with bike technology — argue this question like policy wonks debate Medicare reform. It's really a matter of personal preference.

The price of a bike also depends on the quality of the components, the mechanical doodads that enable your bike to move, shift, and brake. High-end components tend to be lighter, stronger, and more efficient, but in many cases, you won't notice the difference from one set of components to the next.

Find a bike dealer you trust, someone who's more interested in pairing you with the right bike than just making a sale. (This isn't always easy.) The salesman should take great pains to make sure that your bike fits. The height of your bike's top tube isn't all that matters. Also check out the height and angle of the seat and the distance from the seat to the handlebars. Tell the salesman what sort of terrain you plan to ride so that you buy a bike with appropriate gears. Don't feel pressure to make an instant decision.

Go shopping with a knowledgeable friend and keep in mind that bike prices are negotiable. Ask the salesman if he'll throw in extras for free, like a bike computer to measure your speed and distance or a seat bag to carry food and tools.

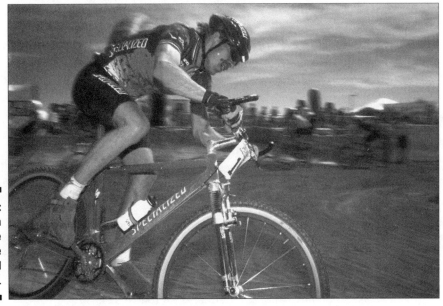

Figure 9-3:
Mountain bikes are comfortable and versatile.

A helmet and other critical bike equipment

Don't even think about pedaling down your driveway without a helmet snug atop your noggin. Don't even think about being *friends* with someone who would cycle without a helmet. You can buy a good helmet for $30.

Also important: gloves designed for cycling (they stop just above your knuckles). Gloves make your ride more comfortable and protect your hands when you crash. (If you ride on mountain trails, you are practically guaranteed to crash.) Cycling glasses are important to protect your eyes from the dust, dirt, and gravel. Besides, squinting requires energy that could be better spent on powering yourself up the hills. Finally, buy a pair of padded cycling shorts and a brightly colored cycling jersey so that you can be easily seen.

Cycling tips for rookies

Get to know your gears so that when you come to a hill, you won't panic, shift into the wrong gear, and tip over because you can't spin the pedals. Ride with friends who are more experienced and ask them to give you pointers on when to shift gears.

Learn how to fix a flat tire so that you don't get stranded miles from home. As far as we know, there's no cycling equivalent of the auto club to come save you. No matter where you're riding, always carry water and emergency food such as an energy bar or fruit. Cycling jerseys are made for such occasions; they have pockets deep enough to hold half a grocery store.

Special road-biking tips

Follow the rules of the road. Stop at all stop signs and use those hand signals you learned in Driver's Ed. Don't trust a single car, ever. Assume the driver doesn't see you, even if he appears to be staring you in the face.

Cheaper bikes come with *toe clips* (pedal straps) that enable you to pull up on the pedal as well as push down. But we recommend *clipless pedals* — special pedals without straps that allow you to pull up even more efficiently and more comfortably. You wear shoes with cleats that click into the pedal itself. These pedal systems are like ski bindings: You're locked in, but your feet pop out easily when you fall. To clip out, you simply twist your foot to the side.

Beginners usually have an accident or two with toe clips because they haven't developed the instinct to twist sideways. We know one woman who tipped over with both feet clicked into her pedals. We won't describe the injury in detail, but let's just say that she was injured in such a way that she had to visit her gynecologist. You also can buy clipless pedals specially designed for mountain bikes, but they're not as essential as for road bikes.

Special mountain-biking tips

Before you head for the dirt trails, get familiar with your bike on the road. Then when you go off-road, start on wide dirt roads rather than narrow trails that require technical skill. And don't think that because there are no cars, you're immune to injury. More crashes happen on mountain trails than on the road because there are more obstacles and because riders get careless and cocky. Be courteous when you cycle off-road. You're usually sharing the trails with hikers and horses.

When you navigate a steep, winding downhill, look 20 yards in front of you, always scouting out potential obstacles and planning that next turn. If you do crash, roll out of it, rather than impersonate Superman, which is a great way to break your wrist or collar bone. You can cut down on the number of crashes by spending about $200 for shock absorbers. With *front suspension,* you won't bounce around as much, and you'll feel more in control of your bike.

Mountain biking is great for building leg strength, but if you spend all your time negotiating obstacles and carrying your bike over ditches and streams, you won't get an aerobic workout. Professional mountain bike racers spend at least 60 percent of their time riding on the road.

Cycling the right way

Although cycling doesn't pound your joints as much as many other sports, it still can be hard on your knees. You reduce the possibility of injury by positioning your seat correctly (ask your sales guy for advice) and by pedaling at any easy cadence. *Cadence* refers to the number of revolutions per minute that you pedal. Inexperienced cyclists tend to use more tension than they can handle, which forces them into a slow cadence; their legs tire prematurely, and they cheat themselves out of a good workout. Professional cyclists train at a cadence of 90 to 100 rpm, which means that they go round and round really fast, a technique called *spinning.*

Road cycling can wreak havoc on your lower back because you're in a crouched position for so long. Keep your upper body relaxed and your arms loose. Grasp your handlebars with the same tension that you'd hold a child's hand when you cross the street. Pedal in smooth circles rather than simply mashing the pedals downward. Imagine that you have a bed of nails in your shoes, and you have to pedal without stomping on the nails.

Head into a turn at a slow enough pace that you maintain control and never let your eyes wander from the road or trail. Never squeeze the brakes — particularly the front brake — with a lot of pressure. You'll go flying over the handlebars, a maneuver known as an *endo,* and go right into a *face plant,* a maneuver we think is self-explanatory.

In-Line Skating

In 1980, RollerBlade introduced a new kind of skate: Instead of two wheels at the toe and two wheels at the heel, the four wheels were positioned in a single-file line (see Figure 9-4). This was the biggest innovation in skating since a 16th-Century Dutchman patterned the first pair of roller skates after ice skates. Now in-line skating — often called rollerblading — is the skate of choice for more than 15 million people.

Skating is fun because it isn't as linear as running, walking, and cycling. You can curve, turn, glide, sprint, and spin. Skating is also a terrific tush toner because you push your legs out to the side, which works several seldom-used hip muscles. Skating is a good calorie burner, too.

But in-line skating is also dangerous. Nearly 183,000 skaters — one in every 150 skaters — visited an emergency room in 1994. The injury rate is so high because the sport requires a lot of balance and concentration, and it's tough to stop on in-line skates. You have to simultaneously lean forward from your waist, tilt the braking skate up, and exert pressure on the heel pad while maintaining your balance. Stopping is actually an advanced move. The best a novice can hope to do is slow down.

Skating isn't something most people can pick up on their own. To find out if this is the sport for you, take a few lessons to familiarize yourself with the basics. You can find an instructor through a skate shop, or call the International In-Line Skating Association for a referral. Definitely rent skates several times before you buy.

Essential skating gear

Skating equipment isn't cheap. A good pair of skates costs between $100 and $400. Try on several pair at the store and wear each for at least 10 minutes, until your feet start to get hot. Tilt your feet to the inside and the outside, putting plenty of pressure on your foot to make sure that nothing hurts. Otherwise, you're asking for blisters. The boots should feel snug in the toe and heel. If your heel is loose, you won't have enough control when you skate.

In-line skates have more on conventional roller skates than just wheel placement. The wheels are faster, smoother, and more durable. Most skates have a plastic shell and foam-lined bootie, so they breathe more easily and conform to your feet much better than leather skates. You typically can get a more comfortable fit with skates that buckle rather than lace. Make sure that you wear synthetic socks; cotton fibers retain moisture, which can irritate your feet.

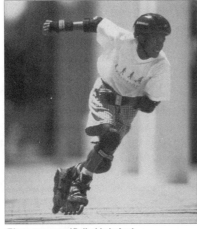

Figure 9-4:
With in-line skates, you can curve, turn, glide, and spin.

(Photo courtesy of Rollerblade, Inc.)

A helmet is as essential for skating as it is for biking. A cycling helmet will suffice, but you can buy special in-line helmets with more protection at the rear of the head. Also crucial: wrist guards, knee guards, and elbow guards (about $20 each or $30 to $50 for a pack that contains all three). Purchase safety equipment before you buy your skates so you won't be tempted to take a quick spin before suiting up.

Skating tips for rookies

Learn to balance by walking on the skates on your living-room carpet or your lawn. Then head to a parking lot to practice skating, turning, and stopping. Stick to bike paths until you're quite comfortable skating, and when you do head for the open road, always skate with — not against — traffic. Remember: You're responsible for abiding by the same rules as motorists. Skip hills until you've mastered stopping, and always skate slowly enough that you feel like you could stop at any time. Don't expect brakes to bring you to a complete halt.

Walkers, runners, and cyclists — groups that ordinarily scorn one another — have formed an unholy alliance against in-line skaters, so pay attention when you skate. Respect other exercisers' personal space. Don't go careening around the park just to see how many runners you can take down.

And in case you had any ideas, don't skate with your dog. You'll get a sore wrist, your dog will get a sore neck, and you'll have a good chance of becoming an injury statistic. In fact, don't skate while holding anything in your hand, even a can of Coke. When you fall, your reflex is to save what you're holding, not to protect your body.

Skating the right way

Keep your hands in front of your body at all times, with your elbows in, your forearms straight ahead, and your palms down, as if you're placing your hands on a table. If you move your hands off center, your body is likely to follow. Keep your arms as still as possible; don't pump them back and forth as if you're on a cross-country ski machine.

Travel in a modified squat position, bending at the knees as if you're about to sit down. Keep your weight on your back wheel and push off straight with your heel. Pull your abdominal muscles inward and don't round your back. If you start to lose your balance, crouch lower — don't stand up straighter. If you veer off the pavement and onto mud or grass, run on your skates rather than stopping cold.

Swimming

Swimming is truly a zero-impact sport. Although you can strain your shoulders if you overdo it, there's absolutely no pounding on your joints, and the only thing you're in danger of crashing into is the end of the pool. You can get a great aerobic workout that uses your whole body. Plus, water has a gentle, soothing effect on the body, so swimming is helpful for those with arthritis or other joint diseases. (See Figure 9-5.)

Swimming is great for people who want to keep exercising when they're injured and for people who are pregnant or overweight. That extra body fat helps you glide along near the surface of the water, so you don't expend energy trying to keep yourself from sinking like a stone.

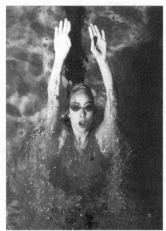

Figure 9-5: Swimming is a no-impact sport.

(Photo courtesy of Richard Lee.)

Lap swimming has the reputation of being drudgery — after all, the scenery doesn't change a whole lot from one end of the pool to the other. The trick is to use an array of gadgets that elevate swim workouts from forced labor to bona fide fun.

Essential swimming gear

Obviously, a body of water is helpful — preferably one manned by a lifeguard. And in most (legal) instances you must wear a swim suit. By the way, we said *swim* suit, not bathing suit. You don't want a suit that looks good while you're sunbathing but creeps up your butt when you get in the water.

If you swim in a chlorinated pool, goggles are a must to prevent eye irritation and to help you see better in the water. Cheap goggles — $5 to $10 — tend to be just as good as the $40 kind. You can buy prescription goggles for about $75; ask your eye doctor about them. Buy goggles from a store that lets you try them on. You should feel some suction around your eyes, but not so much that you feel like your eyes are going to pop out. You also need a cap — so that your hair doesn't get plastered on your face as you swim or turn to straw from the chemicals.

As for the fun swimming gadgets: Many pools let you borrow equipment, but you can buy a whole set for less than $75. We especially like rubber swimming fins, which give you a lot more speed and power in the water. If you are a beginning swimmer, you may feel like you're going nowhere, and you may have trouble moving fast enough to get your heart rate up. Slip on a pair of fins and you'll feel like you're powering across the pool like an Olympian.

You can use fins when you kick with a kickboard and when you swim freestyle, backstroke, or butterfly. But don't use fins so much that they become a crutch. As you get in better shape, you may want to switch from long swim fins to short fins, which make you work a lot harder. Don't swim with scuba fins; they're too big and too stiff.

You might also want to invest in a pair of plastic paddles, which are slightly larger than your hand and give your upper body an extra challenge. However, use hand paddles sparingly. Overuse can lead to shoulder injuries. When you swim with paddles, put a pull-buoy (a foam gadget) between your thighs. This keeps your legs buoyant so that you can concentrate on paddling.

Swimming tips for rookies

Even if you're the queen of your aerobics class or a champion at cycling uphill, you might still tire quickly in the pool at first. More than any other aerobic activity, swimming relies on technique. It takes time to develop the specific skills you need to swim efficiently.

Beginners waste a lot of energy flailing and splashing around rather than moving forward. Take a few lessons if you haven't swum in a while, just to refresh your memory on stroke technique and breathing. Good swimming technique is especially important if you plan to swim in an open body of water like the ocean or a lake, which we don't recommend until you've got a month or two of pool swimming under your belt.

Break your workout into intervals. For instance, don't just get into the pool, swim 20 laps, and get out. Instead, do an easy 4 laps for a warm-up. Then do 8 sets of 2 laps at a faster pace, resting 20 seconds between sets. Then cool down with 2 easy laps, and maybe a few extras with a kickboard. Mix up your strokes, too. The four basic strokes — crawl, backstroke, breaststroke, and butterfly — use your muscles in different ways.

If you find swimming a big yawn, but enjoy being in the water, try water running or water aerobics. Don't assume that water aerobics is for little old ladies in shower caps. With the right instructor and exercise program, you can get a challenging water aerobics workout. Water running can be even tougher.

Swimming the right way

You probably will spend the bulk of your workouts doing the crawl stroke, also called freestyle. It's generally faster than the other strokes, so you can cover more distance and get the maximum aerobic benefit from your workout. Pay attention to your freestyle technique. Don't cut your strokes short; reach out as far as you can and pull all the way through the water so your hand brushes your thigh. Elongate your stroke so that you take fewer than 25 strokes in a 25-yard pool. The fewer strokes, the better. Top swimmers get so much power from each stroke that they take just 11 to 14 strokes per length of a 25-yard pool.

Kick up and down from your hips, not your knees. Don't kick too deeply or allow your feet to break the water's surface. Proper kicking causes the water to boil rather than splash.

Breathe through your mouth every two strokes, or every three strokes if you want to alternate. You need as much oxygen as you can get. Beginners sometimes make the mistake of taking six or eight strokes before breathing, which wears them out quickly. To breathe, roll your entire body to the side until your mouth and nose come out of the water. Imagine that your entire body is on a skewer and must rotate together.

Part III
Building Strength

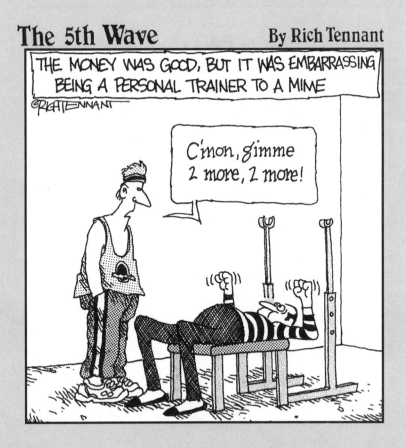

In this part . . .

We give you the know-how to tone and strengthen your muscles, whether you work out at home or at the gym. Chapter 10 gives you five great reasons to lift weight and explains how long it takes to firm up your muscles. In Chapter 11 we run down your major muscle groups so that you can go around saying things like, "I worked my lats and pecs today." In Chapter 12 we explain the differences between barbells, dumbbells, and weight machines, and we help you choose the best equipment for *you*. Chapter 13 helps you get started on a weight-training program. We discuss how much weight to lift, how many exercises to do, and how often to use good form so you don't get injured.

Chapter 10
Why You've Gotta Lift Weights

In This Chapter

▶ Five important reasons to pick up a dumbbell

▶ How long it takes to get strong

▶ Your chances of looking like Sylvester Stallone or Linda Hamilton

▶ Myths about bulking up

▶ What happens if you stop lifting

*M*aybe you've never considered yourself the weight-lifting type. Maybe you suspect that the size of one's muscles is inversely proportional to the size of one's brain. Maybe, when you see a hulking guy on the street, you think, "He may be able to bench press my mini-van, but I have a degree in French literature."

The truth is, weight lifting is an incredibly smart thing to do. It's not just a form of narcissism, and it's not just for body builders. Heck, these days even 80-year-olds are pumping iron. In this chapter, you learn why you should, too. If you think lifting weight seems too boring, too dangerous, too much trouble, or too likely to transform you into an East German swimmer, we hope this chapter changes your mind.

Throughout this book, we use the terms *weight lifting, weight training,* and *strength training* interchangeably, even though you don't necessarily need weight to build strength. *Resistance training* means the same thing, but we spare you that bit of verbiage.

Five Important Reasons to Pick Up a Dumbbell

People who start lifting weight regularly will tell you how much more fit, powerful, and energetic they feel . . . but enough about feelings. There's plenty of good, solid evidence that strength training will transform you into a healthier human being. We're betting that at least *one* of the following reasons will get you to hoist a little iron.

Stay strong for everyday life

People who don't exercise lose 30 to 40 percent of their strength by age 65. By age 74, more than one-fourth of American men and two-thirds of American women can't lift an object heavier than 10 pounds, like a small dog or a loaded garbage bag. These changes are *not* the normal consequences of aging. They're a result of neglect — of experiencing life from your La-Z-Boy recliner and the front seat of your Winnebago. If you don't use your muscles, they simply waste away. This gradual slide toward wimpiness can begin as early as your mid-twenties.

Fortunately, strength is one of the easiest physical abilities to retain as you get older. In other words, you can do a lot more to halt strength loss than you can to prevent wrinkling skin or fading eyesight. One study, which included men up to age 96, found that by lifting weight, most seniors can at least double — if not triple — their muscle power.

So if the heaviest thing that you've been lifting lately is a can of beer, it's time to build enough brawn to get along in the real world. Increased strength is what you need to rip the top off a stubborn jar of ketchup, hoist your kid onto the mechanical horsey, and close a suitcase that's too full. Even if you have the stamina to sprint the full length of an airport to catch your plane, it's not going to do you much good if you can't lug along that overstuffed luggage.

Keep your bones healthy

Keeping your bones healthy, we admit, is not a sexy reason to lift weight. Magazine covers do not scream, "Maintain Your Bone Density!" because, let's face it, most people don't *care* about their bone density — until it's too late. *Bone density,* by the way, refers to how thick your bones are. Picture strong, dense bones as poles of steel. As you lose density, your bones become more porous and fragile, like chalk.

Roughly 25 million Americans have *osteoporosis,* a disease of severe bone loss that causes 1.5 million fractures a year, mostly of the back, hip, and wrist. Many of these fractures lead to fatal complications. When a bone is extremely weak, it doesn't even take a fall to break it — bending over to pick up a baby can be enough. In addition to fractures, bone loss also can cause a hunchback. Fewer men get osteoporosis than women because men's bones are denser to begin with, but as more men live longer, osteoporosis will become a widespread problem for them, too.

Osteoporosis isn't something that happens to you overnight, like becoming eligible for a senior discount at the movies. Around age 35, most people begin to lose about $1/2$ to 1 percent of their bone each year (for women, bone loss accelerates after menopause). But if you do everything right, you can slow your rate of bone loss significantly — by about 50 percent. If you've already lost a lot of bone, you may even be able to build some of it back. Strength training alone can't stop bone loss, but it can play a big role. Also important are calcium, vitamin D, and land-based aerobic exercise such as walking.

Strong muscles and strong bones go hand in hand. The more weight you can lift, the more stress you can put on your bones; this stress is what stimulates them. If you never tax your bones, they have no incentive to stay strong. The first astronauts to spend time in space experienced significant bone density loss. In space, not only does no one hear you scream, but you're weightless — there's no load placed on your muscles and bones. Today's astronauts prevent bone loss by exercising several hours a day.

Bone, like muscle, is much easier to preserve than to restore. Still, it's never too late to start lifting weight. Studies show that bones benefit from strength training at any age. In one study, women ages 50 to 70 who did two 45-minute weight-lifting sessions a week for nearly a year increased their spine and hip density by 1 percent, which might not sound like a lot, but actually is; nonlifters lost 2.5 percent. The sooner you start lifting, the better. (See Figure 10-1.)

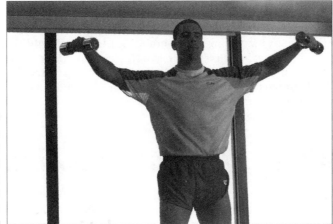

Figure 10-1: The sooner you start lifting weights, the better.

(Photo courtesy of Dan Kron.)

Look better, but not necessarily bigger

Now let's talk about pure, unadulterated vanity. Aerobic exercise burns lots of calories, but weight lifting firms, lifts, builds, and shapes your muscles. A marathon runner may be able to go the distance, but he won't turn any heads on the beach if he has a concave chest and string-bean arms.

We want to be clear here: In the workout world, there's no such thing as *spot reducing*—that is, selectively zapping fat off a particular part of your body. But you can pick problem areas, such as your butt or your arms, and reshape them through weight training. And if you have wide hips or a thick middle, you can bring your body more into proportion by doing exercises that broaden your shoulders and back.

Prevent injuries

When your muscles are strong, you're also less injury prone. You are less likely to step off a curb and twist your ankle. Plus, you have a better sense of balance and surefootedness, so you're less apt to take a tumble during a weekend game of touch football.

Lose fat

This is an area of controversy. Some scientists suspect that weight training can help you lose fat by increasing your metabolism. However, only a handful of researchers have tackled this subject, and the results of their studies have been mixed. Still, we're inclined to believe that weight training can contribute to fat loss and help prevent weight gain. Read Chapter 27 to find out more about what affects your metabolism.

Building Muscle: Your Questions Answered

There sure are a lot of misconceptions about weight training. Many people have no idea what changes to expect when they begin lifting weight, so they ask some not-so-dumb questions, like the ones that follow.

How long does it take to get stronger?

You may be able to lift more weight after just one weight-lifting workout. This isn't because you've built up more muscle; it's mainly because your weight-training skills have improved. The first time you try the bench press, you waste a lot of energy trying to balance the bar, keep it steady, and move it in a straight line. But once you get the hang of the process — typically after one weight-lifting session — you're able to put all your energy into only lifting the weight.

Another reason you develop strength after just one workout is that, in a sense, your muscles have memory. Your nerves, the pathways that link your brain and muscles, learn how to carry information more quickly — much like the speed-dial feature on your telephone. So after learning an exercise, your brain tells your muscles, "You know what this is. Go for it."

During the first six weeks you lift weight, most of the strength you gain is due to skill and muscle memory. After that time, your muscles begin to grow. In other words, the size of your muscle fibers increase — you don't actually grow more muscle cells. Realize that some muscles gain strength faster than others. In general, large muscles, like your chest and back muscles, grow faster than smaller ones, like your arm and shoulder muscles. Most people can increase their strength between 7 percent and 40 percent after about 10 weeks of training each muscle group twice a week.

Do some people have greater strength potential than others?

How much muscle power you develop depends on a lot of things, including your age, sex, and body type (and, of course, your diligence). Seniors generally do not have the same strength potential as young people, but it's not clear whether this is due to the normal aging process or years of inactivity. However, look at Jack La Lanne, who has worked out all his life. For his 80th birthday, he towed a rowboat across a river with his teeth.

Men typically have the capacity for greater overall strength than women. This is because men's bodies tend to have a high proportion of muscle and more of the strength hormone testosterone.

Also, every body type has a different capacity for building strength and muscle. All the training in the world won't change your body type. If you start out short and narrow, weight training will not miraculously make you tall and broad. Weight training will, however, make you a more fit, muscular version of short and narrow. There are literally hundreds of different body types, but most people fall into one of three broad categories: mesomorph, ectomorph, and endomorph.

✔ **Mesomorph:** This is the most square of all the body types. Mesomorphs tend to have fairly large bones and shoulders that are a little wider than their hips. Mesomorphs are neither fat nor skinny; they tend to be muscular. People with this body type typically gain more strength and size from weight lifting than do people with other body types. Mesomorphs include Linda Hamilton, Madonna, Arnold Schwarzenegger, and Sylvester Stallone.

✔ **Ectomorph:** The beanpole type — skinny, wiry, and small-boned. An ectomorph's shoulders and hips are about the same width. Weight training tends to increase an ectomorph's definition and shape, but ectomorphs don't have the same capacity for size as the other two body types. Examples include Courtney Cox, Audrey Hepburn, Brad Pitt, and Jimmy Stewart.

✔ **Endomorph:** The roundest type. Female endomorphs tend to be curvy; both men and women tend to store more body fat and have larger bones than the other two body types. Female endormorphs typically have hips that are wider than their shoulders. Endomorphs include Kim Basinger, Oprah Winfrey, Jay Leno, and John Travolta.

Strength is one thing, but how long will it take before I see some improvements?

Most people start to see changes after six weeks of weight lifting, but we can't give you an exact answer. Results depend on your body type, your starting point, and the amount of time and effort you devote to lifting weight. In general, those who have the furthest to go make the most dramatic changes.

Everyone notices the biggest improvements in the muscles that they use the least. The *triceps* (the muscles at the rear of your upper arm) are a classic example: You don't use them much in everyday life, so when you start targeting them with weight they become more firm really fast. The same goes for shoulders. Most people don't tend to carry much fat on their shoulders, so shoulders shape and tone relatively quickly.

What if I want to get muscle definition like Linda Hamilton or Sylvester Stallone?

Lifting weight diligently will help shape your body, but you'll never see *muscle definition* if you have a thick layer of fat covering your muscles. Muscle definition means that you have so little body fat that you can see the outline of your muscles. You begin to see a hint of definition when your body fat dips into the

20 percent to 22 percent range. At around 18 percent, muscle definition is really apparent. Below 15 percent, you develop an appearance that body builders reverentially refer to as *ripped*. We tell you all about body fat in Chapter 1.

However, cultivating a defined look is not always healthy. Women with body fat below 16 percent often experience menstrual irregularities, a condition that's considered a major risk factor for osteoporosis. Also, keep in mind that you can still look firm, fit, sexy, and healthy even if you aren't ripped to shreds.

Will weight lifting turn me into Amazon Woman or The Incredible Hulk?

About 99 percent of women — and a significant percentage of men — can't develop huge muscles without spending hours a day in the gym lifting some serious poundage. Even then, most women don't have testosterone to add major bulk to their frame unless they take steroids — in which case, they also end up with acne, a beard, and a voice like James Earl Jones's.

Lifting may actually make you smaller. Because muscle is a very compact, dense tissue, it takes up less room than fat. At first, you may not lose any weight. You may even gain a few pounds, because muscle weighs more per square inch than fat, but your clothes will fit better. As we explain in Chapter 1, that number on your bathroom scale is relatively meaningless.

But what if I want to increase bulk?

Again, developing huge muscles is very difficult for people with certain body types. If you're lean and wiry to begin with, you'll probably add definition but not much size. The people who have the greatest chance of building up their frames are those who have a muscular body type even before they start lifting.

If I stop lifting weight, won't my muscle turn to fat?

Only if silver can be transformed into gold. Fat and muscle are two distinctly different substances. When you look at them under the microscope, fat looks like chicken coop wire and muscle looks like frayed electrical wiring. If you stop lifting weight, your muscles simply *atrophy,* a fancy word for shrink.

We think this myth got started because so many former football stars gain weight later in life. Basically, they eat too much and don't get enough exercise. If for some reason, you do stop lifting weight, your muscles will just shrink.

Should I lose weight before I start lifting weights?

Actually, no. We've already told you that weight training burns calories and may speed up your metabolism. Strength training also makes you look better. You'll have more tone, better posture, and a better proportioned body — even if you don't lose an ounce.

In addition, lifting weight enhances your aerobic efforts. With stronger muscles, you have more staying power on the stairclimber. You can put more oomph into every step, and you're less apt to have a setback due to injury from your aerobic workouts. For instance, you may be working out like gangbusters when, suddenly, you feel a little twinge in your knee. You lay off for a couple of days, which turns into a couple of years. This whole incident may have been prevented if the muscles that support your knees were stronger. Plus, adding weight training to your new exercise program gives you a lot more variety and helps keep you motivated.

Chapter 11

Your Muscles: Love 'Em and Learn 'Em

There are 650 muscles in your body; we are happy to report that you don't need to learn all of them. Consider, for instance, the inferior retinaculum of the long extensor of your big toe. We don't want you to learn that one. In fact, *we* don't even know that one — we had to look it up in our anatomy book. If you have any desire to learn about that muscle, shut this book and apply to medical school.

Meanwhile, in this chapter, we tell you about the 20 or so muscles that any conscientious exerciser should know. What's the point? For one thing, you won't need an interpreter when a trainer, video instructor, or fellow gym member says, "Let's do lats and pecs today." Before you know it, you'll be saying stuff like that, too. And you'll sound really impressive — like wine afficionados who say, "This Chardonnay has a superior bouquet."

But more important, if you can name your major muscles and understand how each one operates, you'll probably get better results from your workout program. You'll understand, for instance, how certain exercises can help you prevent lower back pain. You'll understand why you should do several different shoulder exercises, rather than just one. And you'll be sure to perform your biceps exercises properly; if you know where your biceps *are,* you'll realize exactly where you should feel the tension. With many weight-training exercises, it's easy to emphasize the wrong muscle if you don't understand the purpose of the move. If you simply hop on a machine and pull some lever without knowing which muscle to focus on, you may be cheating yourself out of a good workout. (See Figures 11-1 and 11-2 for a full view of your muscles.)

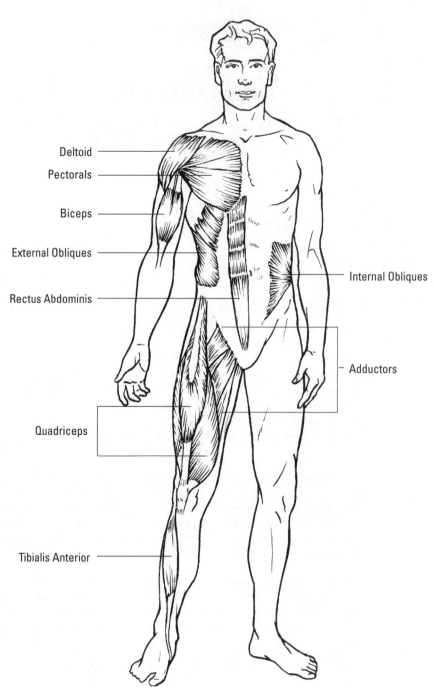

Deltoid

Pectorals

Biceps

External Obliques

Rectus Abdominis

Internal Obliques

Adductors

Quadriceps

Tibialis Anterior

Figure 11-1:
Your
muscles—
front view.

(Illustration by Karen Kuchar)

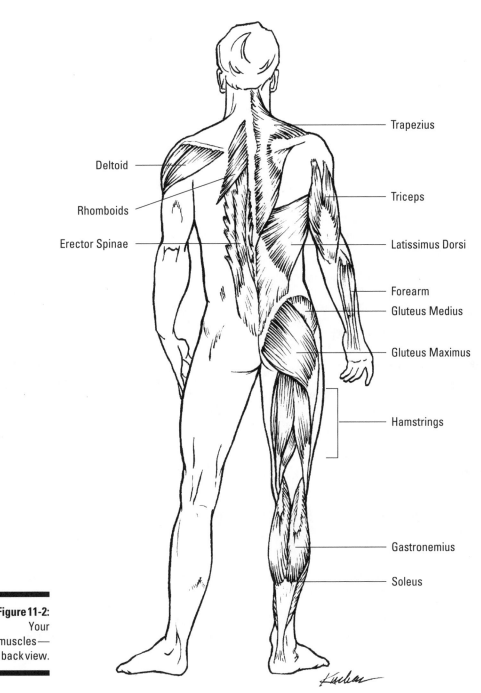

Trapezius

Deltoid

Triceps

Rhomboids

Erector Spinae

Latissimus Dorsi

Forearm

Gluteus Medius

Gluteus Maximus

Hamstrings

Gastronemius

Soleus

Figure 11-2:
Your
muscles—
back view.

(Illustration by Karen Kuchar)

Shoulders

Strong shoulders are the key to building a strong upper body. Just about every major exercise you can do for your chest and back involves your shoulders, too. So if your shoulders are weak, you really limit the amount of weight you can use in your upper body repertoire.

Deltoids

Street name: Delts

What they are: Muscles that wrap completely around the tops of your arms. Cup your hand over your shoulder and you get the idea. Now swing your arm around in a circle, raise it up above your head, and then swing it forward and backward. You can see what a versatile muscle your shoulder is. The front portion of the shoulder muscle is referred to as the *anterior delt,* the side is called the *medial delt,* and the back is called the *rear* or *posterior delt.* Go ahead, toss those terms around and amaze your friends.

What they do: Move your upper arm.

Why work them: You'll never have to wear shoulder pads if, god forbid, they ever come back in style. Also, strengthening your shoulders can help you avoid injuries like shoulder dislocations or muscle tears. And with strong shoulders, you'll have no trouble putting that useless "waist trimmer" gadget that you bought for $19.95 on the top shelf in the closet.

Special tips: Ask your trainer to show you exercises that target the front, middle, and back of your shoulders and the delts as a whole.

Rotator cuff

Street name: Rotators

What they are: Four small muscles beneath your shoulder; together, they're called your rotator cuff.

What they do: Help hold your arm in its socket. You use these muscles for throwing and catching. Baseball pitchers are constantly sidelined with rotator cuff injuries.

Why work them: This is a commonly injured muscle group, even among people who don't play ball. If you have weak rotators, you can damage them simply by carrying a briefcase or reaching across the table for a bowl of Cheetos. Most people don't do exercises that specifically target these muscles — a big mistake.

Special tips: To keep your rotator cuff strong, ask your trainer to show you exercises called *internal* and *external rotation*. Working your shoulders in a variety of directions will also help. If you have chronic shoulder pain, check with your orthopedist to see if you have injured your rotator cuff. Sometimes rotator tears can be corrected with exercise; other times, they require surgery.

Back

It's tempting to neglect your back muscles because you don't face them in the mirror every day. But these muscles are just as important as the muscles in the front of your body, particularly when it comes to injury prevention.

We know a man who injured his back while putting on his underwear in the health club locker room. He was lying on the floor stark naked for a few hours before he let the staff members call a nurse. Trainers had repeatedly reminded him to work on strengthening his lower back muscles and abdominals. After that incident, he finally listened.

Trapezius

Street name: Traps

What it is: A fairly large, kite-shaped muscle that spans up into your neck, across your shoulders, and down to the center of your back.

What it does: Enables you to shrug your shoulders. You also use your trapezius when you lift your arm out to the side, like you do when you're hailing a cab.

Why work it: A toned trapezius adds shape to your shoulders and upper back. Strengthening this muscle may also alleviate the kind of neck and shoulder pain you might get if you sit at a desk all day or if your phone is a permanent appendage to your ear.

Special tips: Give this muscle extra attention if you often carry a knapsack or heavy bag over your shoulder. Ask your trainer to teach you shrugs or shoulder rolls.

Latissimus dorsi

Street name: Lats. Don't make the mistake of saying "laterals," as some less-informed exercisers do.

What it is: Your largest back muscle. Feel the widest part of your back just behind your armpit — you've just found your lats. Your lats run the entire length of your back from below your shoulders to your lower back.

What it does: Enables you to pull, like when you open a door against the wind or drag your Great Dane into the vet's office.

Why work it: Well-toned lats make your hips and waist appear smaller by adding shape and width to your upper body. If you play sports, especially a racquet sport, golf, or hockey, pay special attention to your lats. Runners, walkers, and cyclists also should focus on their lats to help counteract that tendency toward rounded shoulders.

Rhomboids

Street name: None. No one talks about them.

What they are: A small, rectangular group of muscles at the center of your back, hidden beneath your trapezius.

What they do: Help pull your shoulder blades together so that you maintain good posture.

Why work them: To counteract the tendency to hunch your shoulders forward.

Special tips: You won't find a "rhomboid machine" in the gym. That's because you don't need to target your rhomboids specifically — they come along for the ride when you work your trapezius, rear shoulders, and lats. You use your rhomboids during exercises like chin-ups and side shoulder raises.

Erector spinae

Street Name: Lower back

What they are: Muscles that run the entire length of your spine. Focus on the erector spinae muscles at the lower third of your back.

What do they do: Straighten your spine — for example, when you stand back up after tying your shoes.

Why work them: About 80 percent of adult Americans experience back pain at some point in their lives. You can prevent much of this pain by devoting equal time to strengthening your lower back and abdominal muscles. Strong lower back muscles are also very important for posture.

Special tips: The lower back is an injury-prone area. If you have constant lower back pain, ask your doctor to recommend exercises for your specific problem.

Chest

The fibers of your chest muscles spread out like a fan, connecting to your arms, ribs, and collar bone. For this reason, your chest muscles respond well when you work them from a variety of angles. For instance, you can do chest exercises while lying flat on your back on a bench, reclining at various angles, sitting upright, standing, or lying face down (like when you do push-ups). Ask a trainer to show you a several chest exercises so you can vary your workouts.

Pectorals

Street name: Pecs

What they are: Your chest muscles. Place your hand on your chest as if you're pledging allegiance to the flag. You've found your pecs.

What they do: Enable you to push — a shopping cart, a lawn mover, or some jerk standing in your way. You also use your pecs to wrap your arms around something, like when you give your mom a bear hug.

Why work them: You'll look great in tight T-shirts. You also need strong chest muscles for sports like tennis, golf, and football.

Special tips: For women — it's important to understand that your pecs are not your breasts; in fact they reside directly underneath your breast tissue. However, toning your pecs can lift your breasts and make them appear firmer.

For men — don't become obsessed with bench pressing to the point of excluding all other exercises. Men with overdeveloped chest muscles and wimpy legs resemble hard-boiled eggs on toothpicks. Besides, doing too much bench work sets you up for shoulder injuries.

Arms

Take a survey of today's TV stars, fashion models, and music artists, and you'll see that firm arm muscles are in style. Even department store mannequins now have toned arms. Fortunately, firm arms are a realistic goal for most people who work out.

One friend of ours reports that after two months of lifting weights three times a week, her biggest thrill is that her arms no longer look flabby. "I'm so proud of myself that I went out and bought two new sleeveless shirts," she says.

Biceps

Street name: Bi(s) or guns

What they are: The two muscles at the front of your upper arm.

What they do: Bend your elbow. When you picked up this book or when you turned the pages, you used your biceps.

Why work them: It'll be easier to lift a stack of newspapers or carry an armload of wood. Your biceps also help out your back muscles when you pull something. Plus, strong biceps make you look buff.

Special tips: Many people have sloppy posture when they do biceps exercises — they rock their bodies back and forth to hoist the weight up. Not only is this posture dangerous for your lower back, but it also makes life too easy for your biceps. Pay special attention to form on these exercises, and make sure that you don't use too much weight.

Triceps

Street name: Tri(s)

Where they are: The muscle at the back of your upper arm.

What they do: The opposite of what your biceps do; that is, your triceps straighten your elbow. Your triceps help out your chest muscles when you push something.

Why work them: To help firm up *bingo arms*. That's when the back of your arms flap loosely away from the bones — a condition common among people whose main form of physical activity is playing bingo.

Special tips: Working your triceps is especially important if you often hold a briefcase or handbag while your arm is straight. If your triceps are weak — and that's the case for many people, because these muscles don't get much work in daily life — you may be prone to elbow pain.

Forearm muscles

Street name: Wrists

What they are: The many muscles that run from your wrist to the bottom of your elbow.

Why work them: To prevent or alleviate symptoms of carpal tunnel syndrome and tennis elbow. *Carpal tunnel syndrome* is a painful irritation of the nerves of the wrist. It's usually the result of repetitive motions such as typing or certain assembly line tasks, such as tightening a bolt with a wrench. For a description of tennis elbow, see Chapter 24. Strong wrists also give you a stronger grip for weight lifting.

Special tips: If you don't have time during your workout to do wrist-strengthening exercises, grab a can of soup and bend your wrist up and down 10 to 20 times while you're watching TV.

Abdominals

Developing a toned, flat abdomen has become somewhat of a national obsession. Most fitness magazines don't let a month go by without an article titled "Midriff Madness!" or "Flatten Your Tummy in 3 Minutes a Day!" But don't delude yourself: All the abdominal exercises in the world won't make your tummy pancake flat if you've got extra body fat stored around your middle.

Rectus abdominis

Street name: Abs. Don't refer to your abdominals as your stomach, which is the organ responsible for digesting food.

What it is: A flat sheet of muscle that runs from just under your chest down to a few inches south of your belly button. This is one long, continuous muscle; you don't have *upper abs* and *lower abs,* as many people mistakenly think. But you can do exercises that specifically emphasize the *upper portion* of your rectus, and others that emphasize the *lower portion*.

What it does: Enables you to bend at the waist, and keeps your torso stable while you move other muscles. For instance, when you're shoveling dirt in your garden, your arms are moving but you have to brace your body to get enough leverage and to protect your lower back.

Why work it: The obvious reason is so you'll have a firm, muscular midriff. If your abs are really toned and you don't have much excess fat around your middle, you can see six distinct sections of the muscle. This is known as *washboard abs,* or the *six pack.* But having such a firm midriff is really not worth fixating on — for most of us, washboard abs are not a realistic proposition. Even people with relatively low body fat tend to store at least some excess fat around the middle. Appearances aside, strong abs improve your posture by making it easier to stand up straight. Plus, they're important for guarding against lower back pain.

Special tips: Your ab routine should include exercises like crunches, curl ups, or quarter sit-ups. (Ask a trainer to teach them to you, or watch a video led by one of the Dummies-approved instructors we list in Chapter 21.) Those full sit-ups you did back in high school gym class won't do the job, plus they're hard on your back, especially if you lock your feet under a couch. Although many gyms have abdominal machines, we feel that floor exercises like the crunch are more effective. As for those ab-strengthening gadgets advertised on TV infomercials, you're better off spending your money on the Garden Weasel.

Internal and external obliques

Street names: Obliques or the waist

What they are: The muscles that run diagonally down the sides of your rectus abdominis, or abs (see the "Rectus abdominis" section).

What they do: Help you twist from the waist or do a side bend.

Why work them: To strengthen your middle. (But remember . . . strengthening these muscles won't get rid of the flab.) Also, strong obliques are essential for reducing lower back pain. They work with your rectus abdominis and lower back muscles to support your spine.

Special tips: Doing side bends while holding a weight in each hand is not a good idea unless you want to build a thicker waist. In addition, placing a pole across your shoulders and twisting from side to side can wreak havoc on your lower back, especially if you do this movement a zillion times.

Your best bet: crunches with a twist at the waist. This exercise strengthens your obliques without adding bulk or destroying your lower back.

Butt and Hips

If your rear end and hips are larger than you'd like them to be, don't be afraid to strengthen these muscles with weights. If you work out properly these muscles will look firmer and more shapely, not bigger and bulkier. Also, strengthening your butt and hip muscles can help prevent hip and lower back injuries. If your job requires you to sit on your rear end all day, it's a good idea to do exercises that target these muscles.

Gluteus maximus

Street names: Glutes, buns, or butt

What it is: The largest muscle in your body — as if you need anyone to tell you that. Your two glutes (left and right cheeks) span the entire width of your derriere.

What it does: Helps you jump, climb stairs and hills, or straighten your leg behind you. You also use your maximus when you stand up from a sitting position.

Why work it: To lift your butt, make it rounder, and give it more shape. You also need your glutes to get off the couch so that you can go work out.

Special tips: Some glute exercises can be hard on your knees. Always use good form when doing any exercise but be especially careful when you do squats and lunges, two variations of the deep knee bend.

Gluteus medius

Street names: Outer thigh, outer hip, or leg abductors

What it is: The meatiest part of your hips.

What it does: Helps you slide your leg out to the side, like when you go skating or step aside so someone can get past you. These muscles also help your gluteus maximus (or butt) rotate your hips outward, like ballerinas do when they stand with their heels together and toes apart.

Why work it: To firm up your outer thighs and prevent hip injuries. Athletes and seniors should pay special attention to strengthening their hip muscles. You need a strong gluteus medius for activities like running, jumping, pedaling, kicking, and skating — just about any movement that involves your lower body. Strong gluteal muscles also are important for maintaining a natural walking stride. If your hip muscles are weak, you tend to shuffle along.

Special tips: Some exercise programs advise you to do hundreds of leg lifts to tone this area. But, as we explain in Chapter 13, following this advice won't get you anywhere. Work your outer thighs as you would any other muscle group — by doing 8 to 15 moderately challenging repetitions.

You might also hear about two other outer-thigh muscles:

- ✔ Your *gluteus minimus,* a smaller muscle located underneath the medius, assists the medius.

- ✔ The *tensor fasciae latae* runs from your hips to your knees. It also helps the gluteus medius and kicks in whenever you lift your knees toward your chest, like when you're climbing stairs or sprinting to catch the bus.

Leg adductors

Street name: Inner thighs

What they are: Several muscles that run from inside your hip to various points along your inner thigh. There's no need to know each by name.

What they do: Help you move one leg in front of the other. In *The Wizard of Oz,* Dorothy used her adductors when she clicked her heels together and said, "There's no place like home." (She used her outer-thigh muscles as her heels moved apart.)

Why work them: When you sit astride a horse or motorcycle, your inner thighs squeeze inward to keep you from sliding off. You also use your inner-thigh muscles for skating, soccer, and swimming the breaststroke.

Special tips: Forget the ThighMaster and the other "thigh toner" gadgets you see advertised on TV. You can work your inner-thigh muscles more effectively by adding exercise bands to floor exercises or by using machines in the gym specially designed to focus on these muscles.

Don't become fixated on toning your inner thighs; the *New England Journal of Medicine* reported on a woman who had overused a thigh toning gadget to the point that all of the tendons of her inner thighs became inflamed. Ouch.

Legs

Keep in mind that, if all goes well, your legs will be carrying you from here to there for the rest of your life. So treat them with respect. By strengthening your leg muscles, you can head off many common knee and ankle injuries. And by staying healthy, of course, you can stay active. You can work out more and develop lean, toned legs that will power you up a hill *and* look good in shorts.

Quadriceps

Street name: Quads

Where they are: The four muscles at the front of each thigh.

What they do: Straighten your knee.

Why work them: You need strong quads for walking, running, climbing, skiing, skating, hopping, skipping, and jumping.

Special tips: Keeping your quads strong will help prevent knee problems. If you already have knee pain, check with your doctor to find out which exercises are best for you.

Hamstrings

Street name: Hams

What they are: The three muscles at the back of your thigh.

What they do: Work in opposition to your quadriceps. In other words, your hamstrings bend the knee. They also help out your glutes when you move into a standing position (see the "Gluteus maximus" section).

Why work them: Injuries to the hamstrings are pretty common. Weekend warriors are especially prone to hamstring pulls, usually during that crucial touch-football play.

Special tips: Because your hamstrings are susceptible to pulls, make sure they're adequately warmed up before you perform strengthening exercises, and always stretch them after a workout. For tips on warming up and stretching, see Chapter 7.

Gastrocnemius and soleus

Street name: Calves

What they are: Your gastrocnemius is the large diamond-shaped muscle that gives shape to the back of your lower legs. The soleus resides underneath the gastroc, as it's called for short.

What they do: Enable you to stand on your tip toes and spring off the ground whenever you jump for joy.

Why work them: Strong and shapely calves don't just look good; they also give you staying power when you take those long, romantic walks or wait in a three-hour line for Springsteen tickets. Plus, you need strong calves for dancing, jumping, running, and hopping.

Special tips: With calf exercises, some people find it more effective to use slightly lighter weight and do a few more repetitions — say, up to 25 — than with most other muscle groups. The muscle tissue in your calves is very thick and coarse from constant use (walking and standing), so it takes more repetitions to reach the deepest fibers.

Tibialis anterior

Street name: Shins

What it is: The largest of several muscles that run from the front of your ankles up to just below your knee cap.

What it does: Helps you tap your toes or squash a bug.

Why work it: Shin splints — throbbing pain at the front of your ankles — are fairly common among walkers, runners, dancers, and aerobicizers who overdo it. You'll be especially prone to this injury if your shin muscles are weak compared to your calf muscles.

Special tips: If you do get shin splints, stay off your feet for a few days until the pain subsides. Icing and stretching can help speed recovery. For tips on icing, see Chapter 24.

Chapter 12

Demystifying Strength Equipment

· ·

In This Chapter

▶ Figuring out weight machines

▶ Dumbbells and barbells: the pros and cons

▶ How to use cable pulleys

▶ Toning with rubber tubes and bands

▶ Your body as weight equipment

· ·

*I*f you're intimidated by weight-lifting equipment, don't feel like a dummy. Some of these contraptions look like the convergence of a gynecological examination chair, a minimalist sculpture, and an all-terrain vehicle. It's only natural to stare at them and think: Where do I sit? What do I push? Has anyone ever been killed on these things?

As far as we know, no one's ever exploded on the Butt Blaster or been mashed into lunch meat by the leg press. Weight equipment is not as complicated as it looks. Still, you need to know how to use these contraptions safely. In this chapter, we cover the vast array of equipment that you can use at home or at the gym. We explain the pros and cons of each type of machine and help you choose the right equipment for your goals. For tips on *buying* weight equipment, see Chapter 20.

Weight Machines

If you can unfold a lawn chair, you are more than qualified to operate a weight machine. It all comes down to two relatively simple acts: You adjust your seat and then you either push or pull on a bar or a set of handles. These handles are connected to a cable or chain, which, in turn, is attached to a stack of rectangular weight plates. Each plate in the weight stack weighs between 5 and 20 pounds, depending on the make and model, and has a hole drilled in the center. If you want to lift 30 pounds, you stick a metal peg, called a *pin*, into the hole on the plate marked "30." When you pull on the machine's handles, the cable picks up 30 pounds.

Weight machines have been around for more than a hundred years. Back in the '50s, Arthur Jones, inventor of the Nautilus machines, created what is considered the most significant innovation in weight machines to date. Jones realized that, when you lift a barbell or dumbbell, there are certain points during the exercise that feel very heavy and certain points that feel light. (Try a biceps curl with a dumbbell, and you see that the dumbbell is hardest to move when your forearm is parallel to the floor.) Because your muscle is only fully working at the instances where the weight is difficult to lift, Jones concluded, traditional exercises don't give your muscles a complete workout.

Then, Jones discovered, if you use a machine with a kidney-shaped pulley rather than a round one, your muscles will feel resistance during the *entire* exercise and can be strengthened more completely.

Most of today's weight machines still work under the same principles that Jones discovered, but they have become smoother, safer, and more comfortable to use. Most of the top brands, including Body Masters, CYBEX, Hammer, Nautilus, and Galileo, do an excellent job. The brands generally differ in the size and shape of the pulleys; the angles of the bars, seats, and weight stacks; and the type of seat and handle adjustments. You might like the Nautilus chest press but prefer the CYBEX back machine. Try every machine in your gym at least once. Even if the machines are all the same brand, you might feel more comfortable using, say, the vertical chest press rather than the horizontal one.

The weight machines designed for home use — called *multi-gyms* — generally aren't as sophisticated as health club machines, but in many cases, your muscles won't know the difference.

The advantages of machines

Machines are ideal for beginners, because they're really safe. If you can't muster the strength to finish an exercise, you don't have to worry about dropping a bar on your chest.

But one caveat: Don't stick any body part near a weight stack that is being lifted or lowered. We've seen some pretty grim accidents involving crushed hands and — yes — clumps of hair.

Machines require little coordination; they basically hold your body in position and guide you through the motion. Consider the shoulder press machine. You simply sit in a chair and push the handles up — all of your effort goes into lifting those handles. On the other hand, if you're shoulder pressing with a barbell (see the definition of barbell later in this chapter), you not only have to press the bar up but also have to keep it balanced and steady. Initially, your arms will wobble back and forth. Even after you get the hang of it, the exercise always requires a certain amount of balance and coordination. Keep in mind, though, that machines don't guarantee good form while exercising, particularly if you use too much weight or don't adjust the seat properly.

Another plus for machines: They're helpful for *isolating* a particular muscle group. Isolating is just gymspeak for zeroing in on one muscle rather than getting several muscles into the act. This is helpful if you're trying to correct a specific weakness. For instance, if your hamstrings (rear thigh muscles) are underdeveloped, you can use a machine that holds your whole body still while you bend your legs to target your hamstrings. With free weights, you generally can't strengthen your hamstrings without working your front thigh and butt muscles, too.

Finally, machines let you get in a quickie workout. If your gym has 10 or 12 machines arranged in a *circuit,* you can move from one right to the other, exercising your whole body in less than 20 minutes. A circuit simply means that the machines are arranged in a row or a circle in the order that you're supposed to use them. Typically, machines that work your larger muscle groups (chest, back, butt, and thighs) come before machines that work your shoulders and arms.

The drawbacks of weight machines

You might want to stick to machines initially, but plan to mix in some free weights after a month or two of working out two or three days a week. Machine circuits get pretty boring — for you and your muscles. You need to stimulate your muscles with at least occasional changes in your workout. Typically, a gym has only two or three machines for each muscle group; with free weights, you can strengthen each muscle with dozens of exercises.

Realize, too, that every weight machine won't fit every *body*. Most machines are designed for people of average height, so if you're shorter than 5-foot-4 or taller than 6-foot-2, you might not be able to adjust the seat to fit your body. (Figuring out which machines don't fit might take you a while, however. Unlike amusement parks, gyms don't post height-requirement signs.) Manufacturers have tried to get around the height problems by offering a variety of pads to sit on or stick behind you, but they don't work for everyone. If a machine feels uncomfortable to you — even if you're of average height — try another machine that targets the same muscle group or head for the free weight area. No need to feel like you're about to tear off a limb.

Another drawback of machines is that they isolate each muscle group. We know we said this was an advantage, but it's also a flaw. Because you rarely isolate your muscles in everyday life, some experts believe it doesn't make sense to train them that way in the gym. These experts speculate that if muscles become used to working as separate entities, they stop cooperating with one other to the extent they should — a situation that might set you up for injuries.

For instance, consider the *lying leg curl*, a popular hamstring machine. You lie flat on your stomach and then bend your knees until your heels approach your rear end. This exercise does a nice job of focusing on your hamstrings, but when in real life do you lie on your stomach and kick yourself in the butt? Actually, we have relatives who do this when they throw a tantrum, but apparently they don't need to train for it.

Some experts believe you're better off strengthening your hamstrings with exercises such as squatting, a motion you use often in daily life, like when you pick up a heavy box. Because each has its advantages, we recommend doing both free weight and machine exercises.

One final reason to venture beyond machines: You can't take 'em with you. If you're on vacation and your hotel gym has nothing more than a pile of free weights, you need to know what to do with them. Don't give yourself another excuse to blow off a workout.

Special tips for machines

✔ **Make the adjustments.**

Don't just hop on a machine and start pumping away. If the last guy who used it was a foot taller than you, you might find yourself suspended in midair in the middle of the exercise.

To adjust a machine, you usually have to pull out a pin, shift the seat up or down, and then reinsert the pin. Adjusting the seat is a hassle at first, but if you don't do it, you set yourself up for an injury. Also, you cheat yourself out of a good workout. If you don't adjust the biceps curl machine correctly, you might compensate by using your back muscles, thereby defeating the whole purpose of the exercise.

Let a trainer teach you to adjust each machine to fit your body. In general, line up the joint that you're trying to move (your knees, for instance) with the joint of the machine that's moving. You shouldn't have to strain in any way to do the movement.

✔ **Check the weight stack before you lift.**

Never begin the exercise without checking where the pin has been in-serted. If someone has *racked* the machine (put the pin all the way on the bottom so the entire weight stack is captured), either your eyes are going to pop out of your head or you're going to be mighty embarrassed when you can't budge it. When you first learn to use a machine, write down the weight and seat adjustment ("leg extension; 30 lbs.; second setting") on a card or in a workout log. Carry these notes with you and update them regularly.

✔ **Learn the name of each machine.**

You should not refer to the lat pulldown as "that one where you pull down that bar thingie." Knowing what to call each contraption reminds you what the heck you're doing — you'll remember that you're working your lats, assuming you remember what those are. (If you don't, see Chapter 11.) Most machines have some sort of name plaque or label. Check that the name of the machine you're using corresponds to the name of the machine on your workout card.

✔ **Stay in control.**

If the weight stack bangs and clangs, you're lifting too fast. Many machine manufacturers recommend taking two slow counts to lift the weight stack up and four slow counts to lower the weight stack down. You may feel more comfortable speeding it up to a 2-2 count.

✔ **If the machine has a seat belt, use it.**

We're not aware of any gyms that enforce seat-belt laws, but that belt is there for a reason: to keep you still while you move through an exercise. Not every machine has one, so check carefully.

Meet your trainer: Ty the Thigh

If you're one of those people who relate better to your computer than a cold, hard weight stack, you'll love the new computerized weight machines found in some larger gyms. They're basically souped-up Nautilus-type machines, and they offer some innovative features. They help you determine how much weight you should lift and give you encouragement to push harder when you're slacking off. One brand, Powercise, gives each machine a name, like Curly Arm Curl or Ty the Thigh. If you're doing a good job, Ty will say something like, "This set rates an A!" Also, the machines share information. If you're working at half capacity, Curly will let Ty know about your feeble efforts. "Push harder than you did with Curly," Ty will say.

Computerized machines also chew you out for lifting too quickly and failing to complete the entire range of motion. Some even remember your name and last workout. The most common brand you'll see is LifeCircuit, brought to you by the same company that makes the LifeCycle.

Free Weights

Free weights are bars with weight plates on each end. The long bars are called *barbells* and the short bars are called *dumbbells*. It takes two hands to hoist a barbell. You can lift a dumbbell with one hand (although you might do some exercises using two hands on a single dumbbell).

Barbells and dumbbells are called *free* weights because they're not attached to any chains, cables, or weight stacks. You are free to do with them whatever you want, although we recommend using them for strength training rather than, say, banging nails into a wall (see Figure 12-1).

At most gyms, you find a wide array of dumbbells, lined up from lightest, usually 3 pounds, to heaviest, as much as 120 pounds. At larger gyms, you also find a selection of bars with plates welded to each end, starting with 20 pounds and increasing in 10-pound increments.

Virtually every gym has bars *without* weight plates on each end. The bar alone usually weighs 45 pounds. To increase the weight, you attach round plates with a hole drilled through the center and secure the plates with clips called *collars.* An assortment of these weight plates — typically from $2^1/_2$ pounds to 45 pounds — sits on a rack near the bars. If you want to lift 75 pounds, you add a 10-pound plate and a 5-pound plate to each side of the 45-pound bar. After you're finished, be sure to remove these plates and put them back in their proper place. Otherwise, you risk unfriendly stares from the staff and the guy who uses the bar after you.

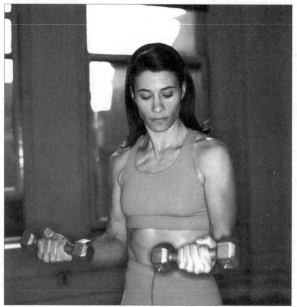

Figure 12-1:
You can use dumbbells for hundreds of exercises.

(Photo courtesy of Richard Lee.)

The advantages of free weights

Free weights are a lot more versatile than machines. Whereas a weight machine is designed for one particular motion, a single pair of dumbbells can be used to perform literally hundreds of exercises. For instance, you can push dumbbells overhead to work your shoulders, press them backward to tone your triceps, or hold one in each hand while you squat to work your thighs and butt muscles. You can change the feel and emphasis of an exercise by simply changing the way you grip the bar or dumbbell.

Another important benefit of free weights is that they work your muscles in a way that closely mimics real-life movements. As we mentioned earlier in this chapter, machines tend to isolate a particular muscle so that the rest of your muscles don't get any action; free-weight training requires several muscles to move, balance, and steady a weight as you lift and lower it. Free-weight exercises allow you to strengthen muscles that wouldn't get much work if you were doing isolation exercises with machines. Some people find that they gain strength and increase in size faster when they do the majority of their exercises with free weights. Finally, you'll never look more impressive than when you're slinging around massive hunks of metal.

The drawbacks of free weights

For some novices, free-weight exercises are hard to get the hang of. You need more instruction than you do with machines — there are a lot more mistakes to make and injuries to avoid. Also, free-weight exercises require more balance than machine moves.

If you're short on time, a free-weight workout probably will take you longer than a machine workout. Instead of simply putting a pin in a weight stack, you might have to slide weight plates on and off a bar.

Special tips for free weights

Don't think that barbells and dumbbells are for advanced weight lifters only. Beginners can use 'em, too. However, anyone using free weights needs to be very careful, even with light weights.

Debbie Bacon of Phoenix, Arizona, learned this lesson the hard way. While waiting for her husband to come home late one night, Debbie decided that exercising might help her stay awake. She was doing shoulder exercises with 7-pound dumbbells when she got so tired that she lost control of the weights and they crashed together. Unfortunately, her right index and ring fingers got in the way.

The incident involved a fractured finger tip and a piece of acrylic nail that got lodged where it shouldn't have been. But we'll spare you the gory details. Suffice it to say that free weights require your full attention. Here are a few other tips to make free-weight training safe and fun:

✔ If you are using very heavy weights, enlist a spotter (see Figure 12-2 and the sidebar "How to spot and be spotted" later in this chapter).

✔ Be careful when you lift a weight from the racks and when you put it back. You're as likely to injure yourself getting into and out of an exercise as you are actually performing it. Never pick a weight up off the floor without bending your elbows and bending your legs. Never drop the weights carelessly when you've completed a set.

✔ Don't be embarrassed to lift the 3-pound dumbbells. They're not there for decoration. And don't be scared off by the trash barrel-sized dumbbells sitting on the racks. Virtually nobody uses them.

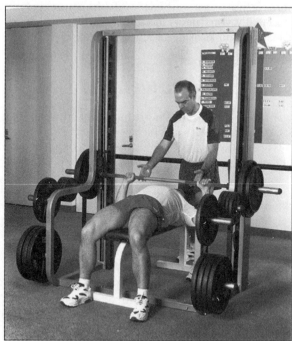

Figure 12-2:
Spotting the
bench
press.

(Photo courtesy of Dan Kron.)

ADVANCED STUFF

How to spot and be spotted

If you spend enough time in the gym, sooner or later someone is going to ask you, "Hey, buddy, mind giving me a spot?" He's not asking you to buy him a puppy; he would like assistance with his next set. You should be flattered at the request, but be aware that spotting is an awesome responsibility. It falls on your shoulders to prevent the weight from, well, falling on the *guy's* shoulders.

By the way, don't hesitate to ask for a spot yourself if you think you might have trouble completing a set. A spotter is particularly helpful when you graduate to a heavier weight. You can enlist help from a health club staff member; or better yet, ask anyone nearby who doesn't look too busy. (This is a good way to make friends at the gym, too.) Fill your spotter in on your game plan. Mention how many reps you think you can do and on which rep you think you'd like to call in the cavalry.

Here's how to handle the job of spotting a fellow weight lifter:

✔ **Pay attention at all times.** Don't get into a heated discussion about the North American Free Trade Agreement; you're supposed to be ready, on a split-second's notice, to lift the bar off your spottee's chest if his arms give out. Politely tune out the rest of the world until your spottee completes his set.

✔ **Ask your spottee where he'd like you to place your hands.** There are several schools of thought on this subject. You can rest a finger tip or two on the bar at all times so that you can give instantaneous help when your spottee calls for it — usually during the last repetition or two. Some people, including us, find that position annoying, because it diminishes the feelings of glory you experience when you complete a set by yourself.

We prefer the ready-willing-and-able spotting technique. That is, have your hands poised a couple inches from the bar; touch the bar only when your spottee begins to struggle.

✔ **Ask how many reps your spottee thinks he can to do on his own.** If he doesn't offer this information, ask so that you have an idea of when he'll need you.

✔ **If you don't think you can handle spotting someone, say so.** This is no time for heroics. In order to spot someone bench pressing 100 pounds, you need not be able to bench 100 pounds yourself — you're just there to help out. However, if you have trouble lifting the 5-pounders off the rack, you're not a candidate for this job.

✔ **Don't over-spot.** You're there to *help* the guy, not do the work for him. When you're spotting someone on the bench press, don't lean directly over the bar, grip it with both hands, and pull it up and down. With a little experience, you'll be able to provide just the right amount of additional effort that the person needs to complete the exercise.

✔ **Always offer encouraging words.** Say things like "It's all yours! You got it! You got it! All you!" This gives your spottee inspiration to squeeze out that last repetition. Plus, it makes everyone else in the gym glance over in admiration.

✔ **No matter which end of the spot you're on, pleasant *breath* is a must.** Remember, you'll be breathing forcefully right into someone's face. You don't want to find a bottle of Scope waiting for you in your locker.

A word about benches

To get a good free-weight workout, you need to use benches in your routine. This goes for home workouts, too. Some benches are flat, and some are upright, like narrow chairs with high, padded backs. Others are adjustable so that you can slide them to an incline or decline position. Here are some tips for using benches:

- **Experiment with the angle of the bench, especially for chest exercises.**

  Inclining the bench a few degrees allows you to work the muscle fibers of your upper chest. Declining the bench emphasizes your lower chest. You can use a slightly different angle each workout if you want.

- **Use a bench for support.**

  When you're doing overhead lifts or bicep curls, adjust the seat so that it's upright, and sit snugly against it. This position will protect your back and prevent you from cheating. You won't be able to rock your body back and forth to build momentum to hoist the dumbbell. You have to rely solely on the muscle power of your biceps.

- **Use weight-lifting benches for one activity only: lifting weights.**

  Don't use a bench to change a light bulb at home and don't use it at the gym to take a nap. Never use a weight bench for step aerobics. You can, however, use your step bench as a weight bench as long as you're not lifting dumbbells heavier than, say, 30 pounds.

- **Keep your feet flat on the floor or flat on the bench — whichever is more comfortable.**

  With your feet firmly anchored, you're less likely to use bad form like arching your back. And you won't accidentally roll off the bench in the middle of an exercise.

Cable Pulleys

At most gyms, you see a box full of ropes, straps, handles, short bars, long bars, V-shaped bars, and bars shaped like a handlebar mustache. This paraphernalia looks like a pile of junk excavated from someone's garage. But in fact, these are the attachments you can clip onto a *cable machine* to do a wide variety of exercises. The cable machine consists of a cable and a round pulley attached to a metal frame.

To strengthen your back, you can pull down a bar clipped to a *high pulley* — one that's attached all the way at the top. To strengthen your biceps, you can pull up on a *low pulley* — attached near the bottom of the frame, typically a few inches from the floor. To strengthen your chest, you can grab a high pulley on either side of you and pull the handles toward your chest, as if you're going to wrap your arms around someone. This exercise works your chest and shoulders in a way that's not possible with machines and free weights.

Cable pulleys are a cross between machines and free weights. On the one hand, the cable is hooked up to a stack of weights, so nothing can come crashing down. On the other hand, the motion isn't guided — you're free to pull the bar down the way you want to, and you're free to make lots of mistakes. Like free weights, cable machines require a certain amount of control and engage several muscles at once.

Don't be afraid to play around with the different types of adjustments. Attaching a new bar is easier than it looks, and you might find that when working your triceps, a V-shaped bar feels more comfortable than a straight bar. When you do make the switcheroo, you might need to adjust the amount of weight you're using. Even if you're doing the very same exercise, you might use more weight pulling down the straight bar than you would pulling down the V-shaped bar.

Tubes and Bands

Exercise tubes are like the thick rubber tubes you can find in a medical supply store — they just come in brighter colors. Some exercise tubes have handles or buckles attached to each end, or they come in a kit with attachable plastic bars and door attachments. You also can buy *exercise bands,* which are long, flat sheets of strong rubber.

You can exercise virtually every muscle group in your body with bands and tubes, although tubes work better for some exercises, while bands work better for others. You just have to experiment. Here's how you can use bands to work both of your biceps at once: You stand on the center of the band and hold an end in each hand, with your elbows by your sides. Bend your arms and curl your hands up toward your shoulders. Lower your arms slowly so the band doesn't just snap back into place.

The advantages: Bands and tubes take up zero space, and they're portable. They give you an instant strength workout, whether you're in a small studio apartment, a hotel room, or on a camping trip in the Mojave desert (see Figure 12-3). Bands and tubes are easy to adjust, too; to make an exercise tougher, just use a shorter or thicker band. They're also cheap: You can purchase a couple of bands for around $10. Even if you go hog wild, you'd have trouble spending more than $60 on a set of bands, a travel bag, and a video explaining how to use the bands.

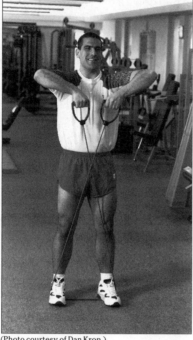

Figure 12-3:
You can use exercise tubes to strengthen virtually every muscle in your body.

(Photo courtesy of Dan Kron.)

The drawbacks: If a band or tube slips, you can get snapped in the face or groin. Ouch. Also, reproducing the same amount of work from one workout to the next is difficult. You know when you're lifting a 20-pound dumbbell or a 50-pound weight stack, but bands and tubes have no comparable measuring system. They simply come in different thicknesses (usually light, medium, heavy, and extra-heavy).

When you are using bands and tubes, keep the following tips in mind:

- Lift *and* lower the band or tube slowly. If you move carefully, you'll feel your muscles working in both directions.

- Don't wrap the band or tube so tightly around your palms that you cut off the circulation to your hands. Instead, wrap it loosely several times so that it forms loops, the way you wind a dog's leash around your hand.

- When you wrap a band or tube under your feet, make sure that it's secure. You don't want a band to slip out from under you.

- Use bands or tubes that are specifically designed for exercising. Inspect them frequently for holes and tears and replace them when they're worn.

Your Body

Yes, your very own body can function as strength equipment. You can lift it, lower it, curl it, twist it, and bend it in all sorts of ways that are designed to increase your strength. We're talking leg lifts, push-ups, pull-ups, and the like. When you move your body weight, you're fighting gravity — and that can be a considerable fight.

The advantages: You don't require any storage space and you certainly can take yourself anywhere. Plus, push-ups and pull-ups are impressive, and they call upon just about every muscle in your body. If you're really serious about building upper body strength, add push-ups and pull-up type exercises to your strength-training routine. (See Figure 12-4.)

The drawbacks: Ever try a pull-up? They're darned hard. Most people can't do pull-ups until they've spent at least a few months lifting weights. And then, eventually, they have the opposite problem: The pull-ups become too easy.

A.

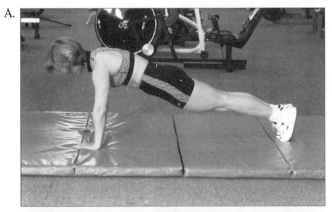

B.

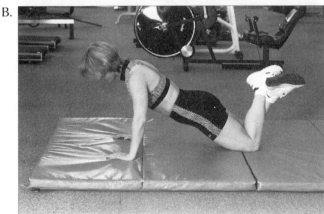

Figure 12-4:
A military
(A) and a
modified (B)
pushup.

(Photos courtesy of Dan Kron.)

Chapter 13

How to Design a Strength-Training Program

Scan the fitness aisle in any bookstore or video store and you'll find fitness experts who claim to have discovered the Secret, the Answer, the world's *best* solution to building a new you. "I can't stand to know a secret that can help others without telling them about it," says one popular instructor, explaining why she wrote her book.

Well, we have a secret, too: There *are* no secrets to weight training. To find a program that works for you, you need to experiment with a variety of training methods. Keep in mind that lifting weight is an art, not an exact science.

In this chapter, we present an array of tools you can use to custom design a strength-training program. We address questions such as, "How much weight should I lift?" "How many exercises do I need to do?" and "How many days a week should I go to the gym?" There's no single answer to any of these questions. You need to decide which techniques you like best — and which ones your body responds to. Also, we recommend consulting with a qualified trainer at least once before you embark on a strength-training program.

The Building Blocks of a Weight Workout

You can't begin to design a strength-training program without knowing two terms: rep and set. *Rep* is short for repetition — one complete motion of an exercise. Let's say you're doing a leg lift. When you lift your leg and then lower it back down, you've completed one rep. A *set* is a group of consecutive repetitions. For instance, you can say, "I did 2 sets of 10 reps on the chest press." This means that you did 10 consecutive chest presses, rested, and then did another 10 chest presses. The number of reps and sets you choose to do will, in large part, determine the results of your workout program.

How many reps should I do?

The number of reps you do depends on your goals. To develop maximum strength and large muscles, do fewer than 8 reps per set. To tone your muscles and develop the type of strength you need for everyday life — moving furniture or shoveling snow — aim for 8 to 15 repetitions. Doing dozens of reps usually doesn't bring good results of any kind.

Why do you build *more* strength doing *fewer* repetitions? Because you use a much heavier weight when you do 6 reps than when you do 15, and lifting heavy weight is what builds maximum muscle strength. No matter how many repetitions you do, always use a heavy enough weight so that the last rep is challenging, but you can maintain good form. After about a month of strength training, you may want to *go to failure*. This means your last repetition is so difficult that you can't squeeze out one more.

If you have a few different goals in mind, you can mix and match the number of reps you do per workout. If you want to get bigger and stronger and also develop more shapely muscles, you can do a heavy workout one day, and a lighter workout the next time out. Your body may respond to one type of training better than another.

Don't lift the same amount of weight for every type of exercise. In general, use more weight to work larger muscles like your thighs, chest, and upper back, and use less weight to exercise your shoulders, arms, and abdominals.

Write down how much weight you lift for each exercise so that next time around you won't have to waste time experimenting all over again. But don't lock yourself in to lifting a certain amount of weight every time. Everyone feels stronger on some days than on others. Just because you can bench press 80 pounds on Monday, doesn't mean you'll be able to do it on Wednesday. Listen to your body. It'll tell you what it can and cannot handle.

How do I know when I'm ready to lift more weight?

It won't take long to outgrow the weights you used during your first workout. When you can easily do the maximum number of reps you're aiming for, increase the weight by the smallest increment possible and drop down to fewer reps. You know you're lifting too much weight if you can't complete your repetitions with good form and if you feel the need to grunt. Not all muscles improve at the same rate. After a month of weight training, you might jump up 20 pounds on a chest exercise but only 5 pounds on a shoulder exercise.

How fast should I do my reps?

Take a full two seconds to lift a weight and two to four seconds to lower it. If you lift more quickly than that, you'll hear a lot of clanging and banging. Plus you'll end up relying on momentum rather than muscle power. Going slow and steady will yield better results because more of your muscle gets into the act.

How many sets should I do for each exercise?

Some research suggests that doing one set per muscle builds just as much strength as doing three or four sets per muscle. However, in order to get the benefits of the one-set method, you may need to push to complete and utter muscle fatigue by the end of that set — and that's harder than most of us are capable of working. So here's the conventional advice: If your goal is to build moderate strength and tone, do at least two sets for every muscle. That's a total of 22 sets, two sets for each of the following 11 muscle groups: buttocks, front of the thigh, back of the thigh, lower legs, upper back, chest, shoulders, back of the arms, front of the arms, abdominals, and lower back. For a rundown on each muscle group, see Chapter 11.

If you're trying to define and shape your muscles, we recommend doing three to six sets per muscle group. This does not mean that you need to do a half dozen sets on the horizontal chest press. We recommend splitting the six sets among two or three different exercises that emphasize different parts of the muscle. For example, you can do two sets of bench presses with the bench horizontal to emphasize the middle portion of the chest muscles, two sets with it inclined to emphasize the upper portion of the chest, and two sets with it declined to emphasize the lower portion. Doing all these exercises can be pretty time consuming; don't fool yourself — reshaping your body is no easy task. It takes about a minute to complete one set, so if you factor in the rest periods between sets, that's more than 90 minutes per workout. Later in this chapter, we explain how you can break up your program into shorter workouts.

If you're aiming for maximum strength — or a physique like the ones you see on ESPN body-building competitions — you need to do at least 10 to 20 sets per muscle group. You'll need to work out for at least an hour almost every day.

How much rest should I take between sets?

The amount of rest you take in between sets is another variable that you can toy around with. Beginners should rest about 90 seconds between sets to give their muscles adequate time to recover. As you get in better shape, you need less rest — only about 30 seconds — before your muscles feel ready for another set. If you follow a chest exercise with, say, a thigh exercise, you typically will need less rest than if you do consecutive exercises for the same muscle group.

After the first few weeks of training, you can fine-tune the amount of rest you take between sets according to your goals. If you're using really heavy weights and doing fewer reps in order to bulk up, you can take up to 5 minutes between sets so that your muscles can pump out their greatest effort each time.

If you're short on time or you like a fast-paced workout, try *circuit training:* You move quickly from exercise to exercise with little or no rest at all. Circuit training does a decent job building strength, but it's not a good substitute for an aerobic workout, even though you feel you're working aerobically. (See Chapter 5 for a definition of aerobic.)

Figure 13-1 contains some guidelines to help you design a weight-training program that suits your goals. These numbers aren't the law — everybody's body responds to weight training differently. Experiment with the different components of a weight program until you find the combination of sets, reps, weight, and rest that works for you.

Table 13-1	Weight Training in a Nutshell		
	Maximum Strength and Size	*Moderate Strength; Maximum Tone*	*Some Strength; Moderate Tone*
Exercises per muscle group	4–6	3–4	1–3
Sets per exercise	4–6	2–4	1–3
Reps per set	2–6	8–12	10–15
Weights	Very heavy	Moderately heavy	Moderate
Rest between sets	2–3 minutes	1–1½ minutes	1 minute or less

In what order should I do my exercises?

In general, exercise larger muscles before smaller ones. Work your back and chest before your shoulders and arms, and your butt before your thighs and calves. Smaller muscles assist the larger muscles. If the smaller muscles are too tired to pitch in and do their job, they give out long before your big muscles get an adequate workout. For instance, your biceps help out your upper back when you do a lat pulldown, an exercise where you pull a bar down to your chest. If you work your biceps first, they'll be too tired to do their job during the pulldown, and your back muscles won't get as good a workout.

As for which muscles to start with — chest, back, or legs — that's up to you. You might want to begin with all your chest exercises then move on to your back. Or you can alternate chest and back moves. You can fit your abdominal exercises in whenever you like.

How many times a week do I need to lift weights?

Work each muscle two or three times a week. If your aim is maximum strength, targeting each muscle three times a week might not give the muscle enough chance to rest. In that case, cut back to two workouts per muscle group per week.

If you really get into weight training, consider doing a *split routine*. You exercise some of your muscles during one workout, and then come back a day or two later to exercise the others. You still work each muscle at least twice a week, but because you don't train every muscle during every workout, you can devote more energy to the muscles you're focusing on that day — and each of your muscles will still get enough rest.

Splitting your routine is a good idea, especially if you are serious about building muscle and if you have free time in small chunks. You'll be fresher and more motivated if you walk into the gym knowing that today, you have to work *only* your chest, triceps, and shoulders. You probably will work these muscles harder than if you try to fit all of your muscle groups into one workout.

You can split your routine in several ways. You decide which you prefer:

> ✔ **Push/Pull:** Work your pulling muscles (your back muscles and biceps) on one day, and during the next session, work your pushing muscles (your chest and triceps). You can fit in your leg, shoulder, and abdominal exercises whenever you want. Following is an example of a push/pull routine. Ask a trainer or experienced friend to teach you exercises for each muscle group.

Monday	push	chest, triceps, lower-body exercises
Tuesday	pull	back, biceps, shoulders, abdominals
Wednesday	REST	
Thursday	push	chest, triceps, lower-body exercises
Friday	REST	
Saturday	pull	back, biceps, shoulders, abdominals
Sunday	REST	

✔ **Upper Body/Lower Body:** You work your upper body one day and your lower body the next. You fit in your abs two to four times a week whenever it's convenient.

Monday	upper body	back, chest, shoulders, triceps, biceps
Tuesday	lower body	gluteals, quadriceps, hamstrings, calves, abdominals
Wednesday	REST	
Thursday	upper body	back, chest, shoulders, triceps, biceps
Friday	REST	
Saturday	lower body	gluteals, quadriceps, hamstrings, calves, abdominals
Sunday	REST	

✔ **Big/Little:** You work your larger muscles and your smaller muscles on separate days. If you do the big/little split, you need to take a full day of rest between workouts. Don't work your triceps on Sunday and then come back Monday to train your chest; your triceps won't have recovered enough to help out with the chest exercises. Here's how a big/little split would work over an eight-day period.

Monday	big	gluteals, quadriceps, hamstrings, back, chest
Tuesday	REST	
Wednesday	little	shoulders, triceps, biceps, calves, abdominals
Thursday	REST	
Friday	big	gluteals, quadriceps, hamstrings, back, chest
Saturday	REST	
Sunday	little	shoulders, triceps, biceps, calves, abdominals
Monday	REST	

All about abs

There are more theories about abdominal training than there are about the Kennedy assassination. Here's our take on getting your midsection into shape. Read Chapter 11 to learn the names and functions of your four abdominal muscles.

✔ Don't do abdominal exercises every day. Your abs, like all of your other muscle groups, need a day of rest between workouts.

✔ Ask a trainer to teach you abdominal exercises that you do on the floor, such as crunches and reverse curls. We're not fond of most abdominal weight machines because they tend to bring the lower back or hip muscles into the act. As for those abdominal infomercial gadgets you can strap over your knees or stick under your butt, most of them don't work.

✔ If you can do more than 25 reps of an abdominal exercise, you're either doing the reps too quickly or with poor form, or the exercise is too easy for you. As with any other exercise, you should be struggling on the last repetition. Doing 100 continuous reps of any ab exercise is a waste of time.

✔ To make abdominal exercises more challenging, you can do them on a slanted bench, so that your head is below your legs. This is more effective than holding a weight plate on your abdomen.

✔ Don't devote too much of your workout time to abdominal exercises. Sure, do a few extra ab moves if you want, but don't neglect your other muscles. You can do a complete abdominal workout in less than 10 minutes.

Whatever you decide to do — your whole body on the same day or your own creative version of the split routine — make sure each muscle group gets at least one full day of rest. (You can do aerobic training every day, because it's much easier on your muscles than weight training.) Lifting weight literally shreds your muscles apart. They need those 48 hours to recover and rebuild. That rest day is just as important to the building and toning process as the actual lifting. If you don't rest, you'll wind up sore and more prone to overuse injuries. Besides, overworking a muscle may weaken it, defeating your purpose for training.

Lifting Weights the Right Way

The way some people lift weights, you'd think they were either in labor — or imitating that moment in episodes of "The Incredible Hulk" when Bill Bixby turns into Lou Ferrigno. Grunting, screaming, and rocking back and forth — these are *not* indications of proper weight-lifting technique. We've seen people invent some pretty outrageous exercises. One guy bent over, picked up a very heavy dumbbell, lifted it straight over his head so that he almost fell backward, and then threw it to the ground so hard that it bounced and broke a mirror. He seemed quite pleased with himself. (See Figure 13-1 to see proper form for a free weight exercise.)

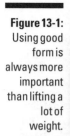

Figure 13-1:
Using good
form is
always more
important
than lifting a
lot of
weight.

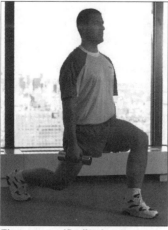

(Photo courtesy of Dan Kron.)

No matter which muscles you train, how much weight you lift, or what type of machinery you use, the following rules always apply:

✔ **Always warm up.**

Before you lift a weight, do at least five minutes of aerobic exercise to get your muscles warm and pliable. If you're going to do arm exercises and there aren't any upper body aerobic machines around (such as a VersaClimber, rower, or cross-country skier), do a few minutes of arm circles to get the blood flowing through your arm muscles.

✔ **Good form is always more important than lifting a lot of weight.**

Don't arch your back, strain your neck, or rock your body to generate momentum.

✔ **Increase your weight gradually.**

Jumping from a 5-pound weight to a 10-pounder doesn't sound like a big leap, but think about it: You're *doubling* the load on that muscle. If you're using a 5-pound weight, move up to a 6-, 7-, or 8-pounder.

✔ **Don't forget to breathe.**

In general, exhale forcefully through your mouth as you lift the weight and inhale deeply through your nose as you lower it.

Although proper breathing is important for speeding oxygen to your muscles, don't get hung up on the mechanics. Some people spend so much time trying to get the correct breathing pattern down that they lose track of what they're doing. Whatever you do, don't hold your breath. You can bring about sharp increases in your blood pressure, and you can even faint from lack of air.

You should, however, hold your breath during extremely heavy lifts. This protects your spine by bracing it with the pressure from the held breath. We mention this information on the outside chance some world-class power lifter reads this section and becomes incensed by the omission of it. Don't hold your breath unless you're aiming to lift world-record amounts of weight.

✔ **Don't get married to your routine.**

Frequently varying your exercises keeps your muscles guessing. By alternating exercises, you engage more muscle fibers and work them from a variety of angles. You can alternate squats with lunges, for instance. Both exercises work your butt and thighs, but the squat emphasizes the butt, whereas the lunge shifts the focus to the thighs. Some people change some or all of their exercises every time they work out. Try different exercises at least once a month. You can expand your repertoire by asking a trainer to teach you new exercises, watching an exercise video, buying a fitness book, reading magazines, or talking to members at your health club.

✔ **Use full range of motion.**

In other words, pull or push as far as you're supposed to. (If you're not sure, a trainer can show you the correct range of motion for each exercise.) Using the full range of motion prevents you from tightening up and may actually enhance your flexibility.

✔ **Pay attention.**

Remind yourself which muscle you're working, and focus on that muscle. It's easy to do abdominal crunches without really working your abs. It's easy to do lat pulldowns without challenging your lats.

Advanced Weight-Training Techniques

We call the following techniques *advanced,* but novices can use them, too. Most of them, anyway — we let you know which ones are off limits for beginners.

✔ **Super Set:** You do two consecutive sets of different exercises without resting in between.

For instance, you do one chest exercise immediately followed by a different chest exercise and *then* take a rest. The idea is to completely tire out the muscle — to work it so hard that you reach the deepest fibers.

You also can do a super set with exercises that target different muscle groups, like a chest exercise followed by a leg exercise. With this type of super set, you don't rest between exercises — the purpose is simply to save time.

✔ **Giant Set:** This a super, super set: You string three or more exercises together and then rest. Try this technique when you haven't worked out for a few days and your muscles are very well rested.

✔ **Pyramids:** You do multiple sets of an exercise, increasing the weight for each set while decreasing the number of reps.

You might do a light warm-up set for 10 reps, then a heavier set for 8 reps, then an even heavier set for 6 reps, and so on, until you reach a weight at which you can do only 1 rep. You don't have to go all the way down to 1 rep for your workout to be considered a pyramid. The idea is to work up slowly and tire out the muscle.

✔ **Negatives:** Someone helps you lift a weight and then you're on your own for the lowering, or *negative,* phase of the lift. (This phase is also referred to as the *eccentric* phase; the positive, or lifting, phase is called the *concentric* phase.)

Your muscles generally can handle more weight when you lower a weight than when you lift it, so this technique gives you a chance to really tire out your muscles. Beginners shouldn't try negatives. They can cause significant muscle soreness.

✔ **Breakdowns:** You lift a heavy weight, and as soon as you've exhausted the muscle — however many reps that may be — you pick up a lighter weight and squeeze out a few more reps. You might do 10 reps of an exercise and then drop 2 to 5 pounds and try to eke out three or four more reps. This is just another way of tiring out the muscle.

✔ **Super Slow Training:** You take 15 to 30 seconds to do each rep. The idea is to take all the momentum out of the movement so that you use pure muscle power. This technique is done primarily on machines, and it's very hard — you should be able to do only 3 to 5 reps. Super slow training requires more patience than most of us have. It's best if you're coached through your reps by a trainer with experience using this technique.

✔ **21s:** You do the top half of any exercise for 7 reps, the bottom half for another 7 reps, and then move through the full range of motion for your final 7 reps.

The theory is that you zero in on more fibers if you isolate parts of the movement. Here's how it works for bicep curls:

- The first 7: Lower the dumbbell until your forearm is parallel to the floor and then curl it back up toward your shoulder.

- The second 7: Start with your arm hanging by your side and then lift the weight until your forearm is parallel to the floor.

- The final 7: Start from the full hang and lift the dumbbell all the way up to your shoulder.

✔ **Periodization:** You organize your training program into several periods, each lasting about four weeks. Each phase has a different emphasis.

The first month you might simply get in shape, doing only very basic exercises, using moderate weights, and performing one set of 8 to 15 reps of each exercise. In the next period, you might go for maximum strength, lifting heavy weight, doing fewer repetitions, and taking more rest between sets. In the third phase, you might focus on building stamina, doing more repetitions, and taking less rest between sets. Periodization is great if you are a beginner because it helps you focus on one goal at a time.

Part IV
Braving the Gym

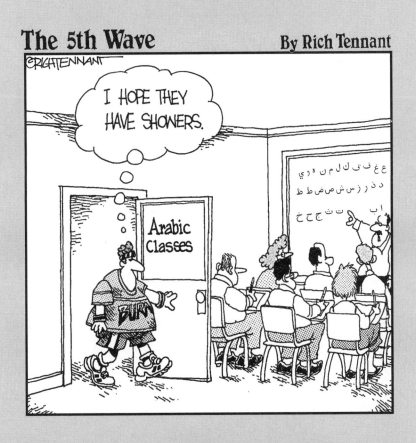

In this part . . .

*W*e prepare you to take the health-club plunge. After all, we don't want you to bolt out the door at the first sight of a guy with biceps bigger than his head. Chapter 14 explains how to choose the best gym for you and how to recognize slimy sales tactics; we also update you on the latest health club trends. In Chapter 15 you learn how to choose a first-rate trainer and how to spot a quack. Chapter 16 covers the unwritten rules of the gym — what to say, what to wear, and what to do about that pool of sweat you may have left on the leg-press machine. Chapter 17 helps you sort through the wide range of classes you're likely to find — from Ab-Solutely Fabulous to Yoga-Robics to Step 'N Slide.

Chapter 14
Choosing a Health Club

. . . .

. . . .

*W*hen it comes to health clubs, we're biased: We like 'em. There's always someone around to give you help and encouragement, and you get a much wider variety of workout choices than you would in your living room. Of course, to reap the benefits of a health club, you have to actually show up. The reality is, most people don't. If every member of your gym worked out regularly, the place probably would look like the floor of the New York Stock Exchange. About half the people who join a club quit exercising within two months, and only 20 percent work out three times a week.

To boost the odds that you'll become a regular, it's important to choose a gym that suits your schedule, your goals, and your personality. This chapter will help you decide whether to join a gym and how to pick the *right* one.

Should You Join a Health Club?

A health club isn't for everybody. Before you shop around, consider whether or not you're the sort of person who will thrive at a gym. This will save you plenty of money and guilt in the long run. If you decide a gym isn't for you, that's fine. There are plenty of other places to get fit (see Chapter 9).

Three reasons to sign up

Joining a gym requires a fair amount of guts. It took our friend Chivas Clem two years to venture into his neighborhood health club. "I almost turned around and walked out," recalls Chivas, who's a very svelte 5-foot-8. "The room was full of these tanned, perfect bodies in spandex cat suits, and I'm totally emaciated. Finally, I get the nerve to ask this hulk-like man behind the counter if I can join. He says, 'So, you've never been to a gym before?' I say, 'No, is it *that* obvious?'"

Don't be put off by insensitive comments like that. If you're debating whether or not to join a gym, remember the following great reasons to sign up.

You need inspiration

At home you can always drum up an excuse not to exercise, even if it means dusting your electric can-opener or reading your VCR manual. But at the gym, what else is there to do but exercise? Even if you never talk to a soul, you can feed off the energy of those around you. You might even find a workout partner. Some gyms will scout out a buddy for you.

You want variety

Even if you can afford $10,000 to build an elaborate home gym, you'll still find more options at a health club. At home, you may have a stationary bike, a treadmill, *or* a stairclimber; at a gym, you have all three and more. The same goes for weights. You can strengthen your triceps just fine with a pair of dumbbells in your living room, but at a gym you also have the option of using machines, barbells, and cable pulleys. (See Figure 14-1.) Gyms constantly update their equipment, so you can try strength and aerobic machines that haven't yet hit the home market or are still too expensive. You also can choose from a long list of classes.

You want expert advice

At a good gym, a trainer is always on hand to help you figure out the chest machine or tell you how to firm up your butt.

Three reasons to say, "No thanks"

Some people collect gym memberships like Elizabeth Taylor collects husbands — with about as much success. They figure that if they keep joining, one of these days they will actually *go*, but inevitably the affair is short-lived. Don't bother buying a membership if you have no serious intention of using it. If you fit the following categories, you're better off finding an alternative way to work out:

You want to exercise alone

If you can't bear the thought of working out in public, start off at home and consider a gym again in a few months when you feel more confident.

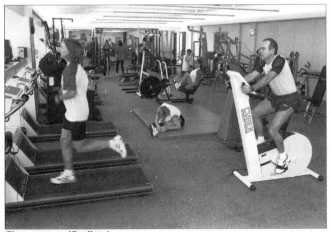

Figure 14-1:
Health clubs
offer a
variety of
exercise
equipment.

(Photo courtesy of Dan Kron.)

Your schedule won't allow time

If you simply don't have the time to drive to a club or if you can't find one to accommodate your work hours, don't force the issue. Exercising at home makes more sense.

You hate exercising indoors

If indoor workouts make you feel like a hamster in a *Habitrail,* head outside and walk, run, skate, or cycle. But keep in mind that it's tough to get a great strength-training workout outdoors.

How to Judge a Gym

Walking into a health club for the first time is like meeting your future in-laws: No matter what, the experience is going to be awkward. But at least you get to choose your gym, so shop around before you part with any money. Don't join a club simply because your accountant goes there or because the club is promoting a special discount. Here are ten factors to consider (some might matter to you; others won't).

Location

This is probably the most important consideration. If your gym is on the other side of town, you won't go — even if it's the *Taj Majal* of health clubs. Ideally, join a club within a ten-minute walk or drive from your home or office.

Size

The big trend here is the super club, the health club equivalent of WalMart. You can find low prices, a wide selection of equipment and classes, plenty of energy, and a large staff of trainers. For an experienced exerciser, a super club can be as fun as an amusement park.

If you're a beginner, however, these four-story clubs can be overwhelming. You can get lost trying to find your way from the locker room to the body-sculpting class. In that case, a smaller, cozier gym might be a better choice. You'll get to know the entire staff on a personal basis, and they might even notice if you don't show up for a while.

Super clubs tend to take a jack-of-all-trades, master-of-none approach. These clubs may have a small yoga room, a limited boxing program, and a single climbing wall. If you're trying to learn a specific skill or technique, a megaclub isn't the place to get in-depth knowledge. Yoga, for instance, is best learned at a studio that teaches only yoga. But if you want a smorgasbord of activities, a super club is the place to be.

Cost

Membership fees vary greatly. Large clubs often charge less than small ones because they have more members. (They also tend to pay their staff less.) But the dollar figure doesn't mean everything. Fifty bucks a month might seem outrageous for a small neighborhood club with old equipment; on the other hand, if the club is half a mile from your house, it's actually a bargain because you'll go. It's a much better investment than a $20-a-month club that's 20 minutes away.

Consider these other money matters when you choose a gym:

- ✔ **Hidden costs:** The monthly membership may be reasonable, but will you pay up the wazoo in extras? A $20-a-month club won't be so cheap if you have to pay $1.50 for parking every day. Some gyms charge extra for specialty classes, such as boxing. Other clubs don't have membership dues but rather charge hefty fees for trainers; the catch is, you can't use the club without one. This type of club could run you $9,000 a year. On the other hand, you're bound to get plenty of attention.

- ✔ **Initiation fees:** In addition to the monthly membership fee, many clubs require an initiation fee. At least they *claim* to require it. If you insist strongly enough, many clubs waive this fee. Or clubs use this initiation fee as a marketing ploy — something they don't really intend for you to pay. Some salesperson might say, "*just* because you seem like a terrific person, and I *really* want you to get in shape, I'll waive the initiation fee. But *shhh* — don't tell my boss. He'll kill me." Initiation fees can range from $25 to $1,500.

✔ **Bargaining:** Many clubs will make special deals if you ask, although they don't advertise this fact. The best time to ask is during slow periods like summer, when clubs are hungrier for sales. You might also get a break if you join with a family member or friend. If you have friends who are already members, ask what they paid; if the sales rep cites you a higher fee, don't be afraid to say, "My friend Jane Smith paid $25 a month, and I'd like the same deal."

✔ **Trial memberships:** If you're unsure about the club, ask for a two-week free trial period before joining — or at least a day pass.

✔ **Long-term memberships:** Don't even think about it. You don't know where you're going to be in three years — or whether the club will even be in business. One club in New York was selling lifetime memberships until the day before it closed its doors. Never sign up for more than one year.

✔ **Cancellation policies:** Sales people won't always tell you this, but in most states the law requires a three-day cooling-off period. In other words, if you change your mind within three days, the club must refund your money in full. If the club won't, get your lawyer to shoot off a letter; that should do the trick. Also, ask what happens if you quit three months after joining. Some clubs will refund your money for any reason. Others will give you a refund only if you prove you are moving more than 25 miles from the club. Most clubs will freeze memberships for medical reasons or long-term travel as long as you let them know in advance.

Equipment

You might not consider yourself qualified to judge the equipment at a gym, but even a novice can make some important assessments. If you wouldn't know a hamstring machine even if you were sitting on one, ask your tour guide specifically about the following factors:

✔ **Variety:** Do you want three varieties of stairclimbers, or will you settle for one? Some clubs have 10-, 15-, and 20-pound dumbbells; at other clubs, you'll also find 12-pounders, $17^1/_2$-pounders, and $22^1/_2$-pounders. Some gyms have a single hamstring machine; others have four, so you can work these muscles standing, sitting, leaning forward, or lying face down.

✔ **Quantity:** Is there enough equipment to support the membership? You don't want your wait for the treadmill to be like the line at the Department of Motor Vehicles. Take a tour at the same time of day you'll be working out, and notice whether the machines are overbooked.

✔ **Quality and upkeep:** Is the place in a state of disrepair? Is the stuffing coming out of the weight benches? Lots of duct tape is not a good sign. Get on a couple of weight machines and see how smoothly the weight stacks work. Pick up a few free weights and see if the ends are loose. Listen to the cardiovascular equipment: Are the treadmills loud and whiny? That noise means that the motors need a tune-up. Don't be afraid to test drive a good portion of the equipment.

Four slimy sales tactics to recognize

Some clubs will try anything to rope you in. Be prepared to combat these sales strategies:

✔ **Limited offers:** "You must join *right now*," the salesperson will say, "or I can't give you this special deal. I'm really sorry, but the sale ends today." The truth is, if you come back tomorrow, the club may offer you an even *better* deal so that you don't walk out again.

✔ **Creating fear or insecurity:** The salesperson may rattle off death statistics for men your age who don't exercise — or tell you that women just a few years older than you disintegrate from osteoporosis because they don't work out. The salesperson may even tell perfectly healthy women that they are fat. They'll try to create an immediate need so you don't know how you can go on living without a gym membership.

✔ **An answer for everything:** If you say that you have to ask your wife, the salesperson may attack your manhood: "What's the matter? You need *her* to tell you what to do about your health?" If you say you can't afford it, they'll say, "How can you *not* afford to invest in your health?" They'll whip out the contract and keep inching it across the desk toward you. Be prepared to walk out, even as they tell you how insane you are for doing so.

✔ **The bait-and-switch:** The newspaper ad tells you one price, but when you go in, the salesperson says, "Oh, *that* sale ended yesterday, but I can give you *this* offer." Or, "You misunderstood the woman on the phone — we can't give you the first three months free." Always ask who you're talking to so you can name names. Bring the newspaper ad along so you can use it for proof.

Among the best brands for health-club weight machines are: CYBEX, Nautilus, Trotter, Hammer, Icarian, and BodyMasters. There are other good makes, but most decent gyms have at least some of these names. On the cardiovascular side, look for LifeFitness, Trotter, Tectrix, StairMaster, Startrek, and Quinton.

Classes

Make sure that the club offers what you want, whether it's beginning step aerobics, body sculpting, water aerobics, or funk. (Some clubs don't offer classes.) See if the classes meet at convenient times. To assess whether classes are any good, ask if you can sample a few before joining. Also, ask other members for their opinions. For more on qualities to look for in specific classes, see Chapter 17.

Members

Do they seem like your type? Some gyms cater to people over 40, others serve women only; if the members look like they could open a door from the *hinged* side, you're in a body-building gym. In general, don't be too judgmental. People are people, and most of them are nice, even if they look like underwear models for Calvin Klein or Victoria's Secret. Don't give the membership factor too much weight, unless you're joining a gym primarily to socialize.

Besides, you might be surprised by who becomes your friends. "The members that I was most intimidated by ended up being just regular guys," says one friends of ours. "One guy had his head shaved except for a rat tail in the back. He looked really mean and scary, but he was a doll when you talked to him. It turned out that he was a nurse."

Staff

If you're inexperienced, the staff is going to play an important role in your success. Ask the same questions you'd ask when hiring a personal trainer. (See Chapter 15 for a list of these questions.) Are the trainers certified by a reputable organization? Are they experienced? Look around: Are the trainers standing around telling jokes to each other while some poor guy is stuck under a weight bar? Is the only visible staff member doing his algebra homework at the front desk? Does anyone acknowledge your existence when you walk in?

Cleanliness

Is the place clean and well ventilated? Pay special attention to the locker rooms: Are the bathrooms spotless, or is it foot fungus city? Open the shower curtains and check the floor, the soap dish, and the walls for gunk and mold. If a club isn't clean, don't join. It's not worth the risk. Ask how often the cleaning crew makes its rounds.

Extra facilities

Is there a Jacuzzi or sauna? Towel service? Day care? Massage? Nutrition counseling? A snack bar? A pro shop? A TV in front of every treadmill? Do you *care?*

Hours

There are 24-hour gyms, and gyms that close at 8 p.m. Check your club's hours, particularly on weekends, when most gyms close earlier. Generally, the larger the club, the longer the hours.

Now appearing at a gym near you

Competition is forcing clubs to offer more and more services. Some are great; some are bogus. Here are four services that we're happy about.

- **Nutritional counseling:** When it comes to weight loss, exercise alone isn't going to cut it. But beware: As with trainers, *anyone* can call himself a nutritionist. Make sure you're dealing with a Registered Dietitian. And don't let your "nutritionist" hard sell you any products — including expensive supplements or prepackaged wonder foods that have been designed "especially for your body chemistry." Prices vary widely, from $200 to $1,000 for a package of three to ten sessions.

- **Family fitness:** Some clubs have full-fledged kid gyms with tyke-sized weight machines. This is great. It's never too early to get kids into the habit of exercising, as long as you don't force them. There's no research proving that exercise can be harmful to kids, as long as it's done in moderation.

- **Spa services:** You can treat yourself to massages, facials, mud wraps, salt scrubs, or meditations. Prices for these services vary greatly, as does quality. Make sure that your massage therapist is board certified. (See Chapter 22 for more tips about massage.)

- **Cybersweat:** Some of the larger, high-tech clubs now feature interactive information kiosks to teach you about weight training, as shown in the following figure. For instance, if you want to know about a particular back exercise, you touch the corresponding button and you watch a short video about how to use the machine and which muscles you're strengthening. Some kiosks even give printouts.

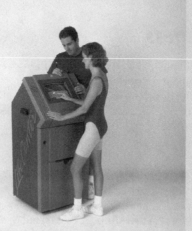

(The Life Fitness interactive information kiosk.)

Chapter 15

Hiring a Trainer

. . . .

In This Chapter

▶ Five smart reasons — and one dumb one — to hire a trainer

▶ How to weed out the posers

▶ How much a trainer should cost

▶ Signs of a quality trainer

▶ How to be a good client

. . . .

*L*ifting weights isn't nuclear physics, but neither is it something you should attempt to figure out on your own. We recommend signing up with a trainer — for at least one session — to get yourself started on a strength and cardiovascular program suited to *your* goals. Even workout veterans have plenty to gain from a session or two with a trainer.

A trainer can teach you the subtleties of using exercise equipment: how to grip a barbell, how far to pull down a rope, and how to adjust a machine to fit your body — stuff that's tough to learn from a book or video. At least a *good* trainer can teach you all of this. The problem is, the industry has its share of quacks. This chapter explains who can benefit from a trainer and discusses how to find a qualified one.

Five Smart Reasons to Hire a Trainer

Trainers do a lot more than just whip wimpy actors into shape for their next action movie, and they don't all charge $200 an hour. (We talk more about trainer fees later in this chapter.) Consider hiring a trainer if you meet any of the following criteria:

- ✓ **You're totally out of shape (or *deconditioned*, as the politically correct like to say).**

  If climbing the ropes in high school gym class was the last time you worked out, a personal trainer is a great way to bring you into the modern age. You don't need to sign up for life; 5 to 10 sessions will get you up and running.

- ✓ **You want to update your program.**

  You can hire a trainer for a session or two to reevaluate your workout regimen. If you're feeling stagnant, a new routine can give you a jump start and ultimately improve your fitness level. (Of course, you actually have to work out for this to happen.)

- ✓ **You're training for a specific goal.**

  Say you want to run your first 5-mile race but aren't sure how long, how far, how often, or how hard to train. A qualified trainer can design a workout program that'll get you to the finish line. Look for a trainer who specializes in the area you want to work on, such as losing weight, building strength, or getting fit for ski season.

- ✓ **You're coming back from an injury or illness.**

  If you have a specific condition such as lower back pain or if you've just had reconstructive surgery on your knee, a trainer can help you get back on your feet. But check with your doctor; he might want you to visit a physical therapist first. Still, more and more physicians are giving the okay for trainers to participate in a patient's rehabilitation. Screen the trainer carefully — ask your doctor for a recommendation — so that you don't make matters worse. A growing number of trainers specialize in conditions such as multiple sclerosis or breast cancer.

- ✓ **You need motivation.**

  If you won't exercise unless a trainer is standing there counting your repetitions, consider the money well spent.

One Reason Not to Hire a Trainer

Don't waste your money or the trainer's time if you need someone to supply 100 percent of your motivation and if you're going to whine the whole time. Nobody can force you to get in shape if you aren't willing to work hard. Get yourself in a positive frame of mind before you hire a trainer.

Weeding Out the Posers

Currently, only Louisiana has any legal requirements for fitness trainers, and even those laws have loopholes. This means anyone who can hoist a dumbbell and print up a business card on a home computer can call himself a personal trainer.

Screen a potential trainer with the same care that you use to screen a potential employee. And don't be afraid to try someone new if you don't hit it off with the first trainer. It's your money, and this is your health we're talking about. The following section tells you what to consider when investigating trainers. Later in this chapter we tell you where to find a qualified trainer.

Certification

As with many other occupations and professions, the fitness industry offers certification tests. A certification is by no means a guarantee of competence. But getting certified by quality organizations is a time-consuming, pain-in-the-butt process. You've got to study for at least a few months and then spend a full day taking a test. At the very least, going through this process shows commitment: You know that the trainer isn't just doing this job because it pays better than his old job as a bike messenger.

However, not all certifications are equal. In fact, some are downright bogus, requiring little more than the ability to write out a check. The following are among the best organizations that certify trainers. The organizations can refer you to certified trainers in your area. The phone numbers for these organizations are listed in the Resources section of this book. Make sure your trainer's certification is current. Most expire after a year or two unless the trainer takes continuing education classes.

- ✔ **ACSM (American College of Sports Medicine):** The ACSM offers several different certification levels. The certification we recommend is the Health/Fitness Instructor. The test is very tough, so many trainers avoid it.

  For personal trainers, we don't recommend the ACSM Exercise Leader certification. It's geared toward teaching group classes and requires less knowledge of physiology than the other ACSM diplomas. The Exercise Leader certification is, however, Dummies-approved for aerobics instructors — see Chapter 17.

- ✔ **ACE (American Council on Exercise):** This organization certifies both trainers and aerobics instructors; again, we prefer certification geared toward trainers. The ACE Personal Trainer certification is the most popular in the industry. The test is much easier than the ACSM Health/Fitness Instructor test, but the certification is very practical and emphasizes program design.

- ✔ **NSCA (National Strength and Conditioning Association):** This organization offers two tough certifications: the Certified Strength and Conditioning Specialist (CSCS), geared toward training athletes, and the Certified Personal Trainer (CPT), designed for trainers who work in gyms. All trainers must pass a three-part written exam that includes a video analysis of exercises. Trainers certified by the NSCA usually know a lot about weight-lifting techniques.

- ✔ **AFAA (Aerobics and Fitness Association of America):** This organization offers a variety of certifications, including Personal Trainer, Aerobics Instructor, and Weight Loss Specialist. Aerobics teachers flock to AFAA— not so with personal trainers. The Personal Trainer tests cover a wide range of topics but require less knowledge than ACSM or ACE certification tests. If the AFAA Personal Trainer is your trainer's only certification, your trainer might be an aerobics instructor trying to make the switch to personal trainer without enough education or experience.

- ✔ **NASM (National Academy of Sports Medicine):** This group offers two well-respected and practical Personal Trainer certifications. Trainers must attend a workshop and pass an exam. Trainers need a strong physiology background going into the workshop, which covers current training techniques.

- ✔ **Specialty certifications:** Some specialty fields, such as yoga and Pilates (a technique we describe in Chapter 17), do have certifications. Others, such as boxing, don't. Don't expect a boxing instructor or a country-western line dancing teacher to be certified as a trainer. But if he does have a diploma from one of the Dummies-approved organizations we list, that's a plus.

These organizations aren't the only ones that offer legitimate certifications. Many colleges and universities offer their own extensive programs, and some health clubs put their employees through rigorous training courses.

However, some organizations will certify any breathing body. These schools are sometimes advertised on late-night TV or in the back of fitness magazines (alongside the ads for legitimate schools). You definitely don't want a trainer who graduated from the National Correspondence School of Diesel Mechanics, TV Repair, and Personal Training. If you're skeptical, ask to see a copy of the actual certificate; if it's printed with a dot matrix printer and riddled with typos (we're not kidding—this happens), find somebody else.

University degrees

Most trainers don't have degrees in physiology or related fields, so don't hold it against them. But a Master's Degree is usually even better than a certification, and a fitness-related BA or BS can be a big plus. Look for degrees in exercise physiology, exercise science, physical therapy, occupational therapy, fitness management, sports medicine, physical education, and kinesiology. If the trainer has a fitness-related university degree but not an industry certification, ask if he keeps up with the latest techniques by going to conferences and seminars.

Many registered nurses and physical therapists are getting into the training business. They tend to know a lot about how muscles work; what's more, they may be able to accept insurance reimbursement if a doctor recommends training for treatment or rehab purposes.

Experience

Pick a trainer who has at least two years' experience at a club or on his own. Be sure to check references. The best way to get the lowdown on a trainer is from other clients.

Brochures

Trainers should have a brochure or packet describing their background and experience as well as their focus and philosophy. The packet also should clearly explain fees, payment schedules, and cancellation policies. Printed materials show a degree of professionalism.

An interview

To make sure that you're compatible with your trainer, talk with him at length and ask questions before hiring him. A trainer may look good on paper but may not be able to speak in complete sentences. Or you may have a personality conflict — the trainer may have too much or too little enthusiasm for your taste.

Don't judge your potential trainer by looks alone. Just because someone's a chiseled workout god doesn't mean he knows which exercises are best for you or even how to teach them to you. And a great teacher can live in a less-than-godlike body.

Liability insurance

Make sure your trainer has insurance to cover any mishaps that might be his fault. Many trainers have you sign a release, but this will not absolve them from responsibility if they do something stupid, like ask you to bench press 200 pounds during your first workout. Chances are, liability won't become an issue, but now's definitely the time to find out if the trainer is covered.

A trial session

Before you commit to several sessions with a trainer, ask for a free or discounted trial workout. Many trainers will comply in the hopes of getting a long-term client.

Trainer Fees

Fees vary from region to region, and from big cities to small towns. In Des Moines, you might pay $25 an hour; in New York, the going rate is about $75, and it's not uncommon to find trainers charging more than $100. Ask friends or call gyms to get a sense of rates in your area so that you know if a trainer's fees are way out of the ballpark.

And on the off chance that someone is charging too little, watch out. Your so-called trainer might just be a pizza delivery guy who happens to work out in his spare time and thinks he can make extra cash on the side.

If you belong to a health club, you'll probably save money by hiring a trainer through the club. Good gyms thoroughly screen their trainers and keep an eye on them. However, follow the rules we listed in the previous section for weeding out bad trainers: Don't *assume* the club hires trainers who are certified and experienced.

You also can cut costs by signing up for joint sessions with a friend. The trainer may charge slightly more than the regular hourly fee, but split two ways, your session is still a deal. You won't get quite as much attention from the trainer, but teaming up with a friend may make a session affordable. Try to pick a friend who's at the same level as you or has similar fitness goals. If you're training for a marathon and your friend is a linebacker getting ready for football season, the trainer is going to have a tough time serving both of your needs at once.

Finally, ask whether your trainer charges by the hour or by the session. Typically, sessions last 45 to 90 minutes. If you're paying by the hour and your session runs over, you may wind up paying a lot more than you expected.

Signs of a Quality Trainer

Trainers have different philosophies and use a variety of techniques. Some come from the drill-sergeant school of motivation; others prefer the cheerleading approach. Still, there are some characteristics that all trainers should share. Make sure your trainer does the following:

✔ **Evaluates your fitness and goals.**

Before anything else, your trainer should assess your current physical condition. (See Chapter 1 to learn what's included in a fitness evaluation.) Then your trainer should have a long talk with you about your expectations for the training sessions — your hopes, your dreams, and your specific goals. All of this is crucial: To really be of help to you, a trainer must know where you're starting from and where you want to go. (See Figure 15-1.)

✔ **Gives you a balanced program.**

Unless you specifically ask otherwise, your sessions should include three components: cardiovascular exercise, strength training, and flexibility exercises. Some trainers prefer that you do your cardiovascular training on your own, but if you ask they should help you design a program and keep tabs on your workout and intensity.

Many trainers skip the stretching and cool-down portions of a workout; that's a real no-no. For details about the importance of warming up, cooling down, and stretching, see Chapter 7.

✔ **Watches you closely.**

Your trainer should pay attention to your form and give you pointers throughout the session. On the other hand, you don't want a trainer who blabs incessantly.

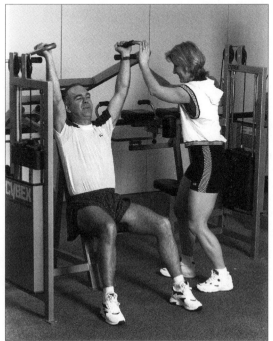

Figure 15-1:
A quality trainer should keep your fitness goals in mind.

(Photo courtesy of Dan Kron.)

Your trainer also should *spot* you — in other words, stand poised to grab the weight and give you some help if your muscles give out. For tips on the proper way to spot a friend and be spotted, see Chapter 12.

✔ **Reassesses your goals and measures your progress.**

A good trainer will retest you after the first six weeks of training and, if you've been working out consistently, every two to three months thereafter. A trainer who is really on the ball will reassess your goals even more often to keep you motivated.

✔ **Listens to you.**

If you mention that an exercise doesn't feel right, your trainer should figure out why and show you an alternative move for the same body part. There's no single exercise you absolutely must do. If you tell him you're feeling stagnant, overtrained, or underchallenged, he should alter your program.

✔ **Teaches you to be independent.**

Ironically, good trainers train themselves out of a job by teaching you how to do everything on your own. After a few months, you should be able to set the correct amount of weight, adjust the machines, use proper form, and modify your routine as needed. Of course, if you'd never exercise by yourself, you're welcome to hire your trainer for life; he'll be glad to accommodate you. Regardless, you should know how to do everything on your own. This way, if you're out of town on business or vacation, you'll be able to keep up your workouts at a hotel or local gym. And if, heaven forbid, your trainer goes on vacation, you won't have an excuse to stop working out.

✔ **Speaks English, not jargon.**

Some trainers say things like, "Your patella edema is a limiting factor in increasing your volume of oxygen uptake." Translation: "You can't run faster because you have bad knees."

If you can't understand what your trainer is saying, find someone new; you shouldn't expend extra energy just trying to figure out what the heck you're being asked to do. Trainers with *jargonitis* tend to be really insecure. Occasionally, however, a small dose of fitness verbiage is good for you; a trainer might be trying to teach you something that you actually should know, like where your hamstrings are. (By the way, if you don't know where your hamstrings are, read Chapter 11.)

How to Be a Good Client

You have the right to demand a lot from your trainer, but your trainer can also expect a certain level of courtesy, attention, and effort from you. Keep in mind the following rules of client etiquette. Some of these tips apply just to home trainers; others apply to those trainers at a gym.

✔ **Don't show up at the door in your pajamas.**

Your trainer shouldn't have to serve as your alarm clock or wait a half hour for you to get your act together. Like you, the trainer has a schedule, and time is money. If you're late getting started, the trainer has every right to cut your session short or charge you extra.

✔ **Don't answer the phone.**

This just wastes the trainer's time and distracts you from your workout. Also, if you have kids at home, make sure that someone is watching them. Your trainer won't be happy if your five-year-old runs into the room screaming, "Mommy! Mommy! My Power Ranger broke!"

✔ **Schedule in advance.**

You'll have a very happy trainer if you schedule a month in advance. At the very least, don't call in the morning and ask for a session that afternoon if you can help it.

✔ **Speak up.**

Just because you've hired a trainer does not mean you've lost the power of speech. If you don't understand why you're doing something, ask. If something doesn't feel right, say so. Your trainer isn't a mindreader.

One woman we know severely pulled her inner-thigh muscles because a trainer went overboard on a stretch. Afterward, she said she felt pain for nearly a minute before she heard a loud pop. Why didn't she say anything? Because she didn't want to question the trainer. Granted, the trainer should have paid better attention, but he couldn't have been expected to know how the woman felt.

✔ **Keep the relationship professional.**

Your trainer is not your therapist. Inevitably, you'll get into personal stuff; after all, this is your *personal* trainer. But don't take your bad day out on your trainer and don't expect your trainer to fix your life. And never make a pass at your trainer.

Chapter 16

Gym 101: The Unwritten Rules

- -

In This Chapter

▶ Your first workout with a trainer

▶ Going it alone in the gym

▶ Packing the perfect gym bag

▶ Health club etiquette: the unwritten rules

- -

*Y*ou won't find any technical stuff in this chapter. It's all about how to feel comfortable at a health club — how to get through your first workout, what to wear, what to bring, and how to act when you can't figure out how to operate the Gravitron.

Your First Real Workout

Take advantage of the free training session that most gyms offer. This session is separate from your free fitness evaluation described in Chapter 1. During this complimentary session, the trainer should set you up on a program, give you the lay of the land, and show you how to work the fancy gizmos. (For tips on making sure that your trainer has a clue, see Chapter 15.)

But even with the guidance of a trainer, your first session may be a little awkward. Our friend Jean Thornton from Alabama says she just had to swallow her pride while trying out the weight machines for the first time. "Here was this cute, young trainer helping me climb onto the hamstring machine," she remembers. "I felt like a 40-year-old woman trying to get on a horse for the first time. I'm lying on the bench with my butt in the air, and the trainer's saying, 'Keep your butt down.' And I'm saying, 'That's as far down as it goes. It's just big.'"

Having a good sense of humor can get you through a first workout session without any ego damage. Here are a few other tips for your first workout with a trainer:

- ✔ **Sign up for a session during off-peak hours.** Gyms usually are busiest from 7 a.m. to 9 a.m., 12 p.m. to 2 p.m., and 5 p.m. to 7 p.m. You might feel more relaxed if other members aren't waiting to use the machines.

- ✔ **Wear comfortable clothes.** Go for maximum comfort and minimum embarrassment. Don't wear something that exposes you to the world when you climb on some strange contraption. You might end up spreading your legs in front of 30 strangers, none of whom are your gynecologist or proctologist. Don't wear anything so baggy that it impedes your movement or can possibly get caught in some moving part. See the sidebar, "The truth about plastic exercise suits," later in this chapter for more information about what to wear.

- ✔ **Bring a water bottle.** Every gym has a drinking fountain, but you'll drink a lot more if you carry a bottle with you. (In Chapter 4, we explain why drinking water is so important.)

- ✔ **Bring a good attitude.** Working out isn't like getting your appendix removed. If you start to feel intimidated or overwhelmed, remind yourself why you're at the gym.

- ✔ **Bring a towel.** If you have any interest in making friends at the gym, wipe the sweat off yourself and the machines.

- ✔ **Ask questions, take notes, and draw pictures.** During your first session, your trainer will fill out a card listing each exercise in your program, how much weight to lift, and how many sets and reps to do. (See Figure 16-1.) But if you supplement this information with your own notes and pictures, remembering what to do when you work out alone will be easier. For example, if your trainer writes "lat pulldown," you can add, "pull bar down to chest; strengthens back muscles; adjust seat to second notch." Don't be afraid to ask lots of questions.

- ✔ **Don't expect to absorb everything your trainer tells you on the first day.** Every time you work out, you'll pick up more information, such as how to adjust each machine and how to stretch each muscle group. You can make things easier on yourself by scheduling a second trainer appointment to reinforce what you learned on the first go around. Some gyms charge for a second appointment; some don't. If you bring up the issue when you join the gym, some clubs will throw in a few extra training sessions.

- ✔ **Don't feel embarrassed if you can't lift much weight.** Hey, you're a beginner. The trainer doesn't expect you to be Arnold Schwarzenegger. One friend of ours lost any such illusions during his first session with a trainer. "I sat down on this machine and pulled the handles back, and the trainer said, 'Do you feel that?' I said, 'Yeah, it's really pulling on my

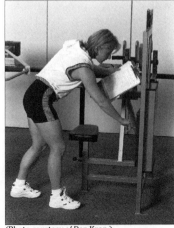

Figure 16-1:
Record the details of each session on a workout card.

(Photo courtesy of Dan Kron.)

muscles.' Then the trainer said, 'Oh, I forgot to put the weight on.'" When stuff like that happens, just laugh and realize that it doesn't take much time to get stronger. (See Chapter 10 for an explanation of just how long it takes.)

✔ **Don't overdo it.** If you push too hard, you'll feel so sore that you won't want to come back. Don't try to show the trainer how tough you are.

The morning after your first few workouts, you should wake up feeling a little achy and tender — but not so sore that you can't stand upright. The discomfort usually is at its worst about 48 hours after your workout — a phenomenon known as *Delayed Onset Muscle Soreness.*

Delayed Onset Muscle Soreness is caused by microscopic rips in the muscles that you exercise. These rips fill up with fluids and waste products, and until the muscles recover, you're going to be in a little pain. The good news is that once the muscles repair themselves, they're stronger and harder to rip. So after a few weeks of working out, you won't get really sore except after especially tough workouts.

Braving the Gym Alone

"When I went to the gym by myself — that's when it was really scary," recalls Jean Thornton. "I told myself, 'Wait a minute. Take a deep breath. You just have to close your eyes and jump off that diving board.'" Here are strategies for getting comfortable in the gym once you've weaned yourself from your trainer:

✓ **Take a friend.** Going to the gym with a buddy can make you feel more comfortable and less self-conscious. You two can pretend to discuss the stock market while you figure out how to start up the stairclimber.

✓ **Go at off-peak hours.** No one will be breathing down your neck to use a machine, and you'll have more attention from the staff if you need some reminders. If you can't come during off-peak hours, choose the morning because most gyms aren't as packed as they are in the evening, and the morning crowds tend to be fairly regular. You'll get to know other faces, and they'll get to know yours.

Monday is always the busiest day in any gym — everyone's trying to atone for sins they may have committed over the weekend, like eating too many Ding Dongs. Things tail off by Thursday or Friday (but don't wait until then to work out).

✓ **Wear headphones.** You don't even need to turn your headphones on. Either way, they create personal space. Nobody will bother you — if that's what you want. Just be careful not to turn the music up too loud, especially during high-impact exercises such as running on the treadmill. Extremely loud music can cause hearing damage. Also, make sure your headphone wires don't get caught in any weight machines.

✓ **Make friends.** Knowing other members can give you more encouragement. One good way to meet someone is to ask for a *spot*. (In other words, ask somebody to assist you while you do a weight-lifting exercise. Smile and look approachable; maybe someone will ask you to spot *them*. For instructions on how to spot and be spotted, see Chapter 12.)

In general, when you talk to people at the gym, stick to topics related to working out. For instance, ask them if they're done using a particular machine or bench. Ask how to do a certain exercise. The worst approach is to go up to people in the locker room when they're naked, stick your hand out, and say, "HimynameisMoreySchmulowitz. Howtheheckareya?"

✓ **Don't worry about people glaring at you.** Despite what you might think, the other members *aren't* staring at you. Most people are far too absorbed in their own workout to pay attention to anyone else.

Packing the Perfect Gym Bag

You'll feel a lot more comfortable at the gym if you come prepared. Using 17 paper towels to dry yourself off after a shower is no fun. Some gyms provide towels, cosmetics — even workout clothes. Check with your gym so you don't overpack (see Figure 16-2). Here's a list of what you typically need to bring:

✔ membership card

✔ a water bottle

✔ a small towel to wipe sweat off the machines

✔ a large towel for the shower

✔ gym clothes: shoes, socks, shorts, tights, sweats, T-shirt, leotard, sports bra, or jock

✔ plastic bag for wet, dirty clothes

✔ toiletries: soap, shampoo, deodorant, and foot deodorant for sneakers

✔ sweat band, ponytail holder, or whatever you need to keep sweat from dripping into your eyes

✔ shower sandals

✔ postworkout snack, especially if you have a long drive home. Eat within an hour of finishing your workout. See Chapter 4 for snack ideas.

The truth about plastic exercise suits

Contrary to fitness folklore, you cannot sweat off your fat by wearing plastic workout suits or 20 layers of thermal underwear. So, do not show up at the gym dressed to go dog sledding in Siberia. You will only lose water — not fat — and the water is simply replaced next time you drink. Clothing that traps your body heat and sweat can cause dehydration, electrolyte imbalances, blood poisoning, and, in extreme cases, death.

Remarkably, you still see these products advertised in catalogs. One vinyl jumpsuit is touted as "the perfect exercise aid to rid the body of excess water and unwanted inches using natural body heat from physical exertion." First of all,

"excess water" is like excess money; there's no such thing. You may have more water than you need at a particular time. But sooner or later (usually sooner, if you're working out), your body ends up excreting that water.

The same company claims that its vinyl shorts "provide a constant, moist warmth for the muscles, helping to lessen the chance of strains and cramps." This ad is misleading, too. Wearing vinyl workout clothes can lead to dehydration, which can *cause* cramps, not prevent them. Besides, exercising in vinyl clothing makes you feel like you're wearing Saran Wrap.

The following items aren't essential, but they can make your workouts more fun or comfortable.

- ✔ **Radio/tape player with headphones, a good workout tape, and extra batteries:** Listening to music can make a half hour on the treadmill fly by. In fact, one recent study showed that women who exercised to music lasted 25 percent longer than those who exercised in silence. The extra batteries are key; we can't count the times we've shown up at the gym with our tape player only to find that the batteries are dead. You might also want to bring magazines or a newspaper to read while you work out on the aerobic machines. For other ideas of how to combat boredom while you work out, see Chapter 8.

- ✔ **Heart rate monitor:** This device instantly lets you know how fast your heart is beating. Monitoring your heart rate (a.k.a., your *pulse*) lets you know if you're pushing your body too hard, or if you're not pushing hard enough. For details about how and why to use a monitor, see Chapter 5.

- ✔ **Weight-lifting gloves:** These are special gloves with padded palms and cut-off finger holes. They prevent your hands from getting blistered and callused, and they enable you to grip the weights better.

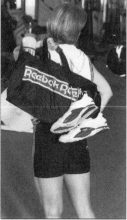

Figure 16-2:
Never leave home without it: the perfect gym bag.

(Photo courtesy of Dan Kron.)

Health Club Etiquette: The Unwritten Rules

Every type of club has its own unwritten customs, like the secret handshake you and your buddies used back in fourth grade. Or the secret code word that Howard Cunningham used to get into the Leopard Lodge on TV's "Happy Days." Health clubs don't have secret code words, of course, but you'll feel more at home if you learn a few of the unwritten rules. Here are some tips on how to act in certain situations.

✔ **If someone's using the weight machine that you want . . .**

. . . ask whether you can *work in.* That's a term for alternating sets with another person. Asking to work in is perfectly legitimate; no one has the right to camp out at one weight machine for a half hour.

Working in with someone is convenient if all you have to do is switch the pin in the weight stack. But it's awkward if you have to readjust the seat or add or subtract weight plates. In those cases, it's more polite to wait until the person is done.

✔ **If someone is standing over your shoulder waiting to use the machine that you're on . . .**

. . . kindly ask that person to work in with *you.* Or tell the person how much longer you plan to use the machine. Say something like, "This is my last set. Then it's all yours."

✔ **If you need help adjusting a machine or you forgot how to use it . . .**

. . . turn to a staffer or a gym member with a kind face and say, "I'm new here. Can you help me?"

✔ **If someone's doing an exercise that you want to learn . . .**

. . . find an appropriate break in that person's workout and ask him to show you the exercise. Most people are happy to help — in fact, they are flattered that you asked.

✔ **If you aren't 100 percent sure that you can safely complete your repetitions . . .**

. . . ask someone to spot you.

If you're embarrassed to ask for a spot, think about a guy named Anthony Clark, whose photo hangs on the wall at Dave's Power Palace, a gym in Carson City, Nevada. Clark lost control while doing an exercise called the *squat.* He dumped his barbell forward, and the barbell landed on the weight rack — with Clark's neck sandwiched in between. Fortunately, Clark's two spotters came to the rescue, and he managed to survive unscathed. Chances are, this isn't going to happen to you; after all, the guy *was* squatting 992 pounds. But the point is, be careful out there.

✔ **If someone's hitting on you and the feeling isn't mutual . . .**

. . . heck, we don't know. You're on your own here.

Major no-nos

- ✔ **Don't forget your towel.** No one likes to sit down in a pool of sweat. Always wipe off your equipment after you're finished.

- ✔ **Don't fill up your entire water bottle when someone else is waiting for the drinking fountain.** Let the other guy get his drink and then resume filling up your bottle.

- ✔ **Don't grunt.** You might as well announce over the loudspeaker, "Hey, everyone, look over here! I'm lifting more weight than I can handle!"

- ✔ **Don't leave your dumbbells on the floor.** Always put weights back on the rack and in the right order. Don't stick the 15-pound dumbbells where the 10-pounders are supposed to go.

- ✔ **Don't sit on a machine or bench that you're not actually using.**

- ✔ **Don't spit or deposit gum in the water fountain.** Many people don't quite grasp this concept.

- ✔ **Don't violate anyone else's personal space.** If someone seems to be jamming through a workout, that's not the time to tap him on the shoulder and ask his opinion on school prayer. This rule applies to the locker room, too.

Locker room rules

Don't do anything you wouldn't do in your own bathroom. You're sharing this space with a lot of other people, so have some consideration.

- ✔ Don't take a marathon shower if people are waiting.

- ✔ Don't leave hair clogging the drain and don't leave empty bottles of shampoo in the stall.

- ✔ Don't use more than one locker.

- ✔ Don't hog the mirror or the blow dryer.

- ✔ Don't shake baby powder all over the floor.

- ✔ Limit the number of towels you use, especially during busy hours, when the club is likely to run out.

Chapter 17

Picking an Exercise Class

*E*xercise classes have made an evolutionary leap since the early 80s. Back then, *aerobics* meant two hours of sadistic military drills — and a steady stream of casualties from the ultra-deep knee bends, jerky moves, and high kicks considered criminal today. Classes are better now because most health clubs and aerobics studios require the instructors to have experience and certification. Many clubs audition teachers, do regular evaluations, and pay attention to participant feedback.

These days, you also have a lot more choices than you used to (see Figure 17-1). Bored with low-impact aerobics? Try Short Circuit, Gospel Aerobics, or The Funky Diva Workout. Classes also have become more equipment-oriented, using dumbbells, tubes, balls, steps, slides, jump ropes — even stationary bikes.

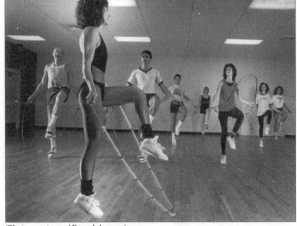

(Photo courtesy of Dean Johnson.)

This chapter covers the classes you're most likely to find at clubs and studios. For each class, we tell you how much you'll sweat, what you'll gain, and how you'll fare if you're a klutz. Plus, you'll learn how to get the most out of a class while suffering the least amount of embarrassment.

Why Take a Class?

Classes are suited to a certain kind of personality. You'll love 'em if you feed off group energy or if you enjoy following someone else's lead. But if you treat exercise as down time you may prefer to exercise on your own.

Beginners will find classes especially valuable. With luck, you'll get an instructor who can teach you a few things about exercise, like how to take your pulse properly and how to use good form when you lift a dumbbell. You'll also develop a certain body awareness that you might not learn from walking on the treadmill or pumping weights. You'll probably make friends, too.

Classes are also a great way to learn a new skill. If you want to buy a step for your home, you can get the moves down in a class. Let the teacher correct you so that you know what to watch for when you do the workout alone in your living room. You can supplement this learning process with exercise videos.

Getting Through When You Haven't a Clue

Make life easier for yourself: Choose classes with the words *beginner* or *basic* in the title. You'll get a much different impression of step aerobics from a slower, simplified beginner class than if you accidentally wander into an advanced class and hear, "OK, we're going to U-turn right, U-turn left, electric slide four times, then step, hop, turn, and repeat. Got it? Let's go!"

Before the class starts, tell the teacher you're a novice. A good instructor will keep an eye on you and correct your mistakes without making you feel like an idiot. If you don't mind the spotlight, stand in the front — the instructor will be more likely to notice and correct you. If you're shy and prefer to make your mistakes more privately, stand in the back or get lost in the middle. Throughout the class, keep your eye on the teacher rather than a fellow student. And don't compete with anyone. This isn't the time to give your ego a workout.

If you get tired, just march in place. Don't stop cold and walk out in the middle of a class — you risk nausea or even fainting. But don't be afraid to bail out if the instructor is a lemon. Always bring a water bottle to class — you'll drink more often, and you'll avoid the long lines at the drinking fountain.

Finally, come back for more, even if the class leaves you feeling like a clod. Skills and fitness take time to develop. You'll feel pretty darn good when you master a class that used to wipe you out.

What to Expect from Your Instructor

Try to watch a few classes before you take one. A good instructor has the class moving in unison and right on cue, even if the steps are complicated. If everyone's bumping into each other or several people have stopped completely and are staring off into space, look for another class. No matter what type of class you're taking, your teacher should . . .

- ✔ . . . ask questions at the beginning of the class, such as "Any newcomers?" "Anyone with an injury I need to know about?" "Is there anyone here who's never tried step before?"

- ✔ . . . include a warm-up and a cool-down period. The cool-down should be followed by stretching exercises.

- ✔ . . . give clear instructions so you always know where you are and what's coming next. Your instructor might say, "Two steps right," and then point right with two fingers.

✔ . . . give you plenty of information on technique — but not so much that you feel overwhelmed.

✔ . . . speak in plain language. The really obnoxious instructors say things like "plantar flex at your ankle joint" — rather than "point your foot." However, a good teacher should educate you. It's perfectly okay for an instructor to say, "Feel this move in your quadriceps."

✔ . . . watch the class rather than gaze at himself in the mirror. He should face the students at least some of the time and occasionally walk around adjusting everyone's form.

✔ . . . do a pulse or intensity check during the toughest part of the workout. This goes for toning and strength classes, too, even if the check is as minimal as asking, "How's everyone doing?"

✔ . . . make the class fun. This isn't boot camp. Don't take your classes so seriously that they become a chore.

✔ . . . have an education. If your instructor is certified by one of the major national fitness organizations, that's a definite plus. Dummies-approved certifications for aerobics instructors include several from the Aerobics and Fitness Association of America (AFAA), the Aerobics Instructor from the American Council on Exercise (ACE), and the Exercise Leader from the American College of Sports Medicine (ACSM).

The certifications for aerobics instructors usually require less knowledge of physiology than personal training certifications, but they're more geared toward the skills you need to lead a group, such as motivation and modifying exercises for different levels. Most specialty fields, such as boxing and tai chi, don't have certifications. However, some of the teachers have aerobic instructor certifications to supplement their specialty.

A Word about Cost

Class fees vary widely. Some health club memberships include unlimited classes. Aerobics studios charge $3 to $20 per class, usually more for the specialty classes we describe later in this chapter. At many clubs and studios, you can buy a package of classes — say, 10 at once — but find out if you must use up the package by a certain date. Another option is to buy a month's worth of unlimited class memberships. Some clubs will let you try out a class for free.

Popular Classes

Two classes that have the same name may be completely different. One "body sculpting" class might use dumbbells; another might use rubber exercise tubes. And, of course, no two teachers have the exact same style. Still, every body sculpting class has a number of common characteristics. The same goes for other types of classes. Here's a rundown of the most common classes around, roughly in order of their popularity.

Step aerobics

What it is: A choreographed routine of stepping up and down on a rectangular, square, or circular platform (see Figure 17-2). Many classes combine step aerobics with body sculpting, jumping rope, sliding, or funk aerobics.

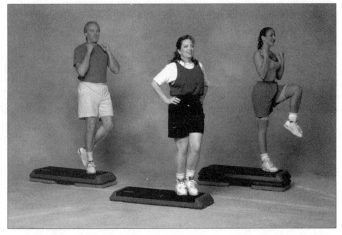

Figure 17-2:
Step aerobics strengthens your heart and tones your tush.

What it does for you: Gets your heart and lungs in shape and tones your tush. Step aerobics is a terrific cross-training activity for runners, cyclists, and walkers.

The exhaustion factor: Depends on the choreography, the pace, and the height of your step. In general, the more complex the choreography and the higher your step, the tougher the workout.

Never use a platform so high that your knee is higher than your hip when you step up. In some classes you hold weights while you step. The jury is still out on whether this is effective or even safe, but as long as you keep the weights light (say, 3 pounds or less), using them probably won't kill you.

The coordination factor: High. Even basic classes can confound the choreographically challenged. Funk Step requires major amounts of coordination — some instructors make everything so dancy that you feel like you're auditioning for a Broadway musical. Clubs are trying to attract the nonaerobics crowd with classes like Stepping for Athletes. (Translation: This is a class for people, like the authors of this book, who are in decent shape but have two left feet.)

Who'll dig it: Most everyone. Step classes draw a lot more men than do regular aerobic classes. And women like step because it's such a great butt toner. However, if you have back, knee, or ankle problems, you might be better off with another type of class — or at least, keep the platform very low.

What to wear: A good pair of aerobics or walking shoes with extra cushioning at the ball of the foot and some ankle support (not as much as basketball sneakers). Don't wear running shoes. You might stumble if the waffle pattern on the bottom of the shoe catches on the top of the platform.

Signs of a sharp instructor: Good instructors will ask if anyone is new to step or has any back, knee, or ankle problems. They'll accomodate newcomers by going over the basics, such as how to place your foot on the platform. Instructors should also alert you before every *transition* — step jargon for any type of change in the routine (such as changing directions). In addition, instructors should make sure that you don't lead with the same foot for more than a minute or two. The music shouldn't be so fast that you have to rush your movements to keep up. Instructors should include calf stretches at the end of the class.

Tips for first-timers: No matter how fit you are, always start with the lowest step — don't put *any* risers underneath. Don't feel intimidated if the guy next to you looks like he's standing on a coffee table. Also, forget about the arm movements and concentrate on the footwork, if you need to. When step workouts start to feel easy, consider adding a riser.

High/low-impact aerobics

What it is: A traditional dance-inspired routine. With low-impact, you always have one foot on the floor — you don't do any jumping or hopping. High-impact moves at a slower pace, but you jump around a lot. High/low combines the two types of routines.

What it does for you: Gets you aerobically fit.

The exhaustion factor: Depends on the class. Classes are too varied to make generalizations.

The coordination factor: Moderate to high, especially if you're a new exerciser or if your parents didn't spring for eight years of tap, ballet, and jazz.

Who'll dig it: Anyone who wants to work out in a group without using any equipment.

Signs of a sharp instructor: Instructors should spell out the terminology, rather than just say, "grapevine left, grapevine right."

Tips for first-timers: Shop around for a teacher you like who plays music you can tolerate. Music can be a great motivator or a major turn-off.

Body Sculpting

What it is: A nonaerobic, muscle-toning class. Most sculpting classes use weight bars, exercise bands, or dumbbells, or a combination of these gadgets. You perform traditional weight-training moves in a class setting.

What it does for you: Gives you strength and muscle tone and lowers your risk of bone loss. For details on the hazards of bone loss, see Chapter 10.

The exhaustion factor: Depends on the instructor, the level of class you're taking, and how much experience you have with strength training. Prepare to be sore if you're a novice or if you usually do different exercises.

The coordination factor: Low. Anyone can do this, although it might take a few sessions to learn proper form.

Who'll dig it: Anyone who wants to firm up. Body sculpting is great if you want to learn the fundamentals before you venture into the gym on your own. We also recommend body sculpting for people who won't lift weights unless they are in a class.

Signs of a sharp instructor: Instructors should tell you to use moderately heavy weights so that you don't do much more than 15 reps per set. (We define *reps* and *sets* in Chapter 13.) Watch out for instructors who do dozens of repetitions with light weights: You're not going to build much strength or tone that way. The instructor should correct your form and remind you where you should feel the exercise. Watch for a warm up and cool down, too. Some instructors skimp on these essential workout components.

Tips for first-timers: Prepare yourself for muscle soreness the day or two after your workout. If you want to focus on a particular part of your body, look for a specialty class like Bodacious Butt or Ab-solutely Fabulous.

Circuit

What it is: A fast-paced class in which you do one exercise for 30 seconds to 5 minutes and then move on to another exercise. It's like a game of musical chairs: Everyone begins at a station, and when the instructor yells "Time!" everyone moves to the next free station. Some classes alternate an aerobic activity (like stepping or stationary cycling) with a muscle-strengthening activity (like using weight machines). Others focus exclusively on muscle toning or aerobic exercise.

What it does for you: Increases your strength and aerobic fitness and burns lots of calories. However, you don't get the same level of conditioning as you would from doing your aerobics and strength training separately. If you take circuit classes, aim to get in an additional 20 minutes of straight aerobic exercise at least three days a week.

The exhaustion factor: Moderate. Circuit training tends to be intense, but it's completely adaptable to the individual. Beginners use less weight and perform simpler moves than more experienced exercisers, but everyone gets a good workout.

The coordination factor: Low. Nothing to worry about.

Who'll dig it: Anyone looking for a good sweat to shake them out of a training plateau. Circuit classes also are popular among busy people who want to combine a strength and aerobic routine into one workout. Anyone who wants a really fun and fast-paced workout will like circuit classes.

Signs of a sharp instructor: Good instructors are aware of each class member's level and modify the moves accordingly. Even though you're moving quickly from station to station, the instructor still needs to focus on proper technique. Look for no more than a one-minute rest between stations. Expect a heart rate check 12 to 20 minutes into the main workout. (Checking your heart rate, or *pulse,* lets you know if you're pushing yourself too hard or if you're slacking off. Chapter 5 explains how to check your heart rate.)

Tips for first-timers: Pay attention to how you feel. Many people are surprised at how challenging circuit work can be.

Funk and Hip-Hop

What it is: An aerobic routine set to funky music with choreography borrowed from club dance moves. Classes range from simple moves with a little attitude thrown in, to what seems like a tryout for an MTV funk-a-thon. At many urban clubs, you'll find funk aerobics, hip-hop step, and even funk 'n slide classes.

What it does for you: Develops heart and lung power and really improves your coordination and agility. You teach your body to move in complex ways and use muscles that you didn't know you had.

The exhaustion factor: Depends on the difficulty level of the class. Some hip hop classes are geared toward beginners. Others expect you to be in awesome shape.

The coordination factor: High. If you're a complete exercise dysfunctional, you'll have a tough time keeping up. Aerobically, you may not be all that challenged, but you'll spend a good deal of the class untangling your feet.

Who'll dig it: Anyone with a dance background or anyone who likes hip-hop music. If you're a Fleetwood Mac fan, you may want to pass.

What to wear: You can wear your typical sweats and T-shirt, but don't be surprised if you're the only one. Funk classes tend to have their own style of dressing: high top sneakers, off-the-shoulder tops, baggy shorts, sexy bras, oversized socks.

Signs of a sharp instructor: Good instructors break down complicated moves into a series of smaller ones before putting them all together. They also show you a variety of interpretations to each move and do the moves more slowly and with less attitude when the class is first learning.

Tips for first-timers: If you don't possess the funk gene, definitely take a beginner class and scope out the class first. More than in any other class, novices tend to get left in the dust, but a really good instructor will give enough instruction so everyone can stay together.

Yoga

What it is: A series of poses designed to improve flexibility and strength and to perfect breathing techniques. So many types of yoga exist that classes vary widely. Some classes have a spiritual aspect to them; the instructor may even light incense and have the class do a chant. Other classes take a more practical approach. Some classes combine yoga with aerobic moves.

What it does for you: Improves your flexibility and posture and calms your frazzled nerves. Yoga also teaches you how to breath properly, using your diaphragm rather than just sucking in air through your nose and mouth.

The exhaustion factor: Depends on your flexibility and your ability to concentrate — and, of course, on the class. Most poses can be modified for all different levels, so virtually anyone can do yoga.

The coordination factor: Moderate. If you're a novice, you might have trouble moving from one position directly into another. But this shouldn't stop anyone from trying.

Who'll dig it: People who are already flexible are natural at yoga; however, the people who aren't naturally flexible are the ones who *need* yoga. If you don't stretch on your own or don't know how to stretch well, yoga is an excellent way to work on flexibility. It's also great for type-A exercisers or anyone stressed out by life.

What to wear: Comfortable clothing and clean socks with no holes because you're not going to be wearing your sneakers. You can do yoga in socks or in your bare feet, although some studios don't allow bare feet. Some people prefer to wear leotards or Lycra so that the teacher can easily see if they are posing correctly.

Signs of a sharp instructor: Good instructors modify the poses for all levels of flexibility, and they offer hands-on repositioning. You're better off with a teacher who specializes in yoga (and has some yoga credentials) than with someone who's just filling time between step classes.

Tips for first-timers: Decide what you want out of yoga, then ask around for the type of class that fits your profile. Classes are often named descriptively — Yoga for Runners or Relaxation Yoga — to help you make choices.

Don't compare yourself to anyone else. Just because the 80-year-old woman next to you can transform herself into a pretzel doesn't mean that you should be able to as well. Expect to be sore for a day or two after the class.

Slide

What it is: With nylon booties over your shoes, you glide side-to-side on a slick board that's about five feet long with rubber bumpers on each end. Classes usually add a variety of arm movements and turns for fun and an extra challenge.

What it does for you: Gives you a great aerobic workout if you can slide continuously for more than 10 minutes. Sliding also emphasizes the often-neglected inner- and outer-thigh muscles. People with ankle problems may experience too much pounding from the push offs.

The exhaustion factor: Very high. Sliding looks effortless; it's not. Some classes alternate a few minutes of sliding with other activities, like step, low-impact aerobics, or marching in place.

The coordination factor: Moderate. Most people catch on to the basic side-to-side after about five minutes.

Who'll dig it: Women like sliding because it tones the hips and thighs, men tend to like it because they don't have to dance. Either you'll feel like an Olympic speed skater or Tom Cruise sliding across the floor in *Risky Business* — or you'll feel like a dork sliding across the kitchen in slippers.

What to wear: Regular workout clothing and shoes — the class will supply the nylon booties. Some booties are more slippery than others. Don't wear running shoes with a waffled pattern on the sole; even when you have booties on, they increase drag along the slide.

Signs of a sharp instructor: Good instructors always start with technique reminders and then do a warm-up *off* the slide that includes side-to-side movements. They explain how to adjust your slide: shorter for the uninitiated and longer for those more skilled and fit. Look for ankle and shin stretches at the end, too.

Tips for first-timers: For more power, swing your arms in opposition to your legs. When you reach a bumper, immediately push off with your inside leg.

Boxing

What it is: A class that takes a boxer's training and boils it down into layman's terms. You'll do some or all of the following: jumping rope, shadow boxing, hitting a bag, sparring with your instructor, muscle conditioning, circuit training, and boxing-style footwork.

What it does for you: Develops anaerobic and aerobic fitness — in other words, power and staying power. (For definitions of aerobic and anaerobic, see Chapter 5.) Boxing also improves your coordination, agility, and balance. Most classes build muscle strength, too.

The exhaustion factor: Very high. Boxers are reputed to be among the best conditioned athletes. After one of these classes, you'll know why. You don't understand just how long two minutes is until you've gone a round with a heavy bag. Most classes are geared toward advanced exercisers, although some clubs offer beginner and multilevel classes, too.

The coordination factor: High. The punching drills require some fancy footwork. So does jumping rope, especially if you haven't done it since fifth grade.

Who'll dig it: Anyone looking for a killer workout with plenty of variety, or anyone who hates his boss.

What to wear: The usual aerobic clothing will do, although some funk aerobics clothing crosses over into the boxing classes. High-top aerobics shoes are better than running and walking shoes. Cross trainers are fine. The teacher will supply boxing gloves.

Signs of a sharp instructor: We recommend classes taught by ex-boxers rather than aerobics teachers, but there are a few caveats. Few ex-boxers have much experience training mere mortals, and they may not be acquainted with standard exercise practices. Many ex-boxers force you through moves that are controversial, such as full sit-ups. The trade off is, they'll teach you real boxing skills and tell great stories about their days in the ring. If possible, look for a class taught by a team: a certified instructor and a boxer.

Tips for first-timers: Pay attention to how you feel. If a lot of the moves are bone crunching or the exact opposite of what other instructors have told you not to do, skip the moves or modify them. Don't give up. Boxing will get easier.

Water aerobics and water running

What it is: Water aerobics classes do traditional aerobics moves in waist-to-neck-high water. You might also come across a water running class in which you wear a flotation vest and run in deep water, sometimes while tethered to the side of the pool.

What it does for you: Water aerobics gives you moderate aerobic fitness. Water running — typically a tougher workout than water aerobics — is a good way to keep from losing too much aerobic ground during an injury or lay-off, but it won't keep you quite as sharp as land workouts will.

The exhaustion factor: Low. Most people won't find water aerobics as hard as land-based aerobics. Although water is thicker and therefore harder to pull through than air, water really is a gentler medium. Still, we recommend an occasional water workout to get you off your feet and to give your muscles a balanced workout. Running on land primarily uses your hamstrings (rear thigh muscles), but in the water, your quadriceps (front thigh muscles) pull an equal amount of weight because your legs encounter resistance no matter what direction they're moving.

The coordination factor: Low. You're forced to move so slowly that you have time to think about each move.

Who'll dig it: Anyone who likes the water, has injuries, or is in physical rehab. Water aerobics is a terrific cross-training activity for runners, cyclists, and maniac aerobicizers. Water aerobics is also great for older people and people with multiple sclerosis, osteoporosis, or other degenerative diseases because moving through the water is much easier on your body.

What to wear: A bathing suit that doesn't creep up your rear end. Wear a pair of old sneakers or special aqua exercise shoes so that you don't scrape your feet on the bottom. Shoes will add more resistance to your workout.

Signs of a sharp instructor: Certification is a definite plus, but water certification programs are few and far between. A good certification program is offered by the United States Water Fitness Association.

Safety should be the first priority in any class. A good instructor will identify nonswimmers and insist they wear a life vest at all times during water aerobics. In water *running*, all class members — even experienced swimmers — wear a flotation vest.

Tips for first-timers: Choosing the right class is essential. You don't want to dive in with a group of 90-year-olds with limited mobility unless, of course, you are one. If you're trying to come back from an injury, look for classes with names like Rehab for Runners. Check with the doctor treating your injury to make sure you have the okay to take a class. Also, realize that your target zone is about 10 beats lower in the water than on land. (We define target zone in Chapter 5.)

Specialty Classes

New types of classes pop up all the time. Some of them require specialized equipment or an instructor with specialized training. Here's a look at some classes that are becoming popular.

Line dancing or country-robics

You do those fun dance moves popularized in country-western bars, where everyone on the dance floor seems to move in perfect syncronicity. In beginning line dancing classes, you learn the moves; in advanced classes, you're supposed to know what you're doing and use the instructor only as a guide. If you're not a lonely trucker whose mama just got out of prison — or at least a country music fan — you might prefer City Jam, Gospel Aerobics, or the Disco Flashback workout.

Pilates

Pilates is a technique invented at the turn of the 20th century by a German named Joseph Pilates (pronounced Pi-LAH-tees). Originally designed to give dancers strength without bulk, Pilates is perfect for anyone who wants to improve posture, strength, flexibility, and body awareness. Some classes are done on a floor mat. Other classes are taught on a group of medieval looking machines, including one called the Reformer that resembles a small bed frame.

Pilates is far more intense than it looks and requires concentration. Pilates is a good wake-up call for weight lifters and aerobicizers: You really have to think about what you're doing — you can't just go through the motions, like many people do at the gym. Also, whereas gym-type strength machines tend to target a single muscle group or area of the body, every Pilates exercise requires control of your entire body, particularly your abdominal and butt muscles.

Exercise ball

Classes also go by the name of Axling, Spiraling, the Well Rounded Workout, Physioball, and Resist-a-ball. You exercise with an oversized ball not unlike a beach ball. Some classes emphasize stretching and flexibility, whereas others focus on balance and coordination. For instance, you might roll over the top of the ball and into a push-up position. The ball is good for abdominal and leg work and for rehabilitating lower back injuries. Ball classes are very creative, but they're not for everyone. Some people are bored by the lack of sweat.

Tai chi

This ancient form of Chinese stress management is the perfect antidote to all the tension in your life. The moves are done in slow motion, as if you're under water. The emphasis is moving your "ball" of *chi* or energy. Your goal is to keep your body loose and relaxed. Martial arts classes are drawing bigger crowds now that instructors are adding music and choreography.

Spinning

You pedal a stationary bike while the instructor talks you through a visualization of an outdoor workout. ("You're going up a long hill now — you can't see the top yet. . . .") During the class you vary your pace, sometimes pedaling as fast as you can, other times cranking up the tension and pedaling slowly from a standing position. Spinning is an intense workout — it's popular among people who want to be pushed very hard. Spinning certification programs are now offered by some clubs and by Schwinn, the company that owns the rights to the name. (See Figure 17-3.)

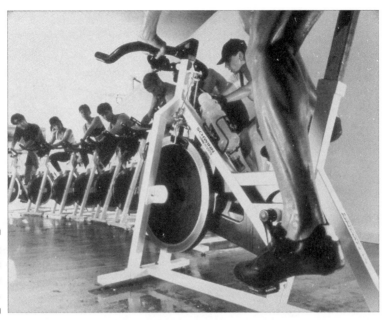

Figure 17-3:
Spinning is
an intense
workout.

Part V
Exercising at Home

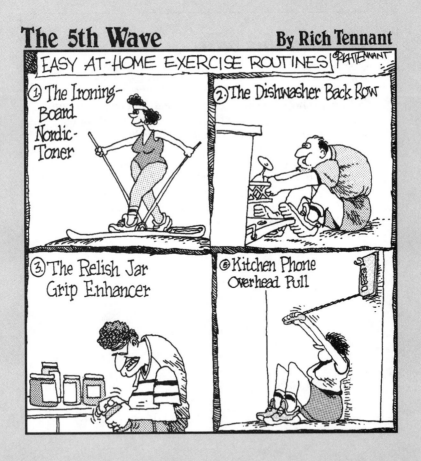

The 5th Wave   By Rich Tennant

EASY AT-HOME EXERCISE ROUTINES

① The Ironing-Board Nordic-Toner

② The Dishwasher Back Row

③ The Relish Jar Grip Enhancer

④ Kitchen Phone Overhead Pull

In this part . . .

You learn how to create the best home gym for your budget and your goals. Chapter 18 covers the basics: where to shop, how to get a good deal, and where to put your equipment so you'll actually use it. Chapter 19 focuses on cardiovascular machinery, and Chapter 20 examines strength and flexibility equipment. We tell you which brands and features to look for, and how to distinguish the quality equipment from the *schlock*. In Chapter 21 you get the lowdown on exercise videos — how to build a first-rate library, which instructors to try, and what to make of the trend that won't die: celebrity videos.

Chapter 18

Designing a Home Gym

- -

In This Chapter

▶ The essentials of a quality gym

▶ Equipment shopping tips

▶ The ten commandments of buying TV fitness gadgets

▶ Strategies to stay motivated at home

- -

*T*he home exercise industry is booming. Americans spend about $1.7 billion on equipment every year, and it's easy to understand why. You can't beat the commute to your living room, and you can work out at 3 a.m. on Sunday if you really want to. You don't have to pay membership fees, wait in line for the shower, or deal with any unidentified biological matter that doesn't contain your own DNA.

Yet, despite all the convenience, home exercisers have a high drop-out rate. The novelty wears off, the bike breaks down, or the 5-pound dumbbell gets used as a doorstop. You can avoid this scenario and the accompanying guilt by planning your home gym carefully. This chapter shows you how.

Planning Ahead

The inspiration to exercise might have come to you suddenly, but don't make any rash decisions when you buy equipment. You'll save time and aggravation by putting some thought into your purchases. Before you even set foot in a fitness store, size up your goals, your budget, and your available space. Here are some specifics to consider before you go shopping.

Think "home gym," not just "home equipment"

If you want to get fit at home, be sure to cover all the bases: aerobic fitness, strength, and flexibility. But your home doesn't have to be a palace with high ceilings, racks of shiny weights, and space-age machinery. A complete home gym can consist of a rubber tube, a step, and a handful of videos — equipment that a student on a budget could fit into a studio apartment.

Before you go shopping, look at the big picture. Think about your aerobic, strength, and flexibility goals, and consider what type of equipment you're going to need to succeed in all three areas. We're not saying you have to buy all of your equipment on the same day. But before you pour big bucks into a super-deluxe stairclimber, consider what you're going to do on the strength-training front. Don't just say, "I'll start with a stairclimber, and maybe eventually I'll buy some weights." If you plan to get your aerobic exercise outdoors—walking, jogging, or skating, for instance—then, sure, spend all of your home-gym budget on weight equipment. Just make sure you have an aerobic exercise plan for the winter. Buying flexibility gadgets needn't be a priority, although in Chapter 20 we do recommend buying a cushy mat.

Choose an inviting spot for your equipment

Where you park your exercise bike can make all the difference between using it to get fit and simply using it as an extra chair for your Academy Awards parties. Put your equipment near entertaining distractions such as the TV or stereo. And make sure that the spot has adequate ventilation, lighting, and climate control; there's a reason only spiders hang out in cold, damp basements.

If you're lucky enough to have a spare room, consider reserving it exclusively for your gym. If you don't have an extra room, at least try to keep all of your equipment in close proximity. Don't store your dumbbells in the bedroom, your treadmill in the basement, and your stretching mat in the coat closet. Also, plan to keep your equipment within reach. You don't want to hunt through 10 drawers to find your favorite video. And chances are, anything you store under your bed will stay there—permanently.

Take careful measurements

Before you buy a major piece of equipment, carefully measure the length, width, and height of your available space. You don't want to bump your head against the ceiling when you press the incline button on your new treadmill. Keep in mind that many equipment stores have high ceilings to accommodate tall equipment.

Measure your door to make sure that you can get your new machinery into the house. One of us ruined a brand new stationary bicycle when we pounded on the handles with a rubber mallet in an attempt to squeeze the bike through a doorway that was too narrow. One of the handles broke off, which served us right.

Equipment Shopping Tips

After you've measured your space, you're ready to hit the stores. The following tips apply to home equipment in general. Chapters 19 and 20 offer suggestions specific to aerobic equipment and strength machines.

Shop around

Prices vary widely, so by all means, bargain hunt. But remember: A machine is not a bargain if it collapses with you on it or gives you a hernia. For fancy equipment with lots of moving parts — treadmills, stairclimbers, rowers, weight machines, and the like — stick with stores that specialize in fitness equipment. They tend to sell sturdier, more reliable, and better designed machines. For simpler equipment like dumbbells, ankle weights, steps, and jump ropes, department stores and sporting goods stores are fine.

If you know the exact make and model you want, you might save money by calling the manufacturer directly. Some will let you buy direct; others will refer you to a local dealer. But do your homework: Sometimes you'll get a better deal from the manufacturer. Other times it's cheaper to go through the dealer. You can often save a couple hundred bucks by making a few phone calls.

Buying used equipment is okay, but keep it simple. Stick to gadgets with no motors or complicated designs. The only exception is buying used equipment through an authorized dealer who will give you a warranty. No matter what type of used equipment you buy, ask for a trial period and be sure to get all of the instruction manuals.

A knowledgeable trainer can save you a lot of research time and may be able to help you purchase equipment. Trainers often get discounts from equipment dealers because they recommend and buy equipment on a regular basis. But ask your trainer if he receives a commission from the dealer or if he'll be charging *you* a commission. If your trainer takes a commission, this may eat away at any potential savings. In other cases, a dealer may give you a discount on top of the trainer's commission.

Take a test drive

You wouldn't buy a car without driving it. The same rule applies to exercise machines. Be sure to test *every* feature. Pull every handle and push every bar. Make sure that a stationary bike pedals smoothly at several tension levels. Try a treadmill on the flat setting *and* at an incline. If the salesperson won't let you give the machine a whirl, say adios.

Ask for a discount

High-tech cardio machines and strength machines tend to be marked up about 40 percent above wholesale, so your salesperson probably has some leeway. It's not inappropriate to ask for a 10 percent discount. You might not get it, but it never hurts to ask. Also, if you're buying several items, ask the salesperson to throw in a complimentary accessory such as a rubber floor mat to place underneath your equipment. A mat saves your carpet from sweat and from grease that drips from the bottom of stairclimbers and treadmills; plus you won't get a permanent depression in your carpet from heavy machines. Depending on the square footage, a mat can cost $50 to $200. Some stores will cut your mat to size.

Check out warranty and service plans

If you're choosing between two similar machines, take the one with the better warranty, even if it costs a bit more. Both aerobic and weight machines should have at least a one-year warranty.

Find out who's responsible for repairs and maintenance: A good warranty is worthless if no one within 3,000 miles can fix the darn thing. If you buy a machine from an equipment specialty store, chances are someone from the store will come to your house and fix it. Some equipment manufacturers, such as Quinton and Star Trek, have repairmen on call throughout the country. If you buy from a sporting goods store or a TV offer you may be out of luck.

The Ten Commandments of Buying TV Fitness Gadgets

An astonishing array of gadgets out there in TV-land claim to transform your beer belly into a washboard with virtually no effort on your part. Unfortunately, the only thing that they're likely to reduce is your bank account. Try to avoid buying exercise equipment from TV. You have no way of judging the quality of a machine or gadget — *everything* looks better on TV. At a recent trade show, we mentioned to an infomercial executive that his company's teal-colored abdominal gadget was cheaply made. "Sure," he told us, "but it looks great on TV."

When you watch exercise equipment ads on TV, keep the following tips in mind.

1. If the advertisement claims that you can tone up while lying in bed watching the tube, save your money for Miracle Mop. There's no such thing as "the no sweat workout that works." If there were, don't you think you'd have done this workout by now?

2. Beware of the phrase *guaranteed or your money back*. Read the fine print: The manufacturers may promise that you'll lose four inches in one month — if you stick to a low-fat diet and a far more extensive exercise program.

3. Don't be impressed by "expert" endorsements. Don't think for a minute that some three-time Mr. Universe built his biceps with some plastic contraption that looks like a model of the Star Ship Enterprise. And never buy anything hawked by an actress who hasn't had a decent gig in more than five years.

4. Don't whip out your credit card just because a product is *not sold in stores.* Truth is, most of these gizmos *are* sold in stores — or they will be in a month or two. Sometimes the product is actually cheaper at the store; plus, you can test out the product.

5. Beware of phrases like *three easy payments.* One gadget claims to cost "Not $60! Not $50!" but "just two easy payments of $19.95." Add in shipping and handling, and it costs $46.85.

6. Don't be impressed that a product was "awarded a U.S. patent." You could patent a nose-hair clipper for mice if you wanted to. To get a patent, you need to have an original idea, not necessarily a *good* one.

7. Don't believe that a gadget will enable you to build strength and lose fat simultaneously. Some product manufacturers make this claim blatantly; others use a more subtle approach. Consider the ThighMaster commercials: A svelte model zips up her pants and says, "Thank you, ThighMaster. I never thought I'd fit into these jeans again." The ThighMaster may help you tone your inner thigh muscles, but it's not going to slim down.

8. Don't be swayed by scientific terminology. Product manufacturers love to throw around big words. Some of these terms, such as *omnikinetics,* have no accepted meaning in the scientific community.

9. Don't believe some new contraption is better than free weights or real weight machines. One product manufacturer claims that "with free weights or machines, getting the right form is impossible," but with its gizmo, "there's no way to use the gadget improperly."

10. Hide your credit card between 12 a.m. and 4 a.m. At that hour, everything kinda looks good. Go to bed.

Strategies to Stay Motivated at Home

Once you've brought your equipment home, it's time to face facts: Now you have to *use* the stuff. Some people hope that the mere act of *buying* home exercise equipment will be enough to get them motivated. But that tactic doesn't usually work. The dumbbells sitting in your family room might remind you to exercise, but they don't have some magical power to make you lift them.

We interviewed a woman who owns more than 200 exercise videos. She had watched them all—from the recliner in her living room. "I've always got these good intentions," she told us. "But most of the tapes just sit in the cabinet." Last we spoke to her, she hadn't given up searching for a video that would push her to exercise. She told us that she had bought a mini-trampoline to go along with one of her new tapes. However, the trampoline was still sitting in the back seat of her Buick.

Even the most motivated and disciplined exercisers sometimes have trouble sticking to their plan. The following tips can help insure that you use the equipment you bought.

- ✔ **Schedule your workouts.** Don't just slip in a few chest presses while you're microwaving spaghetti. Treat your workouts like a regular appointment: Write them down in your daily planner or stick a note on the refrigerator.

- ✔ **Dress the part.** You wouldn't wear jeans at a health club; don't do it at your home gym, either. If you put on a comfortable exercise outfit, you'll feel a lot more like working out. Set out your workout clothes the night before.

- ✔ **Tell your family to get lost — unless they're going to work out with you.** This is *your* time, not the time to help your kids write a book report.

- ✔ **Don't answer the phone.** That's what answering machines and kids are for.

- ✔ **Bring the entertainment to you.** If you can't put your equipment near a TV or stereo, at least wear headphones or read a magazine. For stationary bikes and stairclimbers, buy a plastic rack that fits onto the console and holds reading material and a water bottle. Some brands, such as RackIt, provide space for a radio/tape player, magazine, *and* water bottle. (Plastic racks are sold at fitness equipment stores. Some of them are designed for specific brands of machinery.)

- ✔ **Install a mirror.** A mirror will give your home gym that health-club feel and enable you to keep an eye on your form. (Plus, you can flex your muscles and no one will think you're a jerk.) Over time, you'll watch your body slim down and firm up.

- ✔ **Wear a heart rate monitor.** For about $100, you can know instantly — and accurately — how fast your heart is beating. For details about why you should care and how a monitor works, see Chapter 5. Anyone can benefit from one of these gizmos, but they are especially valuable for the home exerciser. You don't have the roar of the crowd to keep you going, or the wide assortment of equipment to occupy you; your heart rate gives you something tangible to focus on.

- ✔ **Keep a workout log.** Nothing is more motivating than success, and an exercise diary gives you documentation of your accomplishments. Keep your log next to your equipment and record every workout. We recommend buying a log at a bookstore or equipment store, but a notebook will suffice. See Chapter 2 for a sample log page.

- ✔ **Keep evaluating your progress.** Test your fitness when you start your home exercise program and retest yourself about every two months. Chart your results in your workout log. For instructions on testing your fitness, see Chapter 1.

Chapter 19

Buying Aerobic Equipment

● ●

In This Chapter

▶ Stationary bikes

▶ Treadmills

▶ Stairclimbers

▶ Rowing machines

▶ Cross-country skiers

▶ Riders

▶ Cardio bargains: steps, slides, and jump ropes

● ●

*H*ome aerobic machines have gotten pretty fancy, and the array of choices can be mind-blowing. Should you go with the bike? The rower? The bike-rower? The bike-rower-stairclimber-treadmill-automatic slicer-microwave oven? But seriously . . . you should test out several machines before you bring one home.

Don't feel compelled to buy a machine that works your arms and legs at the same time. *Total-body workouts* are the latest fad — manufacturers will stick two rowing arms onto any piece of equipment they can think of. Working your arms and legs simultaneously is a nice idea in theory, but it often gets lost in the translation. Most treadmills with arms are lousy; the rowing motion doesn't match your natural arm swing, so your whole stride is thrown off. On the other hand, many total-body bikes, ladder climbers, and skiers work well. As a bonus, you can choose to use your arms and legs together, or separately when one or the other needs a break

The big selling point with these double-duty machines is the extra calorie burn, but you're not going to burn more calories if the machine slows you down or exhausts you so quickly that you head for the couch after 10 minutes. Many of these machines claim to burn more than 1,000 calories per hour, but at that pace, you're not going to last through an entire commercial break. Also, if reading during your workout is a priority, you won't be able to do it if both your arms and legs are occupied. It all comes down to personal preference.

The best machine is the one you'll use. Don't just go out and buy some contraption because it's cheap or because it looked great on TV. You don't want to end up with a space-eating, dust-collecting monster that you can't wait to unload in your next garage sale. This chapter helps you sort through the different options. After you've bought your equipment, we recommend that you read Chapter 8, which describes how to use good form on each type of aerobic machine.

Stationary Bikes

Biking is a no-brainer: Park your butt on the seat, stick your feet in the pedals, and away you go, so to speak. You can spend up to $3,000 on a fully-loaded, high-tech super cycle — or $200 for a sturdy, no-frills workhorse. Just keep in mind that every cool feature you opt for jacks up the price.

Before you buy, test drive both upright and recumbent bikes. *Recumbent bikes* position you in a bucket seat so that you pedal straight out in front of you. If you have lower back discomfort, you might appreciate the back support. Recumbents target your butt and rear thigh muscles better than *upright bikes* (the traditional kind, which resemble a regular bicycle). (See Figure 19-1.)

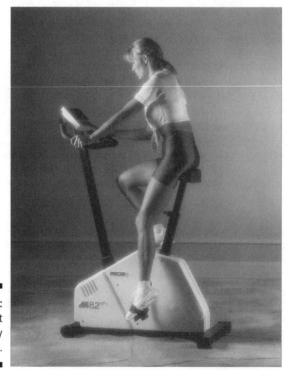

Figure 19-1:
An upright
stationary
bike.

Ride 'Em, Cow Person

You've seen the TV ads and probably wondered, what the heck *is* that? We're talking about those contraptions that look like a stationary bike, only they rock up and down like a mechanical bull. Their names invariably contain the word "rider."

Now for the real question: Can they really get you into shape?

We have our doubts. Few reputable studies have been conducted on these machines, and we're concerned with how much stress that rocking motion places on your body. At a recent trade show, we saw one brand demonstrated in a series of elaborate, choreographed presentations. During the break between performances, nearly all of the demonstrators ran for ice packs to place on their knees and lower backs.

There's also the issue of quality: Though riders generally cost between $300 and $700, they're little more than pieces of cheap metal loosely bolted together.

One brand claims its rider is "3 machines in one: a total aerobic workout, a total strength building workout, and a total flexibility workout." That, we can tell you, is a total exaggeration. You can get your heart pumping on a rider, but don't count on this baby to build or stretch your muscles in any meaningful way.

 Whichever style you prefer, don't buy a bike from a department store. Quality isn't normally a big consideration in their designs, which means a risk of achy knees and a sore lower back. Some cheap bike seats have been known to collapse with a rider in midworkout. You don't want to know where the seat pole winds up. Besides, specialty stores carry plenty of inexpensive models.

Important bike features

Two stationary bikes that look similar might feel very different to your derrière and offer different electronic options. It's important to test-ride every bike and do a thorough check of the features.

- **A comfortable, sturdy seat:** Make sure the seat is compatible with your rear. Fancy features don't help if you can't sit on the thing for more than five minutes. Some people like a seat that's hard and narrow; others prefer one that's wider and softer. Don't assume that a wide, cushy seat is going to be more comfortable. Extra padding under your rear end is nice to have when you watch TV, but when you exercise, the wider surface area can cause chafing and discomfort. Whatever seat you prefer, it should lock securely into place.

- **Seat and handlebar adjustments:** Make sure that, when you sit on the seat, your leg is almost straight at the bottom of the pedal stroke; otherwise, you're asking for knee troubles. The handlebars and width of the pedal straps should be adjustable, too. For more details about stationary bike adjustments, see Chapter 8.

✔ **Feedback:** At the very least, your bike should have a speedometer that displays revolutions per minute and miles per hour, an odometer to measure distance, and a timer to keep track of those minutes as they fly by. Other fun — but expensive — features: preset workout programs, a heart rate monitor, and games that let you race against the computer. We explain all of these features in Chapter 8.

✔ **A way to vary the difficulty:** Look for a knob or button that indicates resistance levels, such as 1 through 12. This way you can accurately measure every workout and keep track of your progress. If 10 minutes on Level 1 used to wear you out, but now you can breeze through 20 minutes on Level 3, you know you've come a long way.

Dummies-approved bike brands

✔ Non-computerized uprights ($200 to $500): Monark, BodyGuard, Schwinn, and Tunturi

✔ Computerized uprights ($500 to $3,000): LifeCyle, Tectrix, Precor, Combi, and Cateye

✔ Computerized recumbents ($500 to $2,000): Precor and LifeFitness

Treadmills

Treadmill prices have dropped considerably in the past few years, but you still need to spend at least $1,000 — usually more — for a safe, well-made machine.

We think *self-powered* treadmills, the ones without motors, are a waste of money. You typically can't get the walking belt moving unless you incline the machine, but that makes the exercise too challenging for many beginners. Running on these treadmills is impossible — you need an even steeper incline, and the belt tends to stick. These days you see many treadmills with arm attachments — ski-pole type mechanisms that you push and pull while you walk or run on the treadmill. We're not fond of this type of treadmill; we think that even the models designed by reputable companies such as NordicTrak tend to be of poor quality and uncomfortable to use.

Important treadmill features

Treadmills used to be large, noisy, cumbersome contraptions. Now most of them are smooth, streamlined, and quiet. Still, you need to thoroughly inspect any treadmill before you buy it. Here's what to look for:

- **A motor to move the walking belt:** Make sure the belt moves fluidly.

- **Safety features:** Don't look twice at any model that doesn't have an emergency stop button and an automatic slow-start speed. A front hand rail is helpful for maintaining balance and is probably safer than side rails, which may actually disrupt your balance if they impede your arm swing. Consider a machine that requires a security code or special magnet to make it go, especially if you have young children.

- **Feedback:** Your machine should display the time, distance, speed, and calories burned, preferably on a digital control panel. Many treadmills now come with a heart-monitor hookup and a set of preprogrammed workouts. (We explain the value of these features in Chapter 8.)

- **An incline capability:** You might not need this feature, but walking uphill adds intensity and variety to your workouts. With most machines, you either turn a crank or press a button to simulate hills.

Dummies-approved treadmills

Trotter, StarTrek, BodyGuard, Precor, and Quinton all make solid treadmills with good warranties and service. (See Figure 19-2.)

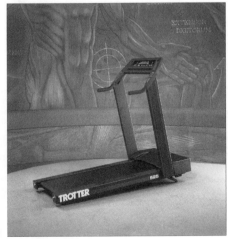

Figure 19-2:
Try the Dummies-approved Trotter treadmill.

Stairclimbers

You're talking about two foot plates you pump up and down to mimic the action of climbing stairs. Stairclimbers, also called steppers, usually have front or side rails that you hold onto for balance. Their consoles display time, distance, number of flights climbed, and calories burned.

Most steppers have an *independent* action; that is, the movement of one pedal is not affected by the other. With *dependent* models, the act of straightening one leg to lower the step causes the other pedal to rise. This isn't just a technical detail: usually you like the feel of one and hate the other.

Almost all steppers in the $200 to $1,200 range use hydraulic pistons or air pressure to power the pedals. These cheaper steppers are nowhere near as smooth moving as the stair machines people line up for at the gym. But some people don't mind the way they feel. At least look for one that doesn't wobble from side to side as you climb. Precor and HydraFitness make decent ones. Department store offerings are generally too flimsy to bother with.

If you want a gym-quality climber, go with the StairMaster 4000, an independent-action machine that uses chains and cables to move the steps — and carries a price tag of nearly $2,500. Tectrix makes a respectable clone for less than $1,500 (see Figure 19-3). LifeStep manufactures the most popular dependent home climber in the same price range.

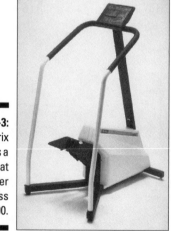

Figure 19-3: Tectrix makes a great stairclimber for less than $1500.

(Photo courtesy of Tectrix Fitness Equipment.)

Rowing Machines

Forget the rowers with two arms that you pull toward you as you slide the seat backwards. You can never get the tension in the arms quite even, and the entire rowing movement feels sticky and unnatural. If you already have one of these, we're betting it's the most expensive coat hanger you own.

A newer breed of rowers has a chain or cable that wraps around a flywheel. The chain is attached to a handle you pull in a smooth movement toward your chest as you straighten your legs and slide the seat backwards. These new rowers do a much better job of capturing the feel of rowing on the water.

Concept II makes an excellent rower that is available only by mail order. This machine is so good that the U.S. Olympic Rowing Team trains on it during the off-season. And at $800, it gets a Dummies Best Buy rating. (See Figure 19-4.) Water Rower makes a good machine that costs about $400 more. The flywheel churns through a tub of water and makes a sound that's relaxing.

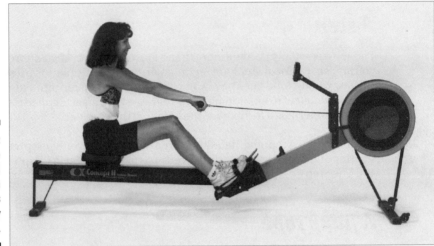

Figure 19-4: The Concept II gets a Dummies Best Buy Rating.

Cross-Country Skiers

Here's one category where we can recommend something that's aggressively advertised on TV. NordicTrack makes the best skiers on the market. You can buy one by calling NordicTrack's toll-free number listed in the back of this book under "Resources" or by visiting one of the company's stores.

NordicTrack skiers have two metal or wooden skis that slide along a track in a gliding movement. You lean against a hip pad and, depending on the model, you either swing a chord as you pump your arms, or push and pull two rowing handles by bending and straightening your arms. The coordination of upper and lower body movement might take a while to grasp, but once you do, the motion feels very much like the real thing. Just make sure that the dog isn't sleeping nearby because the skis require about a foot of clearance at both the front and the back.

NordicTrack skiers start at about $400 — another Dummies Best Buy. The cheaper models do just as good a job as the more expensive ones, so if you don't want extra features such as computerized programs, resist the high-pressure sales tactics that the phone operators use. For about $300, you can buy skiers that are easier to learn but not nearly as effective as NordicTrack. You simply put your feet on two thick pads and shuffle them back and forth.

Three Cardiovascular Bargains

Yes, it is possible to improve your stamina with equipment that costs less than $100. Here are three types of dirt-cheap yet very effective aerobic conditioning gadgets.

A step

Though essentially nothing more than a glorified milk crate, a step can whip you into shape. Most steps are rectangular, hard plastic platforms; some are springy wood. Good ones have some sort of rubber covering on the top to prevent your feet from slipping. Look for Lego-type inserts called risers that snap on underneath to increase the height of the step.

If you're new to stepping, definitely buy a couple of step videos, preferably starring one of the Dummies-approved instructors we list in Chapter 21. Reebok and The Step Company make good steps. Be sure to buy a step that feels sturdy.

A jump rope

Basically, we're talking about a cord between two handles, but a really good jump rope is more involved than that. A plastic or leather cord is better than a flimsy cloth or rope line like the one you used as a kid. The handles should be made of a material that's kind to your hands, like soft rubber or foam. When you turn the rope, you shouldn't feel any hesitation between the cord and handles.

Choose a light rope if your goal is to increase speed, agility, or stamina. You can get a perfectly good one at a sporting goods store or department store for as little as $3, although you may want to spend $15 to $30 for the fancy features we describe in Capter 22. If you're looking to strengthen your upper body while you get your heart and lungs in shape, choose a "heavy" rope that weighs $1/4$ to $1/2$ pound. The weight should be in the cord, not the handles. Good rope brands include the Spalding Sports Rope, LifeLine, Ropics, and The Super Rope.

To size your rope correctly, stand on the center of the cord and pull the ends straight up along your sides. The handles should just reach your armpits.

A slide

Slides are slick plastic boards with a piece of thick rubber padding called bumpers affixed to each end. You wear nylon booties over your shoes so that you can glide side to side over the board, pushing off the bumpers. Sliding is actually harder than it looks — it's a tough workout for your butt and thighs, and it gets your heart pumping fast. But sliding can be boring, and it's hard not to feel silly wearing those booties. (See Figure 19-5.)

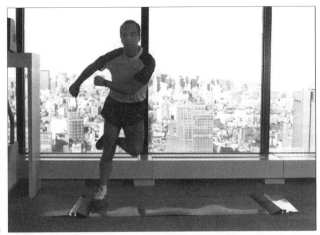

Figure 19-5:
Sliding gets
your heart
pumping
fast.

(Photo courtesy of Dan Kron.)

A slide is convenient for home use because you can roll it up and stick it in a closet. (Just don't forget that you're supposed to take your slide out once in a while.) Make sure you get a high-quality board. It should be at least 5 feet long and should not make an annoying, tearing sound as you glide back and forth. When you hit the bumper, the slide should stay put; some of those late-night TV versions travel across the floor as you travel across the slide. And some real cheapos don't have high enough bumpers, so when you really get going, it's possible to sail up and over the end. Test glide your board at the store.

A good slide has a mat or grip underneath to hold it in place and bumpers that won't come unglued with usage. The inside edges of the bumpers should be angled slightly downward to reduce impact on your feet and ankles. A decent slide with booties costs at least $50. You may want to pay a little more for a travel bag or movable bumpers so you can adjust the slide length. (The longer the slide, the tougher the workout.) We think Reebok makes the best slide.

Chapter 20

Buying Strength (and Stretching) Equipment

· ·

In This Chapter

▶ Free weights: barbells, dumbbells, and ankle weights

▶ Exercise bands and tubes

▶ Multi-gyms

▶ Flexibility devices

· ·

*T*here's no shortage of great gadgets to build muscle at home. There's also, regrettably, no shortage of junk. This chapter covers all of your legitimate strength-training options — from $3 rubber tubes to sophisticated, gym-quality machinery. We introduce you to some innovative new products and help you decide which type of equipment is best for your home and your budget.

If you're going to lift weight at home, we urge you to read Chapters 10 through 13. In those chapters, we explain how to *use* all types of strength equipment and how to design a strength-training program that'll get you results.

Free Weights

Free weights — dumbbells and barbells — are excellent investments: They're simple, they're versatile, and they're relatively inexpensive. They do, however, have the highest accident potential — just ask anyone who has ever dropped a weight on his foot or gotten pinned under a heavy bar. If you're new to free-weight training, *please* take a few sessions with a trainer. And never do any heavy lifting when you're alone.

On the up side, you won't compromise safety by buying the cheap weights sold at department and sporting goods stores. Weight is weight. There's not much difference between one brand and another. Like meat, free weights are usually sold by the pound. You can pay up to $2 a pound for shiny chrome dumbbells and bars. Gray or black steel will run you $.35 to $1 per pound.

Dumbbells

For a beginner, *dumbbells* (the short weights that you can lift with one hand) should be a higher priority than *barbells* (the long ones that require both hands). Dumbbells give you more exercise options, and they force each side of your body to pull its own weight.

When it comes to buying dumbbells, you have two options. The best, most convenient option is to buy several pairs of dumbbells — 5-pound weights, 10-pounders, 15-pounders, and so on. The cheap choice: Buy an adjustable dumbbell kit. A kit comes with two handles and several weight plates you clamp onto each end of the handles with a clip or screw-type mechanism called a *collar.*

Owning a whole array of dumbbells saves you lots of time. Let's say that you're alternating shoulder exercises with 5-pound weights and chest exercises with 15-pound weights. All you have to do is put down the 5s and pick up the 15s. With adjustable dumbbells, you constantly have to remove the collar and add or subtract weight plates, which is a huge pain. You may be tempted to use the wrong weight because making the switch is a hassle. Also, it can be tough to lock the weights on securely; they can jiggle around or, worse, slide off in the middle of your workout.

If you choose to buy separate dumbbells, realize that you'll need about 8 different pairs. Some people use the same 10-pound dumbbells for every exercise. This is not a good idea: A weight that's heavy enough to challenge your back muscles is much too heavy for your arm muscles; a weight that's just right for your shoulders is too light to do your chest any good. If you want to see results, you need to give each muscle the right challenge

For most beginning women, we recommend buying dumbbells weighing 2, 3, 5, 8, 10, 12, 15, and 20 pounds. Even if you can't use the 15s and 20s right away, you'll grow into them pretty fast. The whole set costs between $50 and $150. As for beginning men, start off with 8, 12, 15, 20, 25, 30, 35, 40, 45, and 50 pounds. This set runs $200 to $600.

A terrific new product called PlateMate can save you a lot of money on dumbbells. PlateMates are magnets that you stick onto each end of a dumbbell to increase the weight. The magnets come in two weights: $1^1/_4$ pounds and $2^1/_2$ pounds. With PlateMates, you cut down on the number of dumbbells you need to buy. For instance, instead of buying a pair of 15-pounders, 20-pounders, *and* 25-pounders, you can pass on the 20s, and create your own 20-pound weights by putting a 2¹/₂-pound PlateMate on each end of the 15-pounders. You can stick the PlateMates on the 25-pounders to create 30-pound dumbbells, and so on. PlateMates come in different shapes to accommodate different styles of dumb-bells. A pair of 1¹/₄-pound PlateMates costs about $20; a pair of 2¹/₂-pound magnets costs about $30. We recommend PlateMates in Chapter 22 as one of ten great fitness investments under $100.

Shop around and try out different brands of dumbbells. Some have contoured handles that might feel more comfortable than straight ones. Some dumbbells have foam grips; others are coated in rubber. Dumbbells with hexagonal ends are great because they won't roll away. A dumbbell rack is also a good idea. A rack can cost up to $200 but will keep your weights organized and your home gym looking tidy.

Although traditional dumbbell kits are a hassle, a few companies have come up with innovative alternatives. One kit is called PowerBlocks. Each *block* consists of a series of rectangular, weighted, metal frames, each one nesting inside a slightly larger frame. A series of holes runs along the outside of the frames; you insert a pin inside a hole to select the number of frames you'd like to pick up. You can buy a set of blocks that go from 5 pounds to 90 pounds in 5-pound increments. The blocks don't jiggle around, and you can change the weight instantly. PowerBlocks come with their own stand and take up about the same amount of room as a telephone table. A 40-pound set sells for about $300; the 90-pound set sells for about $600. (See Figure 20-1.)

Another clever product is Smart Locks. These dumbbells have spring-loading collars that pop on and off easily and secure the weight plates better than traditional kits. A set of Smart Locks, including weight plates that build up from 2 pounds to 40 pounds, sells for about $175.

Figure 20-1:
The
PowerBlock
Pro
Aluminum
set.

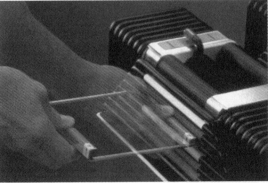

(Photo courtesy of Intellbell, Inc.)

Barbells

Most people can get along just fine with an array of dumbbells, but you can't beat barbells for power lifts like bench pressing and squatting. Plus, barbells add even more variety to your workout. We recommend buying a single bar with a number of weight plates because it's expensive to buy a whole assortment of bars. Bars typically run between $25 and $125, depending on the type of steel and where you buy the bar. Bars tend to cost more at specialty shops than at sporting goods stores.

Bars are typically four to seven feet long and come in two sizes: the skinnier Standard (about 35 pounds) and the thicker Olympic (about 45 pounds). Plates and collars are designed to fit one bar size or the other, so make sure that you're buying plates that match your bar. We prefer Olympic bars because they're more comfortable to wrap your hands around — they're also the standard in most gyms.

It's a good idea to purchase a rack with your barbell. Upright racks take up less room than horizontal ones. A one-bar rack can cost as little as $100.

As an alternative to traditional barbells, you can buy a series of lighter bars from 9 pounds to 27 pounds covered with comfortable rubber padding. One popular company is Body Bar. These bars are good for beginners. They allow you to learn to do barbell exercises without having to use the heavier Standard or Olympic bars. The problem is, you can't clip on weight plates, so you have to buy several bars to accommodate your various muscle groups. They're not cheap: A 12-pound Body Bar runs about $50. Plus, these bars don't come in heavy enough weights for intermediate and advanced exercisers.

Weight benches

When you buy dumbbells and/or barbells, buy a bench, too. A bench lets you do many exercises that you couldn't do otherwise. It's tough to do free-weight exercises lying on your back on the floor; your elbows will hit the ground before you complete the movement. You also can do several exercises while sitting or kneeling on a bench.

If you're lifting dumbbells lighter than 30 pounds, you probably can get away with a plastic step platform rather than a full-fledged weight bench. With two sets of risers underneath, the platform is high enough and sturdy enough for light dumbbell exercises. But if you're lifting heavier dumbbells or using barbells, buy a real weight bench. A bench is higher off the ground and more stable. We recommend benches that can be easily adjusted to incline or decline so that you challenge your muscles at different angles.

Look for a bench with a thick foam pad covered with Naugahyde or imitation leather. The pad should be sturdily bolted to a steel frame and legs. A bench should be at least a few feet high and shouldn't wobble when you get on and off. A basic, flat bench goes for $100 to $300, depending on the quality and thickness of the padding, frame, and legs. We recommend paying a bit more for one that can be set at various inclines. York and Hoist make good ones, but we really love Tuff Stuff benches (about $350) because they both incline *and* decline; most benches do one or the other, in which case a bench that inclines is more valuable than one that declines.

Ankle weights

Ankle weights are great for making floor exercises (like leg lifts) tougher. You'll probably want ankle weights if you like body-sculpting videos because at some point, lifting your own body weight will become too easy. As with dumbbells, you can buy an array of ankle weights, from 2 pounds up to 20 pounds. Or you can buy an adjustable set: You insert small weight bars into pockets along the strap. Adjustable ankle weights are a great way to save money. Just know that the weights tend to rattle around. And, it's easy to get lazy; don't neglect to add or subtract weight when you need to. Use ankle weights sparingly if you have hip, knee, or ankle problems.

Exercise Bands and Tubes

Rubber bands and tubes are the absolute cheapest way to strengthen your muscles — you can buy three or four bands for less than $10. They're also extremely versatile and great for traveling. Even if you own weight machines or an extensive set of free weights, we recommend throwing in a few bands for variety. (See Figure 20-2.)

But exercise bands and tubes have limitations. It's tough to gauge your progress: You can't measure exactly how much weight you're lifting, like you can with free weights and machines. Bands and tubes come in varying tensions: the heavier the band, the more strength you need to pull it. But graduating from a light band to a medium band somehow doesn't offer the same satisfaction as going from 10-pound dumbbells to 20-pounders.

These innocent looking strips of latex definitely can tax your muscles, but you may get to the point where bands don't provide a tough enough workout. Also, many people — us included — find it more satisfying to work with free weights or machines. We like the feel of cold steel in our hands, and we like watching the weight stack move up and down. We don't get the same thrill watching a band expand and contract.

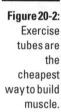

Figure 20-2:
Exercise tubes are the cheapest way to build muscle.

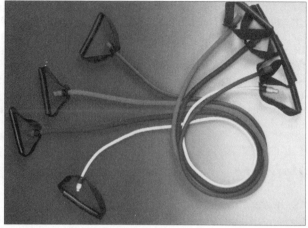

(Photo courtesy of Spri Products, Inc.)

Bands are flat latex strips about six inches wide and about three feet long. Tubes come in different sizes. You'll probably like bands for some exercises and tubes for others; you just have to experiment. Because bands and tubes are so inexpensive, it pays to get a variety.

For a few dollars more, you can buy bands or tubes with plastic or rubber handles — a real plus for getting a firm grip on an exercise. Some bands or tubes have built-in ankle and thigh straps. LifeLine makes nifty band kits that come with a travel bag and several door and bar attachments, priced at under $100. Spri and DynaBand also make quality bands. Because some bands don't come with instructions, we recommend buying a couple of videos with band workouts. The following instructors offer quality band workouts: Lynn Brick, Jody Cohen, David Essel, Donna Richardson, Keli Roberts, and Tamilee Webb.

You also can buy band loops with little foam circles of padding, but you don't really need them. You can just tie your regular band in a circle, which is even more versatile because you can control the diameter of the circle. The smaller the circle, the tighter the tension. You can use a circle to do a number of leg exercises, and a few upper body exercises, too.

Two cautions regarding the use of bands: Check frequently for holes and tears by holding your bands up to the light. Once a band is damaged, replace it immediately. And *never* try to use regular office rubber bands, even thick ones, for exercising. You're just asking to be snapped in the face.

Multi-gyms

Multi-gyms are those contraptions that look like a bunch of health club weight machines welded to each other (see Figure 20-3). Multi-gyms take up a lot of room — usually more than a stereo wall unit — and most require at least seven feet of vertical clearance space. But many people prefer multi-gyms to free weights or bands because they're so safe and easy to use. Besides, you can do several exercises with multi-gyms that you just can't do with weights or bands. Most multi-gyms come with instructions — some even come with videos demonstrating all of the different exercises.

A basic unit has one 200-pound stack of weight plates in 5- to 10-pound increments. This means only one person can use the machine at a time. A multi-gym costs $1,000 to $3,500. If the whole family plans to work out together, you might want a multi-gym with two or three weight stacks, but these can run up to $10,000.

Good high-end brands include Paramount, Pacific, Vectra, and California Gym. For reliable models under $1,000, look at Hoist, Total Gym, and Free Form.

Unfortunately, we haven't yet found a multi-gym sold on TV that isn't cheaply-made. They wobble, they're poorly designed, and the resistance never moves as smoothly as a weight stack. Even some of the TV demonstrators can't help arching their backs on some of the moves. And, sure, you might be able to do 52 exercises with one of these contraptions, but it'll take you about three hours just to make the adjustments, which will give you one more reason to blow off your workout.

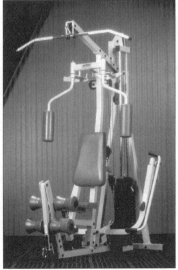

Figure 20-3:
Multi-gyms
are safe and
easy to use.

(Photo courtesy of Richard Lee.)

Take your time shopping for a multi-gym. Try out a whole bunch of different machines, and pay attention to which exercises feel most comfortable. Multi-gyms that look the same sitting on the showroom floor might actually have important differences that you won't notice until you *use* them. For instance, some multi-gyms come with a horizontal chest press; others come with a vertical chest press. You have to decide whether you prefer to lie on your back and press upward, or sit straight up and press forward. Ask the equipment dealer to compare the different ways each multi-gym works each muscle group.

Here's a checklist to consult before you go shopping for a multi-gym. Inspect each machine carefully, and look for the following features:

- ✓ **At least these five exercise stations: chest/shoulder press, high pulley, low pulley, leg extension, and leg curl.** Depending on the brand and model, you might also get a chest butterfly, chin/dip, leg press, and abdominal board attachments. If these attachments aren't included with the basic unit, they're usually available as extra-cost options. Don't buy a machine that requires you to unsnap and rehook cables or arm positions to switch between exercises. Those machines are too much of a hassle; making all of those adjustments can add extra minutes to your workout and interrupt the flow of your routine.

- ✓ **Free assembly.** Pass on any machine that the dealer doesn't put together for you, especially if it comes with an "easy to follow" video on how to build it yourself.

- ✓ **Weight stacks that move up and down smoothly.** Test several exercises in the store to check for sticking points and levers that don't allow you to fully straighten your arms and legs.

- ✓ **A frame made of thick, tubular, or rectangular steel.** The frame shouldn't shake or wobble when you lean against it. Also, the frame should be painted or powder coated to prevent chipping and rusting.

- ✓ **Upholstery that's sewn on securely.** If you see corners that are curled at the edges, the upholstery probably will rip, tear, or unravel.

- ✓ **Plates and cables made of quality materials.** Avoid materials that look like they'll snap, fray, or crack.

- ✓ **Adjustable seats and arms.** If you can adjust the machine, the whole family can work out comfortably.

- ✓ **A good warranty.** The warranty should cover 10 years for the frame, 1 year for moving parts, and 90 days for upholstery. If you ask before you buy the machine, some dealers will give you an extended warranty at no cost. Don't *buy* an extended warranty, however. They tend to be expensive and not worth the money.

Flexibility Gadgets

We didn't devote an entire chapter to stretching products because, strictly speaking, you don't need them. Most people get by just fine with fundamental stretching exercises that don't use anything but your body positioning and gravity. Still, there are some useful tools to help you work on your flexibility. If some of these gadgets get you to stretch when you otherwise wouldn't, they're worth the money. Here's a look at some worthwhile investments:

✔ **A stretching mat:** You can use a thick towel or blanket to pad a hard floor, but a mat is always a good thing to have. A mat is a more formal reminder to do your stretches, and you can use it for abdominal exercises and floor exercises, too. Some stretching mats sell for more than $100, but we have no idea why. Just about any mat you come across will suffice. A top-of-the-line mat — one that's cushiony and long enough so that your head isn't hitting your wood floor — shouldn't cost more than $40. Some can be folded in half for storage; others roll up.

✔ **An oversized plastic ball:** This is a safe way to improve the flexibility of your lower back. You can drape your body over it forward or backward or sideways. (An oversized ball is also useful for abdominal and leg strengthening exercises.) One costs about $30.

The right fit is important. When you sit on the ball, your thighs should be roughly parallel to the floor. However, if you're somewhat inflexible, get a slightly bigger ball. You won't have to bend as far. Also, for stretching, don't fill the ball all the way up; it'll be softer, easier to mold your body to, and less likely to roll away. (See Figure 20-4.)

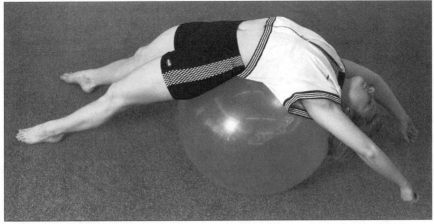

Figure 20-4:
An oversized plastic ball is a nifty flexibility gadget.

(Photo courtesy of Dan Kron.)

✔ **The Stretch-Out Strap:** This four-foot nylon band has large loops sewn along its length. For $10, you may want to own it, especially if you're too stiff to get into certain stretching poses. For instance, if you're sitting on the floor with one leg out and you can't reach your toes, you wrap the strap around your instep and hold a loop in each hand. After holding that position for a while, if you can stretch a little farther, you can let your hands creep up to the loop that's slightly closer to your toes.

✔ **The Prostretch:** This gadget is for stretching your calf and shin muscles and the sides of your ankles. A Prostretch is a shoe imprint cast in hard plastic and mounted on one or two curved rockers (wider versions of the rockers you find on rocking chairs). You place your foot on the imprint and drop your heel back toward the floor. Your toes point upward, giving you a terrific calf stretch. If you're not very flexible, you can do this stretch while sitting down. (See Figure 20-5.)

Because the Prostretch supports your entire foot, you get a better calf stretch than if you just hang your feet off the curb, although most curbs won't run you $25.

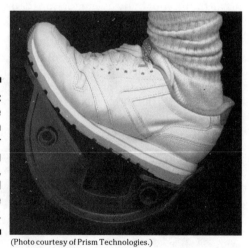

Figure 20-5:
Try the
Prostretch
for
stretching
your calf,
shin, and
side ankle
muscles.

(Photo courtesy of Prism Technologies.)

Chapter 21

Exercise Videos

. . . .

. . . .

*E*xcercise videos won't suit everyone — you might feel silly prancing around your living room alone, mimicking an instructor who says, "You're doing great!" even though he can't see you. But if you're short on time, self-conscious about your body, or looking for inspiration to break a sweat at home, videos might suit you well. You won't feel pressure to keep up with anyone else, and you can build a pretty extensive video library for less than the cost of a yearly gym membership. Plus, you get a lot more instruction from a tape than you can from a book or magazine.

Fortunately, there are plenty of good tapes to choose from. In recent years videos, like health club classes, have become safer, more creative, and more specialized. You can buy tapes for muscle toning, step aerobics, yoga, boxing, pregnancy, post-pregnancy, and chair exercise — the list goes on and on.

Naturally, this being the fitness industry, you also can buy tapes taught by quacks or by narcissistic celebrities who burn more calories talking than exercising. This chapter tells you how to choose the winners and avoid the duds. We offer our best-instructor picks, shopping advice, and important tips for using videos safely.

How to Choose a Video

Choosing the wrong video is hardly the most tragic mistake you can make in life. However, it's no fun getting stuck with some out-of-focus tape taught by an instructor who grates on your nerves. The following tips will help you weed out tapes that aren't right for you and videos that are just plain awful.

Rent before you buy

Large video stores like BlockBuster have a terrific, up-to-date selection. Try out a bunch of instructors. Many have an entire line of tapes, so if you find a teacher you like, chances are you'll be happy with the whole lot. Later in this chapter, we list Dummies-approved instructors.

Video cover-ups

What you see on the cover of an exercise tape is not always what you find when you pop the tape into your VCR. Below are some examples of the dirty, rotten tricks that some companies play. These tapes aren't necessarily bad, but their covers are misleading.

✔ **The tape:** *Aerobics On Location: Have Fun & Get Fit In Florida.* **The cover:** A leggy blonde stands beneath a palm tree on the beach. **The truth:** The workout was taped in a dark studio in Torrance, California. The blonde isn't even in the video; it's taught by a short brunette. And the palm trees? Well, you get a glimpse of them in the aerial Florida footage that's superimposed onto the screen periodically during the workout.

✔ **The tape:** *Anja Schreiner's Lower Body Workout.* **The cover:** Schreiner, a buffed-out bodybuilder, holds a dumbbell in each hand. "Learn Anja's secrets to a new and beautiful you," the box says. **The truth:** The workout doesn't even involve dumbbells. To do this routine, you need a leg press, a hamstring curl machine, and a leg extension — a whole line of gym equipment.

✔ **The tape:** *Gay Gasper's The Next Step.* **The cover:** Has a 1994 copyright. **The truth:** The video is really a re-edited version of Gasper's highly rated 1993 tape of the same name. In 1994, the original program was chopped up and split into a package of two separate tapes that are tough to follow.

✔ **The tape:** *Cosmopolitan's 7 Pounds in 7 Days.* **The cover:** Claims you will "lose 7 pounds in 7 days," a ridiculous statement, to be sure, but one that at least implies that you're getting a tough workout. **The truth:** This calorie-burning program has exactly 7 minutes of beginner-level aerobics — the rest is diet mumbo jumbo.

✔ **The tape:** *The Air Power Workout.* **The cover:** "Breathe your inches away! Lose 4 to 9 inches the first week." The box claims the results are "proven." **The truth:** The star of the video admitted to us that the results are "not scientifically documented."

Inspect the cover

Before you even rent a video — and definitely before you buy — take a good look at the front and back of the jacket. You can't always judge a video by its cover, but you'll find plenty of clues. Pay attention to:

✔ **The type of workout:** Make sure that the workout is what you want, whether that's abdominal toning, funk aerobics, or a stepping/body-sculpting combination. Look for a description of the actual moves — don't go by the title or the hype. *Burns Fat, Pulsating Excitement!,* and *A New Attitude* won't tell you anything.

✔ **The fitness level required:** Look for a box that says "great for beginners." Don't start out with a tape called *For Animals Only.* Some tapes offer modifications for all levels.

✔ **The equipment required:** Do you need a step? A tube? A weight bench? Three sets of dumbbells? Make sure that you either have what's needed or are willing to buy it.

✔ **The length of the whole video and the length of each segment:** A 60-minute step aerobics tape might have only 30-minutes of aerobics. The rest may be a warm-up, stretching session, and cool-down.

✔ **Instructor credentials:** If the teacher is certified by one of the legitimate professional organizations, you can bet that the cover will say so. Be wary if all you can find is "Internationally Recognized Fitness Expert." See Chapter 17 for a list of Dummies-approved aerobics instructor certifications and Chapter 15 for personal trainer certifications.

✔ **The date of the copyright:** Some tapes are timeless classics, but chances are, a video produced in the last couple of years will be more in tune with the latest training techniques. Also, choreography is a lot more creative than it used to be, and safety and instruction are given more consideration these days. Even some of the older tapes led by our Dummies-approved instructors contain moves considered unsafe by today's standards.

Get a sneak preview

Before you try a video workout, sit down on your couch and watch it all the way through. Imagine yourself doing this tape week after week, and consider the following:

✔ **Safety:** Use your common sense. Is the instructor doing anything outrageous, like arching her back so much that you can hear her vertebrae screaming for help?

✔ **The instructor's style and personality:** Is the instructor up-beat and professional, or is he hyperventilating with excitement? Is he kind and encouraging, or does he refer to "the huge butt you may have?" Does he have a clear, resonant voice, or does he sound like he sucked helium? Some instructors sound like the cheerleader from hell, some do the sex-kitten thing, others bark orders like a drill sergeant. One well-known instructor blurts out non sequiturs like "Lose those jigglies!"

✔ **Instruction:** Does the instructor use good form and give adequate directions? Some instructors look great doing the workout but never explain proper technique or warn you about what to do next. Others go on and on about good form but don't practice what they preach. In one tape, an instructor cautions against jumping around on hard surfaces while she leads an outdoor class on cement! Some instructors are so winded that they can't even get the words out.

Don't give up on a tape just because the routine seems too complicated; the first time is bound to be confusing. But go with your instinct: Do you think you'll ever get it, or is the instruction just plain lousy?

✔ **Production quality:** Does the sound warble? Is the video shot in focus? The tape doesn't need to look like an Academy Award-winning feature, but neither should it appear to have been filmed with a handi-cam in someone's garage. At the same time, don't confuse slick production with quality instruction. Cindy Crawford's videos look terrific but, according to most experts, flunk the safety test.

✔ **The music:** Much of the music is bland, synthesized garbage. In fact, the music reminds us of a '70s porn soundtrack. Of course, we don't watch porn, but if we did, we imagine that's what a '70s porn soundtrack would sound like. Exceptions include celebrity videos like Paula Abdul and Cher, who use their own music — which is great, if you like it.

✔ **The hype:** Everyone progresses at a different pace. To motivate you, instructors can and should say things like, "Most people will feel stronger and look better in about six weeks if they do this workout regularly." They should not say, "You'll lose 30 pounds in 6 weeks if you follow my routine and send away for my world-famous protein powder."

Where to buy your videos

At supermarkets or megachains like K-Mart, you can often pick up tapes for a fraction of the cost that you might pay in a retail store. (Videos cost about $7.95 to $29.95.) But these stores don't always have the best selection. They tend to stick to name-brand instructors and celebrity videos, ignoring many first-rate but lesser-known teachers. And beware of return policies: You usually can't get your money back unless the product is defective. You can't just say, "I tried this tape, and it stinks."

One more word about cost: Pay attention to how long a workout you're getting for your money. To boost sales, many companies are producing 20- to 30-minute tapes for $14.95 when a 60- to 90-minute video might cost just $19.95.

Where to get the lowdown on videos

Can't decide among *Ultimate Buns, Lethal Buns,* and *Buns of Steel?*

Here's a simple solution: Call a video consultant.

You've heard of jury consultants, management consultants, and wardrobe consultants — well, now there are folks trained to help you sort through the bewildering slew of exercise tapes on the market. These consultants are the dozen staffers at Collage Video Specialties, a unique company based in Minneapolis, Minnesota.

Collage puts out one product: *The Complete Guide to Exercise Videos* (see the figure). It's the country's only catalog devoted to exercise tapes — and is the only company staffed with operators who have actually sweated their way through *Life's A Bench, Jamaica Me S'wet,* and

THE COMPLETE
guide
TO
EXERCISE
VIDEOS

Including:
- Karen Voight
- Kari Anderson
- Reebok
- Susan Powter
- Donna Richardson
- Kathy Smith
- Tamilee Webb
- Paula Abdul
- Cathe Friedrich
- All "The Firms"
- Gin Miller
- ESPN Fitness Pros
- Karen Alexander

the rest. The consultants have watched hundreds of videos, and they have TVs and VCRs at their desks so they can review the latest tapes between phone orders.

Consultants aside, the Collage catalog is an excellent service. It's published five times a year and features nearly 300 tapes. Each blurb tells you how tough the workout is, how long each segment lasts, what type of music it's set to, how inspirational the instructor is, how the tape was rated by major fitness magazines, and what equipment you need.

If you want to know more, you can call the consultants toll-free. (The phone number is listed in "Resources" at the back of the book.) The catalog's official policy is to accept only defective returns. In reality, they'll take back a tape that you simply don't like — as long as you don't abuse this policy.

You won't find any terrible reviews in the catalog. The company rejects tapes that they consider unsafe or useless, and they tend to use terms like "bubbly" and "enthusiastic" for instructors that we find shrill and annoying. The back of the catalog features a list of mediocre tapes (euphemistically titled "Other Tapes Available") that the company won't promote but will sell if you insist.

In general, you tend to get a more thorough and honest appraisal from the consultants than from the blurbs. When we asked one of the consultants about one instructor featured in the catalog, she said, "She seems so fake. I want to put plugs in my ears and go running the other way."

Your Video Options

Whatever you want to improve, tighten, tone, build, or reduce, there's an exercise video out there for you. Chances are, you'll find dozens. Exercise videos usually fall into one of the following categories:

Aerobic

This category includes high- and low-impact aerobics, step aerobics, slide, funk, jump rope, and some boxing tapes. (For a detailed description of each type of exercise, see Chapter 17.) Look for tips on proper form, how to use the equipment, and how to check your intensity level. These tapes should include an easy warm-up to get your blood flowing. The aerobic workout generally lasts 10 to 45 minutes. The cool-down should last at least 3 minutes and should be followed by a stretching session.

Strength training

Strength-training videos, also called muscle toning videos, use a variety of equipment, including dumbbells, bars, tubes, and bands. Some tapes focus on a particular body area, such as abdominals, thighs, or arms; others tone your whole body. You generally find two types of toning videos: gym-style and choreographed. Gym-style workouts typically work one muscle group at a time, doing 10 to 15 repetitions, and you usually need a weight bench. Choreographed toning routines might work several muscle groups at once or rotate. These routines aren't dancy, but some of them do require coordination; they tend to give you more aerobic conditioning than gym-style workouts, but they won't build as much strength.

Watch these choreographed routines carefully: The instructor should not have you doing a massive number of repetitions. You shouldn't do more than 15 reps per set — perhaps 30 for abdominals.

Toning tapes should explain how to choose the proper weight for each exercise. The warm-up should be well-rounded but have a bit more emphasis on the body parts that you use in the main workout. The instructor should provide tips on proper form, how to make the exercise harder or easier, and how to modify a move if, say, you have a back or elbow injury. The cool-down and stretch segments should be similar to those in aerobic tapes.

Combination videos

These videos combine an aerobic workout with a full-fledged muscle toning routine. The rules for both apply here.

Stretch and yoga

The introduction should cover how to stretch, how to breathe, and what stretching and/or yoga can do for you. You typically start with simple exercises that prepare your muscles for more challenging moves later in the workout. The main workout may not be much different than the warm-up, except that the moves are more advanced. Also, you might hold the positions longer. The instructor should tell where you should feel the stretch and offer constant technique reminders. Expect suggestions for people with back, knee, shoulder, and ankle injuries and for those who are less flexible. The cool-down might include meditation or relaxation exercises.

Specialty tapes

Specialty tapes include country line dancing, pregnancy and post-pregnancy workouts, chair dancing, workouts for those with osteoporosis and arthritis, and routines for those starting out after breast surgery. Some of these tapes are designed to teach you a new skill rather than take you through an actual workout. Use your judgment. If the workout doesn't feel right, return the tape to the rental store.

Dummies-approved instructors

These aren't the only good video instructors around, but they're among the instructors that we think produce high-quality tapes on a consistent basis. (See Figures 21-2, 21-3, and 21-4.)

Beginning

- ✔ Gilad Janklowicz
- ✔ Leisa Hart
- ✔ Cynthia Kereluk
- ✔ Margaret Richards
- ✔ Leslie Sansone
- ✔ Richard Simmons

Beginning/Intermediate

- ✔ Kari Anderson
- ✔ Lynn Brick
- ✔ Gin Miller
- ✔ Donna Richardson

- ✔ Kathy Smith
- ✔ Tamilee Webb

Intermediate/Advanced

- ✔ Jodi Cohen
- ✔ Candice Copeland
- ✔ Victoria Johnson
- ✔ Barry Joyce
- ✔ Keli Roberts
- ✔ Karen Voight

Figure 21-2: Gilad and Margaret Richards are Dummies-approved instructors for beginners.

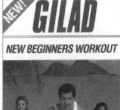
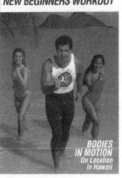
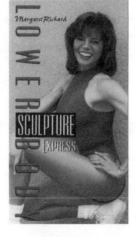

Figure 21-3: Dummies-approved video instructors for beginners and intermediate exercisers: Donna Richardson and Gin Miller.

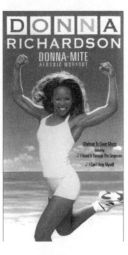
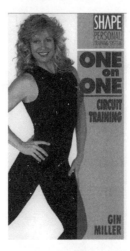

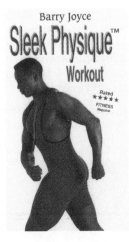

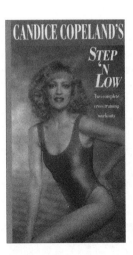

Figure 21-4: Barry Joyce and Candice Copeland are Dummies-approved video instructors for intermediate/advanced folks.

These specialty tape instructors make only a handful of tapes, but we mention them because they teach their specialties so well.

✔ **Jump Rope:** Ken Solis (Ropics)

✔ **Yoga/stretching:** Yoga Journal, Larry Lane, Molly Fox, and Bob Anderson

✔ **Pregnancy:** Madeline Lewis

✔ **Chair exercise:** Maria Serao

Important Safety Tips

Safety is an important consideration, especially when you don't have much exercise experience and you're working out in an unsupervised setting.

✔ Make sure you clear adequate space in front of the TV so that you don't bang your shins on the coffee table or knock over any lamps.

✔ For aerobic and strength-training tapes, wear proper aerobic shoes rather than bare feet or socks. You may want to buy a board made of springy wood similar to what you'll find in good aerobics studios. These boards help absorb impact. Gerstung makes a 30-x-60-inch board for about $160 and a 30-x-30-inch board for about $80. In any case, don't jump around on concrete floors.

✔ Even if the instructor doesn't do it on the video, gauge your intensity by checking your heart rate or taking the talk test during or immediately following an intense portion of the workout. We explain these methods in Chapter 5. All Dummies-approved instructors do intensity checks in their workouts.

✔ Don't try to keep up with the instructors. They practiced the routine for weeks before it was filmed. Look for someone in the video who goes at your pace. Good tapes have demonstrators who exercise at different levels. At the start of the workout, the lead instructor will say something like, "If you're a beginner, keep your eye on Valerie." If you get winded, keep moving by marching in place or walking in a circle.

✔ If you're just starting out, consider buying a video that includes three short workouts rather than one long one. The shorter workouts last 15 to 25 minutes as opposed to 30 to 90 minutes.

✔ Remember that your VCR has a pause button. Use it if you need to get water.

Celebrity videos

"I wanted to be the only actress in Hollywood who hadn't made an exercise video," says Mary Tyler Moore at the beginning of her *Every Woman Workout* tape. Alas, she couldn't resist.

Actually, Moore's tape is pretty decent — you find a solid beginner's workout. But some celeb videos are downright awful. In *Fabio Fitness,* Fabio and his trainer flirt with each other between sets. "You have a great-looking chest," she says; he smiles in agreement. Zsa Zsa Gabor's *It's Simple, Darling* is simply worthless; in between exercises, she offers life and beauty secrets. "Ven you break up your engagement, give up zee ring but not zee stone. Now, vee do leg extensions."

Exercise tapes are often a way for an actor to drum up some cash between gigs, boost a sagging career, or promote a current project. But not all celebrity videos are a mess. Look for celebrities who team up with a real exercise expert. Some celebrities are inconsistent; Jane Fonda, for instance, puts out some fine tapes, but others are tough to follow and include risky exercises. Stay away from her early videos, which are full of bone-crunching moves. Unfortunately, those old tapes are still floating around out there. Here's a list of celebrity tapes we like:

Beginner

✔ Mary Tyler Moore's *Every Woman Workout* series with Laurie Redmond

✔ Kathy Lee's *Feel Fit and Fabulous* with C.B. Yelverton

✔ Lucky Vanous's *The Ultimate Fat Burning System* with Kacy Duke

Intermediate/Advanced

✔ Elle MacPherson's *Your Personal Best* with Karen Voight

✔ Ali McGraw's *Yoga Mind and Body* with Erich Schiffman

✔ MTV's *The Grind Hip-Hop Workout* with Eric Nies

✔ *Frederique Peak 10 Fitness* with Chris Imbo and Kacy Duke

Part VI
The Part of Tens

The 5th Wave   By Rich Tennant

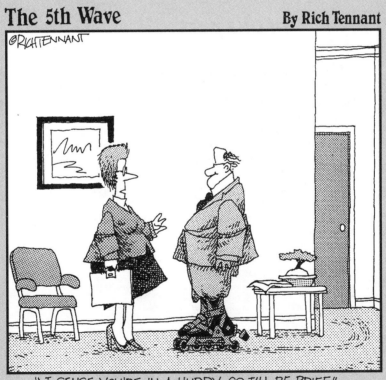

"I SENSE YOU'RE IN A HURRY, SO I'LL BE BRIEF."

In this part . . .

We carry on the Dummies tradition of grouping key information into fun, easy-to-skim lists of ten. Chapters 22 and 23 fill you in on the best and worst ways to spend your fitness dollars. In Chapter 24, you learn how to prevent and treat the most common exercise injuries — and you learn the difference between a sprain, a strain, a pull, and a tear. Chapter 25 explains how to safely exercise through pregnancy, even after you can no longer see if your shoes are tied. Chapter 26 covers how to stay fit when you're traveling. Chapter 27 cuts through the hype about metabolism and answers questions you want to know, such as "What exactly is a calorie, and what does it mean to *burn* one?"

Chapter 22

Ten Great Fitness Investments under $100

*Y*ou can spend thousands of dollars on high-tech exercise machinery (see Chapters 19 and 20 for smart high-end buys), but some of the most valuable fitness products around cost less than $100. In this chapter, we recommend simple products and services that can mean all the difference between pleasure and pain, fun and drudgery. Here are ten cheap fitness investments that are sure to pay you back many times over.

A Personal Training Appointment (or Two or Three)

Hiring a personal trainer sounds like hiring a personal chef — an extravagance that's swell for Oprah but isn't realistic for the rest of us. But we're not talking about a lifetime commitment here. You can hire a trainer for a couple of sessions, either at home or at a health club, to get you started on a program tailored to your goals and your fitness level or to update your current routine. Trainers cost between $25 and $100 per session. If you buddy up with a friend or two, your sessions may cost less.

If you plan to be a short-timer, you need to approach your sessions in a different manner than if you were going to be a regular. Inform your trainer of your intentions so he can cover more in a shorter period of time. And think specifically about your goals for these few sessions. Do you want to learn a routine you can take on business trips? Do you want training advice for a summer cycling vacation? Do you want a program to help you lose fat? Act like you're taking a crash course in French two weeks before you move to Paris: Be prepared to soak up a lot of information. Arm yourself with questions and take notes.

By the end of your final session, make sure you know how to adjust each machine, grip each handle the right way, and perform each exercise using the correct technique. Ask your trainer to write down or print out a program for you to follow when you strike out on your own. One very organized trainer in New York has scanned illustrations and descriptions of hundreds of exercises into her computer. With the click of a mouse, she can print out an easy-to-follow, customized workout plan for her clients — in color, no less. Some trainers charge a bit more for this service, but walking away with a routine on paper is worth the cost.

Even if you plan to take only one or two training sessions, make sure that some of your time is spent on a fitness evaluation, including assessments of your cardiovascular fitness, strength, and flexibility. Any trainer worth his Nikes will use the results to create your program. (For details about fitness evaluations, see Chapter 2.)

Don't pick a trainer because you like the way he fills out his Lycra tights, or because he bills himself as a "Leading Fitness Expert." A trainer should have at least one Dummies Approved certification (see Chapter 14 for a listing) and/or a college or higher degree in exercise physiology or a related field. Ask for references and experience, too.

A New Pair of Shoes

Shoe companies are notorious jargonmeisters. You read about Ground Reaction Inertia Devices and Carbon-Fiber Propulsion Plate Systems, and you feel like you're shopping for a space shuttle, not a running shoe. It's tempting to dismiss the hype and just fit your feet with a plain old pair of sneakers, like you did when you were a kid. But when you cut through the gobbledygook, there *is* some truth in advertising. One of the most important of all fitness purchases is the right pair of shoes for your body and your sport. For the sake of injury prevention and comfort, take your shoe shopping seriously. (See Figure 22-1.)

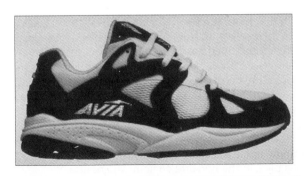

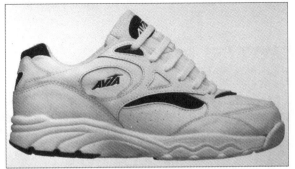

Figure 22-1:
Running and
walking
shoes are
quite
different.

(Photo courtesy of Avia Group International, Inc.)

You may think that a running shoe is fine for your walking program, but walking shoes are more flexible and have firmer heel support than running shoes. Shoes for tennis, golf, and basketball have their own special designs; even sprinters and distance runners have different footwear needs. If you dabble in a variety of activities — walking one day, biking the next, and lifting weight the next — cross-training shoes may suffice. They have an average amount of cushioning, ankle support, and flexibility. But if you spend a lot of time doing one particular activity, invest in shoes designed for that sport.

A decent pair of athletic shoes will cost you at least $40, and in some cases more than double that. But you'll save money down the line; one thing that's always more expensive than a good pair of shoes is a visit to an orthopedist.

Don't try to save a few bucks by buying a knock-off brand from a discount superstore. Bargain brands may look the same, but today's fitness shoes are highly technical. Beneath those swooshes, stripes, and flashy colors, a lot of biomechanical engineering is going on to protect your feet, ankles, and other joints.

It's helpful to buy your shoes at a specialty shop where the sales people are fitness enthusiasts themselves. In New York, runners are blessed with a fine chain of equipment shops called Super Runners. If you're a tennis player, look for a tennis specialty store. Once you find a shoe you're comfortable with, you can save money on future pairs by shopping through a catalog.

No matter what type of athletic shoes you buy, make sure that they feel good from the moment you put them on. Forget this *breaking in* business. Try on several pairs of shoes, and take each one for a test run around the mall. Bounce up and down in them; mime a few quick volleys. If the store won't let you do this, put the shoes back in the box and go somewhere else.

A Library of Exercise Videos

It's hard to take exercise videos seriously when celebrity tapes get all the attention. It's even tougher if you actually *watch* some of these Hollywood videos, like LaToya Jackson's "Step Up Workout," during which the singer prances around in a yellow sequined leotard offering such insights as, "What you have here is a video. So you can always rewind it."

However, you can buy a variety of excellent tapes led by talented instructors you've never heard of, and even a few good videos that feature celebrities. (See Chapter 21 for Dummies Approved videos.) Exercise videos are a great way to learn cutting-edge routines on the cheap.

Even if you're a regular at a health club or have a high-tech home gym, you still may want to own a handful of videos for those days where you need a Simon Says sort of routine. Choose carefully and you'll wind up with a motivating instructor and a safe, effective, creative workout. Most tapes cost around $20, less for shorter videos. For tips on distinguishing the high-quality videos from the schlock, study Chapter 21.

Be aware that exercise videos aren't just for aerobics anymore. You can buy tapes for body building, muscle toning, kick boxing, step aerobics, tai chi, and yoga. And you can find tapes set to the music of your choice — hip hop, disco, pop, new age, and country music. We wouldn't be surprised if an opera tape is floating around somewhere. We recommend building a video library that addresses all aspects of fitness: strength, aerobic conditioning, and flexibility.

A Step

A good step bench is one of the most versatile pieces of exercise equipment you can own. The step was designed to add a challenging dimension to aerobics, but it can easily double as a bench for weight-lifting exercises. However, you need an actual weight bench if you lift more than about 30 pounds in each hand. A step can even be used for many stretching moves. Not bad for a gadget that usually costs less than $75.

You might think a step is a step is a step, but that's not quite true. They come in different shapes and sizes, and some are sturdier than others. Your bench should be long enough for you to safely execute the moves on your favorite step tape and to support you during weight-lifting exercises. Make sure that you can adjust the height of your step. Most steps come with plastic attachments, called risers, that snap underneath the platform. You may want to increase the step height to make your workout more challenging. Besides, you need risers if you're going to use the bench for weight lifting.

The top of your step should be covered with textured rubber so that the platform doesn't get slippery when you start dripping sweat. Look for models made of molded plastic or springy wood. We prefer plastic steps because they're easier to store and adjust. Also, many of the wooden benches have a curved platform, which makes for an uncomfortable weight bench.

Exercise Tubing and Weight Magnets

Rubber tubes and bands are the cheapest and most versatile way to build muscle (see Figure 22-2). Tubes are similar to the surgical tubing used in hospitals; bands are wide, flat sheets of rubber. You can buy a set of both — three tubes and three bands — for less than $20, and you can transport them anywhere since they don't take up much more space than your wallet. Bands work better for some exercises, while tubes feel more comfortable for others. You can learn how to use bands and tubes from a trainer or an exercise video; also, most bands and tubes come with instructions.

You can't build as much raw strength with bands as you can with barbells, but you can get one helluva workout because you're using your muscles in different ways than you do in the weight room. Both bands and tubes come in several different thicknesses, diameters, or widths. The wider, shorter, and less flexible the band is, the more strength required to move it. We suggest buying a whole array of bands. As with dumbbells, the same band won't work for every exercise.

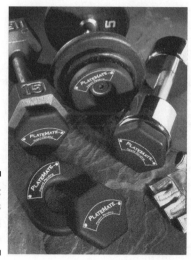

Figure 22-2:
PlateMates
save you big
bucks.

Not everyone has the motivation to pump rubber. If you prefer the feel of cold, hard steel in your hand, we have a fitness bargain to recommend for you, too. A company called PlateMate produces strong magnets that come in two weights: $1^{1}/_{4}$ pounds (a set of two for $20) and $2^{1}/_{2}$ pounds (a set of two for about $30). They're shaped to fit on the ends of your dumbbells, and they work so well that we wonder why no one thought of this before.

Plate Mates can save you big bucks because you need to buy only half as many dumbbell pairs. For instance, instead of buying 5, 8, 10, and 12-pounders, you can simply buy the 5s and 10s, and stick on the PlateMates to fill in the gaps. When you start a weight-training program, it's important to increase your weights by the smallest increment possible. PlateMates are so small you can bring them to the gym to fill in the gaps there, too.

A Massage

Okay, you've been exercising for a solid month. You deserve a reward, and besides, your legs feel a little sore. What better way to treat yourself than with a rubdown?

Massage loosens up kinks in your muscles, relieves stress, and help you relax. Research suggests it may even speed your body's recovery from a workout or injury by delivering more oxygen and nutrients to your muscle cells and restoring muscle and joint mobility. Massage might also make you more mentally alert. In one study, subjects who had been massaged were able to do math problems in half the time, and with half as many errors, as subjects who weren't touched.

While we're not all that motivated to improve our algebra skills, we like massage for a more important reason: It feels soooo good.

Many gyms and spas have massage therapists on call. Depending on where you live, an hour-long massage will run you between $25 and $100. Private sessions in your home usually cost a little more, to compensate for the driving time and the fact that the therapist has to lug a big, heavy table to your door. Most therapists also offer half-hour sessions, but that will feel like a tease. Just when you begin to feel soothed and relaxed, time's up.

There are several different styles of massage. The most popular is Swedish: You lie naked, or close to it, under a sheet or towel while the therapist rubs you with oil or lotion. Shiatzu is similar to acupuncture, only instead of using needles, the therapist uses his hands and feet to stimulate points on your body. You can have a Shiatzu massage lying fully clothed on a floor mat, or you might have a combination Swedish/Shiatzu lying semi-naked on a table.

In most states, massage therapists are required to pass a certification exam. Chances are, any therapist who works at a club or spa will be fully licensed and board certified, but it never hurts to ask. For private home sessions, massage therapy is listed in the yellow pages, but it's best to get a recommendation from a doctor, trainer, or friend you trust. You might think "bad massage" is an oxymoron, but you *can* get rubbed the wrong way. A lousy massage can be ineffective, or even worse, leave you feeling like you've been trampled by a herd of hungry wildebeests.

On behalf of massage therapists everywhere, we offer a bit of massage etiquette.

- **Shower before you hop on to the massage table.** Do not come to your appointment directly from the gym floor, dripping with sweat and wafting a strong, musky odor. No one wants to touch your smelly, icky body. Go hog wild: use deodorant and mouthwash, too.

- **Treat your massage therapists like the licensed professional he is.** Don't confuse him with the people who work in massage parlors. Same word, different meaning.

- **Wear the amount of clothes you're comfortable with.** And only get massaged in areas where you're comfortable being touched. We all have a different tolerance for personal space, and this is, after all, a total stranger rubbing your naked back. Make your feelings known.

- **Speak up.** If your therapist presses too hard or comes to a spot that is especially delicate, tell him to tread lightly. It's not a good idea to kick him. Many therapists have told us that this is a recurring problem. We know one massage therapist who has been kicked so often that he had a sign printed up that reads **DON'T KICK BOB.**

✔ **Arrive on time.** Although this is a laid-back appointment for you, it's your massage therapist's business, and his schedule may be booked tightly. Don't make your therapist so tense that *he* needs a massage.

✔ **Mention any allergies to your massage therapist.** Many use exotic or nut-based oils; some burn incense to aid relaxation. One therapist told us he once used a peanut-based massage oil on a client who was allergic to peanuts. The client's skin immediately developed large purple welts, and the guy had to be rushed to the emergency room.

A Radio/Tape Player

A tape player or radio can be a revelation if you've tried every type of workout in the world and been bored by them all. Listen to whatever keeps you distracted or pumped up — the Weekly Country Countdown, the evening news, Rush Limbaugh, Howard Stern, Dr. Ruth's *Sex For Dummies* on tape.

You can clip your tape player onto your workout shorts, but it's probably more comfortable to wear a sweat-proof pouch that wraps around your waist. If you use cardiovascular machines at home, like a stairclimber or stationary bike, invest in a rack that clips onto the machine and holds your tape player, along with a water bottle and magazine. You can buy these racks at fitness equipment specialty stores. By the way, we haven't had much luck using a portable CD player as a workout companion. They're very sensitive to movement and skip around a lot. They're also bulkier than most tape players or radios.

When you exercise wearing headphones, be aware of your surroundings. This isn't a big deal if you're pedaling the stationary bike at the gym, but you may have a problem if you're hiking through the woods and happen to tune out the growling of a bear. Also, check in with your body from time to time. Are you breathing harder than usual? Are you clenching the stairclimber railings? Are your ankles bleeding from those pricker bushes you just ran through?

Never listen to music while you're riding a road bike or a mountain bike — you need to be able to hear cars and other cyclists at all times. And don't wear headphones while running and walking near traffic. It's not a good idea to cut off one of your most important senses in a high-risk situation.

A Water Bottle

We won't lecture you here about the importance of drinking water; we take care of that in Chapter 4. But we *will* tell you that you're a heckuva lot more likely to down your 8 to 10 glasses a day if you carry around a water bottle — at the gym, at your office, in front of the TV. If water is right in front of you, you'll drink it. If you have to hop off the treadmill and traipse half way across the room, you won't.

Honestly, there's no excuse not to own a water bottle. They're often offered as freebies when you join a gym or buy a bike, and even if you have to break down and pay for one, you're still only out $5. Nevertheless — and this is a curious phenomenon — we happen to know a number of people, primarily of the male persuasion, who consider it a sign of weakness to carry around a water bottle at the gym. One of these guys not only refuses to carry a bottle, but also will not listen to music or read a magazine. He apparently is under the impression that any pleasure he might derive while exercising will reduce his testosterone levels.

If, unlike our friend, you're interested in making your workouts pleasant and safe, any old water bottle will suffice. However, we do prefer clear water bottles; if your bottle is red, you're less likely to notice when moldy grime starts growing inside. That happens when you forget to clean out your bottle periodically. One bottle we like is made by Specialized, a bike company. The spout is covered with a clever valve patterned after the valves in your heart. Water flows easily when you squeeze the bottle; otherwise it stays put and drip free.

Even better than a water bottle is a gizmo called a CamelBak, an ingenious invention that ranks right up there with remote control, the Internet, and the vertical bagel slicer. It's an insulated pouch you can wear like a backpack or a waist pack when you're cycling, walking, hiking, or playing Scrabble with your grandma. To drink water, you suck on a flexible straw that hangs over your shoulder. We resisted the CamelBak for a long time because it looks uncomfortable. We figured, who needs to lug around extra weight on your back? But after 10 minutes, you don't even notice you have the thing on, and you drink twice as much water as usual because it's so convenient. (See Figure 22-3.)

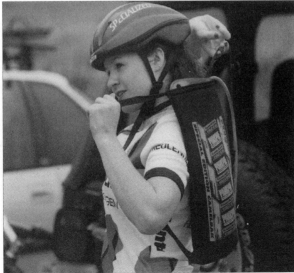

Figure 22-3:
Drinking water the easy way: with a CamelBak.

(Photo courtesy of Tina Gerson.)

A Workout Log

You might think it's obsessive to track your workouts in an exercise diary; after all, who needs extra paperwork? Actually, you might. A workout log offers proof of your commitment to exercise. Nothing is more motivating than seeing your accomplishments on paper.

Jot down as many details as you can think of without making yourself feel like a court reporter at a deposition. Keep track of how long, how far, how fast, and how hard you exercised. At the beginning of each week, write down your goals; at the end of the week, make a note of whether you accomplished them. In Chapter 3, we list a number of other particulars worth noting. We also feature a sample diary page.

A workout diary need not be a fancy affair — a notebook from the drugstore will suffice. Personally, we're partial to store-bought logs designed especially for the purpose of tracking daily workouts. They lend a sense of importance to what you're doing, and many are filled with good training tips, inspirational quotes, and important reminders. They have a fill-in-the-blank format so you don't forget to include essential information.

You can purchase workout diaries for less than $20 at bookstores and sporting good stores or through various catalogs. There are logs designed for specific activities — like walking, cycling, and weight lifting. One of our favorite sport-specific logs is "The Four Seasons Walking and Training Logbook" (Creative Walking, Inc.) by Rob Sweetgall. You also can buy all-purpose logs that provide room to track weight-training exercises *and* cardiovascular workouts. Our favorite in this category is "The Ultimate Workout Log" (Houghton Mifflin), but maybe that's because one of us wrote it. We also like computerized logs such as Bill Rodgers' "Winrunner" and a software program called "PC Coach." These programs spit out charts and graphs so you can easily see trends and patterns in your training.

A Jump Rope

Jump ropes might remind you of pony-tailed little girls in school yards, but don't be fooled: Skipping rope offers some very real, very adult fitness benefits. It strengthens your cardiovascular system, improves your agility, burns tons of calories, and tones your thighs, calves, abdominals, back, chest, and shoulders. You can take your rope with you anywhere; and to use it, you don't need any more space than a small coffee table takes up. Even for a super-deluxe rope, you won't spend more than $30.

Jump ropes have been subjected to a bit of technology in the past few years. Forget about the frayed cloth ropes you used as a kid. Even leather is history. Many ropes are now made of tough, molded plastic, metal wire coated in acrylic, or space-age polymers the names of which we can't pronounce, let alone spell. These materials make for ropes that turn faster and more smoothly. Look for features like soft foam or rubber handles, which prevent callusing, and ball bearing-like swivel action between the cord and handles.

Many people avoid jumping rope because they view it as a high-impact activity. But if you do it right, it's more like a medium-impact activity on the order of a brisk walk. The secret is staying low. Your feet should barely clear the floor, and you should bend your knees just slightly.

Use a light rope if your aim is to work on skill and agility and to jump fast. Fat, weighted ropes work well for building upper body muscular endurance, but using them for fancy foot work or special tricks is a bit like asking a Clydesdale to run the Kentucky Derby. Buy one of each and you can mix up your workouts.

When you use a light rope, keep your arms relaxed and slightly bent, and keep your upper-body movements to a minimum. Rather than turn your arms in big circles, simply let your wrists swivel slightly. Start with a few short sets — about 30 jumps — and rest by marching in place between sets. Gradually increase the number of sets and jumps per set while decreasing the time you spend marching. Eventually, you'll be able to jump 10 minutes or more continuously. Humming the theme song from Rocky helps. It's tough to build up to long periods of jumping rope because it's a very intense activity. It's best used as a cross-training workout.

Chapter 23

Ten Fitness Rip-Offs

. . . .

In This Chapter

▶ Pseudo science

▶ False gods of fitness

▶ Bogus buzzwords

▶ Deceptive infomercials

▶ Gadgets that claim to save the world

. . . .

*F*alling short of your fitness goals can be discouraging, especially when you blame the failure on yourself. Maybe you think your spare tire hasn't disappeared because last week you forgot to wear your "waist trimmer" device. Or maybe your think you didn't try hard enough to follow that expensive diet plan you bought off an infomercial.

Well, the failure might not be your fault. You may have been duped by the unscrupulous segment of the fitness industry. Some companies count on the public's naiveté to keep the money rolling in. They sell "low-fat" foods that actually have plenty of fat and exercise gizmos that, off the record, they admit are useless. Many manufacturers use scientific mumbo jumbo to promote products based on nothing more than wishful thinking. This chapter helps you become a more savvy fitness consumer.

Spot-Reducing Gadgets

One of the most persistent fitness myths of all time is that you can choose a blubbery spot on your body and — by wearing stretchy waist belts or by exercising — melt away that particular hunk of fat (see Figure 23-1). Companies are making a killing perpetuating this lie. One company has sold 15 million "waist trimmers" — thick, neoprene belts that, according to the company's catalog, "melt unwanted inches." (The company also makes "thigh trimmers" and "reducing shorts.") At best, products like this make you sweat more, so you may temporarily lose some water weight, which you gain right back as soon as you take a drink. At worst, these products give the impression that excess sweating is good for you; in fact, dehydration can lead to serious medical problems. When we asked a marketing executive how, in good conscience, his company could sell these products, he shrugged and said, "Hey, that's what middle America wants." He also pointed out that the products do not claim to melt fat; however, we doubt the company was trying to paint the image of "melting" water.

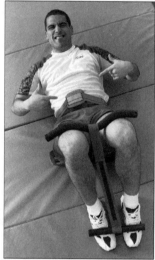

Figure 23-1:
Spot
reducing?

(Photo courtesy of Dan Kron.)

Remarkably, some companies don't even bother toying with semantics to justify their claims; they just come right out and lie. At a recent trade show, we came across another brand of neoprene shorts which, according to the company's literature, cause significant fat loss "around critical areas such as the thighs, buttock, and stomach . . . [through] continuous micro-massage of the fatty tissue." What's more, the company maintains that the "patented interwoven design . . . helps tighten and tone muscles." The company claims to have sold more than a million of these shorts in Europe and is now bringing 'em to the United States.

It's not just these souped-up girdles that cultivate the myth of spot reduction. Many exercise products are guilty, too. In an advertisement for a plastic abdominal gizmo, one woman says, "It took me only three minutes a day to have perfectly flat abs." Another abdominal gadget ad shows two men side-by-side: One has an enormous gut, the other a sculpted waistline. "Go from flab to abs," the ad says. The fact is, abdominal exercises can only tone your abdominals, and many of them don't even do a good job of that. To lose that gut, you've got to reduce your overall body fat with a sensible eating and exercise program.

Pseudo Science

"Scientifically proven" — when it comes to the fitness industry, these two words often translate to "It works because we say so."

Consider the European "weight loss" shorts we described earlier. When we mentioned to a product representative that the company's claims couldn't possibly be true, he became quite excited and said, "Oh, but we have medical studies to prove it!" The man was kind enough to mail us a study, which — we're wondering if he realizes this — actually concludes that the product did *not* cause "any significant difference where the waist or hips are concerned." The women in the four-month study, who wore these shorts 10 hours a day, did lose inches in their thighs, but the study's authors would not attribute these changes to the pants. One thing the researchers did conclude: For best results, the pants should be worn in conjunction with proper diet and exercise.

Many companies cite scientific research without telling you where the studies were conducted. When we asked a representative for one of those "rider" aerobic machines to back up his claims about the machine's calorie-burning potential, he said "laboratory studies" have proven the company's claims. When we asked who did the research, he admitted the studies were carried out by a company he owned. This is like admitting that your mother was the judge of a beauty contest you won; maybe you *were* the best looking, but we need to hear it from an unbiased party.

Furthermore, don't assume that the word "proven" means that *any* studies were conducted — anywhere. An ad for a protein shake that promised miraculous weight loss and muscle building results included scientific footnotes at the bottom of the page. When we went to the library to find these studies, the journals had either ceased publication years earlier or were so obscure that even the New York City Public Library has no record of them.

Other claims try to dazzle you by stringing a bunch of scientific hocus pocus together, rather than explaining what the product does in simple terms. We recently heard one rep say that his machine was "a kinetic, closed-chain, multi-joint, functional modality." Why didn't he just say that it uses your muscles the way you use them in real life?

Celebrity Endorsements

"I've endorsed products that are complete crap," one world-class athlete admitted to us. He has promoted cycling shorts so shabby they don't last more than a few trips through the spin cycle. "I'll wear this stuff in a race once a month and then train in something else," he says. Some top bicycle racers endorse bikes they don't actually ride; the paint job says one brand, but they're actually riding something else.

We're not saying every product endorsed by an athlete or celebrity is junk, but don't think these endorsements guarantee quality. Even celebrities who appear to be so wealthy they couldn't possibly need more money sometimes lend their name to shoddy merchandise. One popular athlete puts his name on a gadget that, off the record, even its manufacturers admit is cheaply made and over-priced. The promotional literature claims that the athlete offered his endorsement because "There is no better fitness product." When we asked a marketing executive the real reason this celebrity endorsed the product, the executive responded, "Why do you *think?*"

Use your common sense: These people are getting paid, in some cases millions of dollars. When that kind money is offered, it's fairly easy to rationalize the endorsement of poor-quality products. Athletes and celebrities tend to have short-lived careers, and at some point their name may be their only asset. "There's a lot you can talk yourself into," one athlete says. "You figure, I'm just a cog in the machine. I've gotta make a living. And if the public's dumb enough to buy this stuff, that's their problem. I mean, they can go read Consumer Reports."

Lifetime Gym Memberships

Lifetime gym memberships are illegal in many states, but that doesn't stop some gyms from offering them anyway. Even if a three-year membership is being dangled under your nose, don't be taken in by promises of cheaper rates and locked-in monthly payments. It's not a good idea to sign up for more than a year. You don't know where you'll be living three years from now, or whether the club will still exist.

A few years back, the New York Attorney General won a $2.5-million judgment against the owner of a company that had closed four health clubs without notice. Washington's Attorney General forced owners of six clubs to pay $20,000 to members who had joined clubs that closed soon thereafter. One New York city gym was selling lifetime memberships up to the day before it closed its doors forever. Duped members were so angry that they broke in and carried away equipment.

False Gods of Fitness

The fitness industry is notorious for hyped credentials. Beware of someone who calls himself an "Internationally Recognized Fitness Expert" but has no professional certification or college degree in the fitness field (see Chapter 15 for a list of legitimate credentials). Some personalities have actually trade-marked tags like "America's Personal Trainer" and "Trainer to the Stars," as if there could be only one person who could claim such a title.

Another trainer whose book jacket refers to him as a "fitness guru" defines an expert as someone who has spent a minimum of ten years in the profession, obtained consistent results over a period of time, and has hands-on experience. He makes no mention of education or certification. Could it be that he has no education himself? At the same time, don't be automatically impressed by university degrees. One best-selling fitness video instructor splashes her Ph.D. in huge letters all over her tapes and books. She does have a doctoral degree, all right — only it's in English literature, a fact you can find in small print on the back of her products.

Keep in mind that terms like "exercise physiologist," "personal trainer," and "nutritionist," which imply a high level of training and education, have no legal meanings. Anyone can use them. To figure out whether someone is a legitimate expert, see Chapter 15.

Bogus Buzzwords

Product manufacturers love to manipulate consumers by spewing jargon. Sometimes they use words that don't actually mean anything; other times they use legitimate words out of context. Pay close attention when you see the following buzzwords.

Cellulite

Hundreds of products claim to banish "cellulite," the puckery fat that tends to form on the butt, hips, and thighs of most women and some men. There are creams, scrubs, diet plans, exercise programs, powders, wraps, and girdles that claim to dissolve this bumpy blubber. These products may have been "used in European spas for centuries," but we assure you not one of them works. Scientifically speaking, cellulite doesn't even exist. It's marketing hype for plain old fat that clumps at various points on your body. The ripple effect is caused by a network of connective tissue fibers that attach muscle to skin and compartmentalize the fat like stitching on a quilt. You reduce cellulite the same way you reduce any fat: through a healthy diet and regular exercise. However, you may never lose the ripples. For some people, they're a genetic fact of life.

Total-body workout

This popular term should refer to any type of exercise that involves most of your major muscles. Some exercise machines do offer legitimate total-body workouts, such as the VersaClimber, cross-country ski machines, rowing machines, and several stationary bikes with upper-body rowing arms. However, these days manufacturers are using the term to describe just about any exercise gizmo, even if it only works those small muscles behind your left ear.

Also, don't assume that because your arms and legs are moving at the same time, you're getting a first-rate workout. Sometimes the arms are just along for the ride; they move because the machine's leg and arm mechanisms are linked together. Furthermore, don't assume that moving more body parts means you're burning more calories. Depending on the type of machine and how well it's built, you may burn more calories by going for a brisk walk or riding a bike. We've found most treadmills with arm attachments to be of poor quality, difficult to use, and not very effective. One more thing to look for is sneaky wording in product claims like "part of a total-body workout." That's like saying "part of a balanced breakfast" when you're referring to a sugar-coated cereal.

Fat burning

There's nothing wrong with the term "fat burning," but its definition gets stretched all the time. Consider a video called *The Fat-Burning Workout.* The tape features a weight-lifting routine and says you "burn fat like crazy." Sure, you burn some fat when you lift weights; in fact, you burn at least some fat calories any time you exercise. But the title implies you're getting an aerobic workout, which burns much more fat and calories than weight lifting. A marketing representative wasn't too apologetic about the use of this term. "The nature of the business — and it's a sales business — is that people will capitalize on any exercise trend that's available," she told us.

"Fat burning" also is commonly used in claims for powders, pills, and other so-called health food products. "Pure fat burning — a revolutionary breakthrough in sports nutrition!" claims one bottle of diet pills. The marketing hoopla for these products implies that they have some magical effect on fat — that you will burn extra fat just by swallowing them. This assertion isn't limited to manufactured products, either. Some people claim that grapefruits and red peppers have the power to melt away body fat.

Just minutes a day

When you hear these four words, ask yourself two questions: Just minutes a day to do *what?* And how *many* minutes a day? One aerobic "rider" advertisement says the machine "takes just minutes a day," but it doesn't specify what benefits you derive from these precious few minutes. An ad for a "5-Minute Body Shaper" uses some sneaky wording, too. According to the ad, one of the benefits of this gizmo is a toned waist; and it's true, most people can do an adequate abdominal training workout in five minutes. However, the ad also maintains that you can get "super aerobic and fat-burning benefits" by using the product for *20* minutes.

Realize that building a new body takes time and patience — a fact that we don't consider depressing. Stick with exercise for a while and you'll find that the process of getting in shape can be just as fun and rewarding as the results. You sleep better, you feel less stress, and you have more energy. It feels good to work out. Really.

Infomercials

In 1984, when the Federal Trade Commission abolished limits on the amount of commercial time a television station could air, the commission unleashed a monster: the infomercial. When it comes to fitness products, there's not a whole lot of info in these half-hour commercials that often masquerade as talk shows. Typically, they're filled with exaggerated claims, shameless testimonials, outlandish stunts, and lots of scientific gobbledygook — all intended to separate you from your dollar.

A few things you should know before you buy that "revolutionary" new gadget, pill, potion, plan, or powder: The audience members — those wholesome folks who whip themselves into a frenzy at the mere mention of the product at hand — are usually paid. The "experts" and individuals who offer testimonials are always paid. Often, the people offering testimonials have never even tried the product they're gushing over. One woman we interviewed gave an emotional testimonial for an exercise video, even though she had never even watched it. "I just wanted to be on TV," she told us. How can the infomercials get away with this? One infomercial host who touts an abdominal toning gadget tells us, "The people you have seen are real!"

We don't think there's anything wrong with inspiring passion and motivation among the masses, as long as you're not selling ocean-front property in Arizona. Unfortunately, many fitness gizmos advertised in infomercials won't do you any good. And on some infomercials, there's no shortage of outright lies. When you hear that the product is "available for a limited time only," it's typically only limited to the time during which people are willing to buy it. If a product is selling like hotcakes, believe us, it's not going to disappear. As for the claim that it's "not sold in stores anywhere," it probably is, and if it isn't, it will be soon — and probably for a few dollars less. The ThighMaster costs $2 less at Woolworth's than it does on TV.

Do not think that the infomercial producers have your best interests at heart. Many of them are counting on you to be suckered into buying some piece of junk you don't need and will never use. At a recent trade show, we mentioned to an infomercial executive that a particular gadget appeared to be a waste of money. "I wouldn't disagree with you," he said, smiling. "But we've sold 20,000 units in the first month." When we mentioned that the product appeared to be extremely flimsy, he agreed and said, "Well, 80 percent of these things are never even used."

The Federal Trade Commission has made an effort to crack down on the infomercials that cross that line from exaggeration to outright lies. The producer of a European diet patch that was supposed to suppress appetite was slapped with a $1.5 million fine because the product didn't work. Several more infomercial health gadgets are currently under investigation.

If you're tempted to buy an infomercial product, jot down the number and *wait* before ordering. You may feel differently about that Ginzu Rider in the light of day. Also, read our Ten Commandments of Buying TV Fitness Gadgets in Chapter 18.

Misleading Food Labels and Packages

While the U.S. Food and Drug Administration has done a pretty good job cleaning up misleading food labels, some label claims still cross the line. The FDA allows for a 25 percent variance in calorie reporting to account for differences between testing methods and differences that may occur from one package of a product to the next. Some manufacturers use this ruling for creative accounting purposes. *New York* magazine once did an expose on low-fat muffins and treats. Many of the products listed exactly 25 percent fewer calories than independent testing found. In some cases, the treats had four times the amount of fat and calories than what was listed on the packaging. The FDA recommends sticking with nationally advertised brands whose fat and calorie contents are subject to more scrutiny and whose manufacturers have a lot more to lose if they get caught in a lie.

Diet Centers Staffed by Unqualified Consultants

There are several reasons to avoid commercial weight-loss centers, including the expensive and unsatisfying prepackaged foods and the fact that an estimated 90 percent of the participants who lose 25 pounds regain the weight within three years. However, the most compelling reason to stay away from some of these places is the lack of qualifications of the staff. While some centers are staffed by registered dietitians and medical professionals, many are run by people who, despite the white lab coats they often wear, have no more nutrition education than you do.

A friend of ours named Stephanie went through a one-week training program to become a "consultant" at of one of the country's largest weight-loss centers. "I felt like the whole program was a con game," she told us. "We learned nothing about nutrition. The whole object was to hard-sell the client. Our instructor wrote on the blackboard, 'Will that be cash, check, or money order?' We had to repeat that phrase over and over and over again. We were told to never, ever take no for an answer."

Stephanie says she was instructed to sell her clients $80 to $100 worth of pre-packaged food each week — even though the clients were primarily low-income. "These people couldn't buy their babies a bottle of milk, but we were supposed to get them to buy every meal from us." Stephanie quit her job after four days. "I just couldn't look the clients in the face," she says.

The consequences of uninformed staffers range from the tragic — many deaths have been attributed to drastic weight loss due to poor supervision — to the ridiculous. Consider the experiences of freelance journalist Laura Fraser, who has written a book about the diet industry called *Losing It* (Dutton, due out in 1997). When Fraser felt her weight creeping up, she went to a popular commercial weight-loss center. During her initial consultation, Fraser, who's 5-foot-6, weighed in at 165 pounds — while wearing thick-soled boots and a heavy winter jacket stuffed with a personal stereo, a book, a wallet, and keys. (Her counselor didn't suggest she remove any of her clothing.) The counselor then punched some numbers into the computer and told Fraser that her goal range should be 120 to 133 pounds. When Fraser said she'd be more comfortable aiming for 145 because she'd once had a serious eating disorder, the counselor said that weight was "not healthy" and completely ignored the eating disorder issue.

A week later — after eating $92.98 worth of prepackaged food — Fraser went back to the center for a weigh-in. This time her counselor instructed her to take off her sweatshirt and running shoes before she got on the scale. The marker settled on 151 pounds. "You've lost . . . 14 pounds!" her counselor said, showering her with congratulations. "That's a new center record!" Fraser went home and weighed her coat, boots, and everything else she had worn the week before: 11 pounds. She then called a well-known obesity expert who told her that the only way she could lose 14 pounds in one week is through catastrophic illness. Either that or amputation.

If you feel you need professional guidance to lose weight, see a registered dietitian (not merely a "nutritionist") who can help you get on a sensible, realistic eating plan that's customized to your lifestyle and food preferences. Programs such as Weight Watchers and Overeaters Anonymous also tend to have better success rates than many of the programs advertised on TV.

Gadgets that Claim to Save the World

One of the latest trends among product manufacturers is to claim that a single machine can do it all. Consider a $200 plastic gizmo that resembles a lawn chair and is designed to strengthen your thighs and abdominals. According to the marketing materials for this so-called cross trainer, "People are tired of the aerobics class scene. Too much impact. Too much hassle. Too much time. But the . . . Cross Trainer solves all of those problems." What we want to know is, *how?* It's impossible for muscle-toning exercises to take the place of an aerobic workout.

Chapter 24

Ten Common Fitness Injuries

Sometimes, exercise hurts. If you never lift anything heavier than a telephone receiver and then start lifting dumbbells, naturally you're going to feel some soreness. That type of pain is nothing to worry about. But, if you wake up the morning after a weight-lifting session and feel like your left arm has been shredded by a combine, that's a different story.

Good pain is achy, dull, and very general. Usually, you feel it throughout an entire muscle or over a large area of your body. Bad pain — the type that signals injury — often tends to be sharp and specific. It usually hurts when you do certain movements, like bending your knee or lifting your arm overhead. This chapter covers ten injuries common to people who exercise. We tell you how to recognize and treat them — and how to prevent them from happening in the first place.

Strains and Sprains

First, let's clear up some terminology. One of your coworkers might hobble into the office announcing he has "strained" a muscle — or maybe he says he has "pulled" a muscle. These terms are interchangeable, but they're *not* synonymous with "sprain."

When you *strain* a muscle, you over-stretch or tear the tendon, the tough, cord-like end of the muscle that attaches to the bone. Strains happen when you push yourself harder than normal, like when you challenge your kid brother to a 100-yard dash. A *sprain* refers to a torn or over-stretched ligament, the connective tissue that joins two bones together. You can sprain a *joint* — like when you turn your ankle while stepping off a curb — but you can't sprain a *muscle*.

Two of the most commonly strained muscles are the hamstrings (rear thigh muscles) and inner thigh (groin) muscles. These muscles often pull because they're tight and because most people don't take five minutes to warm up before working out. You know you've strained your hamstring if a sharp pain shoots up the back of your thigh when you straighten your leg. You have a groin pull if a stabbing pain prevents you from lifting your leg out to the side or in toward your other leg. In both cases, you may feel a lump or a knot where the muscle has tightened up. Stop the offending activity for a few days, until the muscle repairs itself. Otherwise, you may be headed for a full-blown tear. Instead of being laid up for a few days, you could be sidelined for several months. Light stretching may be beneficial.

To speed up the healing process for a strain, apply ice to the injured area. (See the sidebar in this chapter for icing tips.) Gentle massage may help work out muscle kinks. To prevent future pulls, carefully stretch your muscles every day, always after a thorough warm-up, and increase your exercise program on a gradual basis. Check your shoes, too. Athletic shoes with flared heels — heels that are wider on the bottom than on the top — may restrain your foot and ankle from normal movement. That, in turn, may cause your thigh muscles to tighten up. Shoes that are too big cause the same type of problems.

Sprains occur most commonly at the ankle. If you've sprained your ankle badly, you might hear a loud pop or tearing sound when the injury happens. Usually you're left with a bruise and swelling, and you can't place any of your weight on the injured foot without pain. The treatment for a sprain is RICE (see the sidebar "RICE, RICE baby").

Shin Splints

This is a catch-all term for shin pain. You can develop shin splints from doing more exercise than your body is ready to handle, or simply from introducing a new aspect to your training, such as wearing a new pair of shoes, running downhill, or jogging on the beach when you normally jog on asphalt.

To cure shin splints, back off for a few days. When you're free of pain, start back up gradually. Don't increase your exercise time or distance by more than 10 percent a week. Ice helps by reducing inflammation and by dulling the pain. For shin splints, we recommend the ice massage method described in the sidebar "RICE, RICE baby".

To prevent shin splints, strengthen your shin muscles so they work more in harmony with your calves, the muscles that operate in opposition to them. Here's one simple exercise: Stand with your weight distributed evenly over the entire length of your foot, and lift and lower your toes and the balls of your feet 20 to 30 times. Ask a trainer to show you some other shin exercises.

RICE, RICE baby

If your doctor or trainer prescribes RICE for an injury, he isn't suggesting some new-age nutritional treatment. He's referring to the common way to treat sports injuries: Rest, Ice, Compression, and Elevation. Usually, this treatment is all you need to get back on your feet, particularly if you RICE diligently for the first 48 hours after an injury.

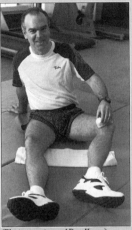

(Photo courtesy of Dan Kron.)

✔ **Rest:** Stop doing activities that aggravate your injury. (If you sprain your ankle, don't try to "walk it off.") Rest can often mean the difference between an injury that heals right away and one that nags you for months. But don't use your injury as an excuse to quit exercising altogether. Simply choose an activity that doesn't hurt. If you pull a hamstring, there's no reason to stop upper-body weight training.

✔ **Ice:** Ice reduces swelling and deadens pain by constricting blood flow into the injured area. Ice for 15 to 20 minutes three or four times a day for as long as you feel pain. It's not true that ice is useless after the first day. You can apply ice with a pack, a plastic bag full of cubes, or a package of frozen corn. Just don't allow the ice to rest directly on your skin; otherwise, you're inviting a whole new list of problems, such as ice burns.

One of our favorite icing techniques is ice massage. Fill a Dixie cup $^3/_4$ full of water and stick it in the freezer. When the water freezes, peel the cup down, so you have what resembles an ice cream cone of ice. Use this to massage the injured area in a circular motion for as long as you can take it, usually 4 or 5 minutes. Ice massage penetrates deeper into your muscles than passively throwing an ice pack over the injured area. Be sure to keep the ice moving.

✔ **Compression:** Put pressure on the injured area to keep the swelling down. Wrap a damp Ace Bandage around the injury, or buy a special knee, elbow, or wrist wrap or brace. Wrap tightly enough so you feel some tension but not so firmly that you cut off your circulation or feel numbness.

✔ **Elevation:** Elevating your injured body part reduces swelling by allowing fluids and waste products to drain from the area, much like water runs downstream. (Waste products are the bits of broken blood cells and other inflammatory agents hanging around the injury.) If your ankle is injured, you don't need to raise it so high that it's perpendicular to the ground. Propping it up on a couple of fluffy pillows will do. Elevation works best when used in conjunction with the rest of the RICE treatment.

Also, be sure to replace your athletic shoes often, so your shins don't take a pounding from lack of cushioning. We know one guy who solved his chronic shin splint problem overnight by buying a pair of shoes with a slightly wider heel. This seemed to suit his running style; a podiatrist or sports medicine specialist can help you find the solution that suits *your* style. If all else fails, he may make a special pair of inserts, called *orthotics,* to properly position your foot in your shoes.

Achilles Tendinitis

Achilles was the mighty Greek warrior whose mother dipped him into the waters of the River Styx to make him invulnerable. The problem was, she missed a spot: the point on the back of his heel where she held him. This area, where the Achilles tendon connects to the heel, is a weak spot for just about anyone who happens to stand or move in an upright position, especially runners, walkers, in-line skaters, cyclists, and tennis players. Once the Achilles tendon gets swollen, sore, or inflamed, you have *Achilles tendinitis.*

The most common culprit is a calf muscle that's too short and tight. A regular stretching program that focuses on your foot, calf, and hamstring muscles may take care of the problem. Our old friend ice also can reduce swelling and relieve pain. If you wear high heels, wean yourself off them and switch to flats; heels can contribute to Achilles tendinitis by keeping your calves in a shortened position for hours on end.

For chronic Achilles inflammation, the remedy that works best is something many diehard exercisers don't want to hear: stop exercising. Give your Achilles tendon a few days off to rest and repair. Ice the spot, but don't do *any* stretching or strengthening exercises that put pressure on your heel. (You can swim, but only if you feel no pain.) If your Achilles problem persists, see an orthopedist or a podiatrist. You may need more aggressive remedies.

Knee Pain

On the surface, the knee seems to be a wonderfully uncomplicated mechanism with a pretty simple job description: to bend and straighten your leg. In reality, the knee is hardwired with more muscles, tendons, ligaments, and cartilage than any other joint in your body. Perhaps that's why it is often the first joint to break down.

Knee pain comes in more varieties than Baskin-Robbins ice cream. It can be caused by a tear in a ligament, a tendon, a muscle, or a piece of cartilage (the cushioning that prevents two bones from rubbing against each other). We can't diagnose your specific ailment, but we can tell you this: Knee pain is often the result of doing the same movement over and over again. Typically, you can't trace it to a specific incident; it's more likely the result of one bike-a-thon or skate-a-thon too many.

Cross training is a good way to avoid knee pain. By varying your exercise activities — jogging one day, cycling the next — you use different muscles, or at least you use the same muscles in a different way. You can still injure your knees with a cross-training regimen, so be careful not to overdo it. If you do feel knee pain coming on, cut back on your exercise routine or switch to an activity that doesn't aggravate the situation. Some people with knee problems from running can bicycle with no pain whatsoever, and vice versa. Ice is always a good choice, too. But don't mess around here. If pain persists, recurs frequently, or is caused by a single incident, get thee to a doctor ASAP.

Stress Fractures

The first modern-day athletes to experience *stress fractures* were soldiers in World War II. The Army took out-of-shape civilians, placed heavy packs on their backs, and sent them off to march for miles and miles. Soon the rookies were complaining about foot pain, but since nothing showed up on X-rays, doctors assumed they were faking it. Often, a second X-ray would be taken several weeks later, revealing a fuzziness along the bone. Bone callus (a build-up of bone material) was forming; the healing process had started. Today, long distance runners, hikers, backpackers, and in-line skaters are the most common sufferers of stress fractures.

Stress fractures are typically not one but a *series* of micro-fractures or hairline breaks that run along the bone. Typically, you don't have a warning sign, like a sudden snap or pop. More often, you wake up one day with pain radiating down the top of one or two of your toes to the center of your foot. You may feel pain when you walk. You may even notice redness or swelling on top of your foot. When you press your finger on that spot, you feel a stabbing pain that immediately grabs your attention.

Don't try to treat this kind of pain yourself. It definitely warrants a visit to your orthopedist or podiatrist, who will X-ray your foot to make sure that your injury is a stress fracture. The doctor will probably prescribe anti-inflammatory medication, ice, and elevation, and implore you to stay off your feet. In extreme cases, he may even put you in a soft or hard cast.

If you think that you have a stress fracture, stop exercising *immediately*. We can't tell you how many times marathoners in agonizing foot pain at mile nine go on to finish the race anyway. When you continue to run on a stress fracture, you transform a minor injury into one that can take months to heal.

Lower Back Pain

Nearly 80 percent of us utter the words "Oh, my aching back," at some point in our adult lives. You may be referring to a nagging stiffness that makes tying your shoes a difficult proposition, or you may be referring to chronic, debilitating pain that keeps you curled up in bed for weeks at a time. While regular workouts (especially abdominal and back exercises) can do a lot to help *prevent* back pain, fitness activities can also *cause* back problems, particularly if you do a lot of pounding or use improper form when you run or cycle. You also can wrench your back by failing to bend your legs when you lift a weight off the rack. (Of course, you also can throw out your back by doing completely nonathletic activities, too, such as improperly lifting a child or a bag of groceries.)

In many instances of back pain, the worst thing you can do is just stay in bed. This weakens the very muscles that need to be loosened up and strengthened. Another time-honored treatment, the heating pad, makes many back conditions worse by further inflaming the nerves.

So what helps back pain heal? Time, for one thing. Many cases of back pain disappear within four weeks without any treatment at all. If that doesn't work, you can see a variety of professionals. Most experts believe that the majority of back pain is muscular in nature and can be treated successfully with nonsurgical procedures, such as exercise, massage, physical therapy, and chiropractic. (To find a good chiropractor, get a recommendation from a friend, or better yet, from a medical doctor.) Swimming, walking, and yoga seem to be the best activities for limbering up tight back muscles. Back and abdominal strengthening exercises supervised by a physical therapist or trainer experienced in dealing with back pain can give you long-term immunity from further recurrence of back pain.

For an episode you're having *right now*, ice and gentle movement are probably your best bet for relief. Some experts recommend seeing a *physiatrist,* a medical doctor who rehabilitates the disabled; physiatrists are more likely to prescribe exercise than medication or surgery. If you experience severe back pain that prevents you from going about your normal activities, see your physician first to rule out any underlying medical causes, such as kidney infections or intestinal disorders.

Tennis Elbow

You don't need to be a tennis player to experience a tenderness on the bony bump on the outside of your elbow or an aching sensation whenever you straighten your arm or pick up an object. Tennis elbow, inflammation of the tendons in your elbow, can be caused by carrying a gym bag or briefcase with a straight arm or by lifting weights with improper form.

When you lift weights or use a stairclimber, take care not to lock your elbows. This is a very common mistake, and the people who do it fail to make the connection between their elbow pain and their sloppy form.

 If you feel pain in your elbow, stop the offending activity. Ice can help, and you can buy a brace or slip-on wrap at the drugstore to help support your elbow. Your doctor might even suggest you wear the brace while you sleep, to keep up continuous compression on your elbow joint. To help prevent future episodes of tennis elbow, strengthen your wrists and your triceps, the muscles at the back of your arm.

Neck Pain

You don't realize how useful your neck is until you can't move it, like when the guy standing next to you asks a question, and answering him requires a three-quarter turn of your body.

Just about anything can cause neck pain — you might sleep on your neck in a funny way or spend too much time cradling the phone on your shoulder. But it's often caused by fitness activities. We're talking about poor weight-lifting technique, such as turning your head to the side while doing a shoulder press, and poor upper-body exercise posture, such as letting your head droop forward when you walk. If you experience neck pain after a traumatic incident, such as getting beaned on the head with a soccer ball, check with your doctor immediately. Also consult a physician if you have constant or recurring neck pain.

Neck pain of the nontraumatic kind usually signals tightness in the muscles of your neck, upper back, and/or shoulders. When you press a finger into the area between your shoulder and your neck and there's very little give or springiness, you have tight neck muscles. One remedy is to gently stretch your neck muscles; if you feel tightness on the right side of your neck, tip your head toward your left shoulder and stretch your right arm downward. Massage is also very useful for freeing up knotty neck muscles. You can give yourself a massage, but somehow that isn't as satisfying as enlisting a friend, significant other, or professional therapist.

Ice, usually an injury-friendly treatment, isn't always the best choice for neck pain. If you're stiff to begin with, applying ice may cause you to tense up even more. If your trouble is a stiff neck, moist heat in the form of a warm wash cloth, shower massage, or whirlpool may be the way to go.

Rotator Cuff Injuries

What's the capital of Belgium? If you can't raise your hand to answer that question, you might have a rotator cuff tear. Throwing, catching, and lifting your arm out to the side may also be painful. (By the way, the answer is *Brussels*.)

The *rotator cuff* is a group of four muscles that surround and protect your shoulder joint. They're particularly delicate and susceptible to injury. They can tear if your arm is violently pulled or twisted or if you fall with your arm outstretched. But the most likely scenario is damage from repetitive movements like throwing, catching, swimming, and lifting weights that are too heavy. Which movements cause pain depends on which rotator cuff muscle you damage and how badly you injure it. Rotator cuff tears are often the reason for the early retirement of baseball players and weekend softball players alike.

These injuries usually are treated with ice, compression, and strength-training exercises using very light weights. Ease up on hard-core weight training exercises, particularly heavy bench pressing both on a flat and an incline bench, and ask a trainer to check your form. Reeducate yourself on throwing, catching, or swim stroke technique — make sure to involve your entire body rather than just your arm and shoulder. In some cases, the rotator cuff is too far gone to strengthen through exercise, and the damaged muscle needs surgical repair or at least physical therapy.

Chafing

You're legs feel great, and you've barely broken a sweat, yet you can't continue your bike ride because your butt is rubbed raw. You've got what's essentially a case of adult diaper rash, an irritation that can crop up anywhere your clothing touches your skin. It's particularly common in hot weather, when heavy sweating contributes to the problem. Every sport has special hot spots to look out for. The bra line and sock line are the most common among runners. But you can also get chafed if your tights, shorts, or shirt rub up against your skin as you move. Only streakers are immune.

To prevent this condition, experiment with fabrics and cuts of clothing that don't irritate your skin. Softer fabrics that include at least some cotton tend to be the kindest to your skin, but it's a matter of personal preference. Try greasing up your hot spots with Vaseline before heading out. Long-distance cyclists slather their butts with udder balm, an ointment made for cows but helpful for reducing chafing in humans. It feels kind of icky, but it usually does the trick. We know one runner who used to get a severe case of irritation on his nipples. He solved this with the strategic placement of Band-Aids. Not very macho, but then, neither were the two spots of blood leaking through his shirt.

Chapter 25

Ten Tips for a Fit Pregnancy

A generation ago, the last place you'd find a pregnant woman was at a health club or a running track. In those days, pregnancy was considered almost an illness — a time to rest in bed, not strengthen your hamstrings. Doctors were afraid that exercise would cause birth defects and increase the rate of miscarriage, but they were just guessing. Now that scientists have actually researched these issues, they know that it's perfectly safe for an expectant mom to work out — as long as she exercises common sense and doesn't try to set a world record in the high hurdles.

Not only is moderate exercise safe for the baby, but it's also been shown to have tremendous benefits for Mom. Compared to unfit pregnant women, regular exercisers tend to have fewer aches and pains, more self-esteem, and more energy and stamina, especially in the third trimester. Regular exercisers also have more confidence — and perhaps strength — during labor, and they seem to tolerate the pain better.

One obstetrician we know says his inactive patients tend to come to the hospital petrified, while his fit patients are fired up and ready for action. "For them, it's like the Super Bowl," the doctor says. "They say, 'Stand back, let me go. I'm going to push this sucker out!'" (By the way, this doctor was hardly the first to notice the benefits of fitness during labor. Biblical writers noted in the book of Exodus that Hebrew slave women had an easier time giving birth than more sedentary Egyptian women.)

Some research even suggests that fit women have shorter labors than unfit women and that they have a lower rate of C-section. But the studies aren't conclusive. Besides, exercise does not guarantee you a free ride in the delivery room. Even if you swim or walk until the day you give birth, you still may have the labor from hell. Some women are simply fated to a prolonged, agonizing labor, while others usher their little ones into the world relatively quickly. However, regardless of the labor experience, fit women do seem to bounce back from pregnancy a lot quicker than their inactive counterparts.

Is it safe to exercise during pregnancy if you're not already in good shape? Yes, as long as you work out moderately and have your doctor's OK. In fact, some doctors believe pregnancy is a terrific time to start working out. Entering labor in poor physical condition, they say, is like running the Boston Marathon without having trained. It only makes sense to prepare your body for the mega-workout to come.

In this chapter, we offer tips for a fit pregnancy, along with several safety precautions. Be sure to get your doctor's permission before embarking on a prenatal exercise program. Some high-risk conditions *do* rule out exercise during pregnancy.

However, if you don't have complications and your doctor discourages you from working out, don't be shy about shopping around for an exercise-friendly physician. Unfortunately, many obstetricians aren't aware of the benefits of prenatal exercise — they may not have studied the subject in medical school, and they may fear being sued if something goes wrong while a patient is following an exercise plan.

When Nancy Trent asked her doctor if she could continue her walking program during her pregnancy, the doctor accused her of being obsessive. Nancy found a different doctor who encouraged her to walk — and later delivered her healthy, 8-pound baby (on the same day that Nancy played a round of golf and did a pregnancy workout video).

Monitor Your Intensity

Until 1994, the American College of Obstetricians and Gynecologists (ACOG) insisted that a pregnant woman should not let her heart rate exceed 140 beats per minute. Many fit women found this guideline too restrictive; well-trained athletes have run marathons during pregnancy with heart rates as high as 190, and without complications. However, most physicians, fearing malpractice suits, were reluctant to approve more demanding exercise programs. In 1994, ACOG released new guidelines, eliminating the heart-rate limitation and making many pregnant jocks happy.

However, for a fitness novice, the 140 heart-rate guideline is a good one. (See Chapter 5 for details about monitoring your heart rate.) Pregnancy is not the time to figure out how fast you can run on the treadmill. If you don't want to be bothered with heart-rate calculations, simply use the talk test: Don't exercise so hard that you can't hold up your end of a conversation. In general, let your body dictate how hard you push yourself. Ask your doctor for guidelines tailored to your fitness level.

Read Fit Pregnancy Magazine

If you expect to stay fit when you're expecting, you can find no better source of information than *Fit Pregnancy,* a glossy, three-times-a-year magazine created by the editors of *Shape. Fit Pregnancy* is the only magazine completely devoted to the concerns of pregnant women who exercise, and it typically vanishes from the newsstands as soon as it arrives. (See Figure 25-1.)

Fit Pregnancy shows you in great detail how to safely lift weights, stretch, and stay aerobically fit for the nine-month haul, and it provides the latest news on the research front. (Many *Fit Pregnancy* readers learned about the new ACOG guidelines before their doctors did.) Diet and nutrition are regular topics, as

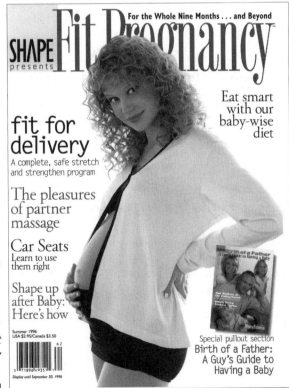

Figure 25-1: Active women practically inhale *Fit Pregnancy* magazine.

(Photo courtesy of *Fit Pregnancy*)

are sex and health issues such as genetic testing, breast feeding, and infant vaccinations. *Fit Pregnancy* rates exercise books and videos, maternity workout clothes, and baby joggers. The magazine also includes a regular humor column. Our favorite installment was by a writer who chronicled the mortifying moments of her girthing process. "With three weeks left," she says, "I realized I was dangerously close to resembling one of the peasants in 'Fiddler on the Roof.'"

Join a Prenatal Exercise Class

Many health clubs and hospitals offer exercise classes specially designed for pregnant women and brand-new moms. Some classes stick to aerobic workouts; others include strength training, even yoga. Naturally, the exercises are adapted to the limitations of a pregnant body — including the loss of balance, shifting center of gravity, and reduced stamina.

Participants love these classes because the atmosphere is so much more supportive than it tends to be in regular classes. You don't find a maniacal drill sergeant instructor yelling, "Okay, today's leg-lift-til-you-drop day." And you don't find class members in two-piece leotards showing off their sculpted abs. Prenatal exercise classes offer camaraderie, and a chance to swap war stories about hemorrhoids, swollen ankles, and husbands who — try as they might — just don't get it.

Guzzle Water and Don't Overheat

Pregnant or not, you shouldn't exercise without a water bottle close at hand. But when you're responsible for someone else's life, too, it's especially important to stay healthfully hydrated. Dehydration is the number-one cause of cramps, particularly in your legs, and it can increase your blood pressure and heart rate, among other things. Always drink before you get thirsty — by the time your body demands, "Water, now!" you're already at a fluid deficit.

Exercise in a well-ventilated area and make sure that you wear clothes that breathe. Your baby's temperature depends entirely on your ability to cool your body. Pregnant women do have a built-in mechanism that allows them to reduce exercise-related heat stress — but only to a point. Extra-high body temperature irritates the fetus and can lead to premature labor.

Interestingly, research has found that women in great physical shape may have a very efficient built-in mechanism for protecting the fetus from overheating. Fit women tend to begin sweating at a lower temperature than inactive women; in other words, they're much more effective at getting rid of heat. When scientists discovered this (and a few other nifty adaptations), they stopped worrying that prenatal exercise might harm the fetus.

Go for a Walk — or a Swim

Walking and swimming are two of the best workouts an expectant mom can do. They're both relatively gentle on the joints (swimming more so) — and the mind. Most pregnant women find that when they're feeling lethargic, going for a walk or a swim gives them a surge of energy.

Walk this way

Some women walk for exercise until the day of delivery. Runners may want to switch to a walk-run program or an all-walk routine if they find that running is just too hard on their lower back and knees. As your pregnancy progresses, avoid steep hills, which make your heart rate soar and may put more pressure on your lower back.

Pay special attention to your walking posture. Stand tall, with your back straight, and your shoulders back and down, not hunched. Lead with your chest. Keep your arms relaxed, and move them forward and back instead of swinging them across your body. Don't walk in very hot or humid weather, because your heart rate elevates more quickly. And don't walk when the ground is icy, because your sense of balance is not what it used to be. If the weather sends you indoors and onto a treadmill, hold on to the rails (but not with a death-grip); treadmills require more balance than walking on the ground.

Make sure that you wear supportive walking shoes (see Figure 25-2). Because you weigh more than usual, your joints are under extra stress, and they need all the shock absorption they can get. Your feet may swell to the point where you need shoes a half size bigger than usual.

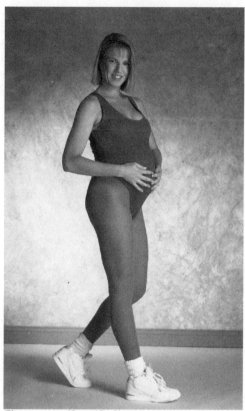

Figure 25-2:
Wear
supportive
shoes.

(Photo courtesy of Buns of Steel.)

Getting into the swim of things

Some pregnant women find walking uncomfortable, particularly in the third trimester, so they switch to lower-impact activities such as swimming. In fact, some pregnant women say that the only time they feel really comfortable is in the water.

Water workouts are great because you don't have to worry about your balance. The water supports your weight and the weight of your baby, too, taking the stress off your lower back. Water also reduces the effect of gravity, lessening pressure on your joints. And nothing is more calming and soothing than gliding through the water; swimming can even help reduce pregnancy-related swelling. Plus, there's no way that you can possibly fall.

Meanwhile, you can still get a great workout. You can run in the pool, swim laps, and tone your muscles with special equipment like webbed gloves and foam dumbbells. As your pregnancy progresses, you may need to modify your water workouts. Using a kickboard may become uncomfortable because it forces you to arch your back, which can trigger back pain. The frog kick (used in the breaststroke) might also cause discomfort. Don't forget to drink water — you can get dehydrated even in the pool.

Continue Lifting Weights

If you've never lifted weights before, pregnancy isn't the time to start an unsupervised strength program. But if you know what you're doing in the weight room or you're experienced using dumbbells at home, you have no reason to quit your routine. And as long as you make the appropriate modifications, there are plenty of great reasons to stick with it. (We don't want to discourage novices from strength training during pregnancy, but you need to work with a trainer who's very experienced with pregnant women or join a supervised, prenatal weight-training class at a health club.)

Lifting weights during pregnancy helps cut down on general aches and pains and may even counteract some of the shoulder and back pain that can be caused by enlarged breasts and a growing uterus. Everyday activities won't take as great a toll, and when the big day comes, you have more strength to pick up your new bundle of joy (not to mention the diaper bag, stroller, car seat, bottles, and toys that you'll be lugging around).

You do need to adapt your weight-training program to your ever-changing body. You may prefer machines to free weights, because they offer more support and require less balance. Of course, some machines won't fit you anymore. When you're seven months pregnant, you can't exactly lie on your stomach and do hamstring curls. A couple of equipment manufacturers have taken care of this problem by designing a hamstring curl machine that you use on your side. But most gyms don't have special pregnancy equipment, so ask a trainer to show you more practical alternatives to your regular routine. Many gyms have standing or seated hamstring machines.

Give special attention to the muscles that are bearing the brunt of your temporary burden, such as your knees, ankles, and lower back. But if any exercise starts to feel uncomfortable, stop doing it. Any time that you feel dizziness, nausea, or a pulling in your abdomen, hips, pelvis, or elsewhere, choose a different exercise.

When you're pregnant, your goals in the weight room should change. Don't focus on sculpting your muscles or setting a personal best in the bench press. Instead, aim to maintain your strength and enjoy the movement. Your last few repetitions of each set should be somewhat challenging, but they shouldn't require all-out oomph. Expect to reduce the amount of weight you lift toward the end of your pregnancy, when you may have less energy. Breathe steadily and pay close attention to your form. Don't grip the handles too hard. Gripping too hard raises your blood pressure, which shoots up anyway when you exercise.

Stretch — But Not Too Far

Regular stretching helps counteract the muscle tightness that typically comes with pregnancy (particularly in the thighs). Tight muscles can throw your posture off kilter, leading to pain in your back and pelvic joints.

Stretching also helps relieve tension in your muscles and teaches you to relax (and what mom-to-be couldn't use a little relaxation?). Always do an aerobic warm-up before you stretch, and make sure that you don't stretch too far. Don't bounce or jerk up and down and don't hold your breath or attempt to stretch beyond your capabilities. You may find that some joints, particularly at your pelvis, are looser than usual due to an influx of pregnancy hormones. For more stretching tips, see Chapter 7.

Don't Lie on Your Back after the First Trimester

Starting around the fourth month, you may feel dizzy when you lie on your back. This means that your little one is pressing on your *inferior vena cava,* a major vein that carries blood to your heart. You can modify exercises in a number of ways to avoid this dizziness. For instance, if you'd like to do abdominal exercises on your back, you can place a folded towel or small blanket underneath one hip. This shifts your body slightly, rolling the baby off the vein. Also, there are plenty of pregnancy exercises you can do with your back against the wall or while standing or sitting in a chair. In addition, you can do gentle exercises with a *physioball* — a large, inflated ball that looks like a sturdy beach ball.

One friend of ours took a ball with her into the delivery room. When she went into *back labor* (when the baby presses heavily against your spine, creating agonizing back pain), she placed the ball against the wall and pressed her back against it. By rolling the ball around on the wall and allowing it to massage her back, she was able to work through most of the pain. She did get some funny looks from the nurses, but once they saw it was working, they thought it was a great idea.

No Risky Business

Pregnancy, in case you were wondering, is not the time to audition for a roller hockey team or take up full-contact karate. As you lose agility and coordination, back off from activities that carry a risk of falling, like bicycling, skating, and skiing. The same goes for sports that involve sharp changes in direction, like tennis and volleyball.

You may think that active pregnant women have a higher injury rate than pregnant women who don't exercise, but research suggests that's not true. And when fit women do get injured, it usually doesn't happen when they're working out; instead, they get injured when they're vacuuming the living room or when they bend over to pick something up. Researchers suspect that this is because pregnant exercisers tend to take extra precautions when they work out.

Keep Exercising after the Baby Arrives

Working out might seem like a pretty tall order when you're getting two hours of sleep a night and your body feels like it's been through the spin cycle. But even short, easy workouts like a 10-minute walk help you sustain energy (at a time when you *really* need it), and exercise may help you sleep better at night. Exercise also can help you cope with the depression that sometimes results from sleep deprivation.

But don't rush back into exercise. There's no need to force yourself into anything at a time when a walk to the bathroom might seem like an athletic feat worthy of an Olympic medal. As soon as you feel ready (a few days or weeks after delivery), try to start a simple routine, such as daily walking. Gradually work up to brisk walks with your baby in the stroller. Consider buying a baby jogger or a special cart that will attach to your bicycle so that you can safely take your screamer along for the ride.

Six weeks after an uncomplicated birth — or sooner if your doctor OKs it — you can begin more vigorous activity, like swimming, jogging, or lifting weights. Just make sure you start back slowly. Your abdominal muscles have been stretched, which means they aren't supporting your back as much as they were before you got pregnant. Check with your doctor before you begin your routine again.

Postpartum exercise makes you feel better, but don't expect it to speed up the weight-loss process. The research is inconclusive, but it appears that if you eat regularly and exercise after giving birth, you go through the same weight-loss patterns as women who don't exercise. In other words, it still takes about six months to a year to return to your pre-pregnancy weight and body composition. But you *can* start regaining your fitness a lot faster.

Chapter 26

Ten Fitness Travel Tips

*B*usiness trips and vacations can sabotage even the best laid plans to exercise and eat right. Just when you've made this fitness thing a habit, your boss sends you to Dubuque for a week to salvage an important deal. Airports, hotels, conference rooms, and steak joints — these aren't the easiest places to stick to your program. But going out of town doesn't have to mean getting out of shape. In this chapter, we offer strategies for staying fit on the road.

Book a Hotel with a Gym

Not long ago, a typical hotel fitness center consisted of a couple of rusty barbells and a stationary bike that, if you were really lucky, may actually have had a seat. But these days, in an effort to stay competitive, many hotels offer mini-health clubs with high-tech machinery and an array of free weights. Some hotel gyms can rival a small health club in terms of equipment and service. New York City's Regency, for instance, has TVs to ease the boredom while you walk on the treadmill — and trainers on call in case you forget how to do squats or want some encouragement. But fitness amenities aren't limited to four-star hotels. On occasion, when staying in the sort of hotel where the seascape oil paintings are bolted to the wall, we've been surprised to discover a passable fitness center just past the ice machine.

Some hotel gyms are free to paying guests; others charge a small fee or, in some larger cities, a fairly hefty fee of up to $25 a visit. Trainer fees are the same as you'd find anywhere, $30 to $100 a session. Some hotels let you use the pool at no cost but charge you for workout rights in the weight room, or vice versa. Be prepared to sign a waiver essentially stating that anything you drop on your head or fall off of is your problem.

To find out which hotels have gyms, talk to your travel agent, who probably has reasonably updated listings. Ask how much the gym costs, what type of equipment it has, and what time it opens and closes. Clarify in advance whether the hotel gym is on the premises. Some hotels have arrangements with local gyms — which might be a problem if your company isn't forking over the bucks for a rental car. It's not out of line to ask what sort of credentials the hotel gym trainers have. Don't lower your standards just because you're away from home.

Another service to ask about: equipment delivery to your room, as in "Room service — I'd like to order a club sandwich, a Caesar salad, and a StairMaster." Some hotels save you the phone call by equipping special fitness traveler rooms with a bike, a rowing machine, or a step aerobics platform. In New York City, the convenience capital of the world, several hotels have cut deals with the Gym Source, an equipment dealer: Guests can call up and order a treadmill or weight machine to be sent to their rooms.

Check Out the Local Gym Scene

Sometimes you're stuck in some dive motel that doesn't have hot water, let alone a gym. That's the time to check out the local health clubs. Some travelers make it a hobby to find a gym in every city that they visit. The search can be an adventure in itself. While bicycling across the United States, one of us became adept at hunting down barbells in rural towns that didn't even have a stoplight. We'd go to the local high school and politely ask to borrow the weight room for 45 minutes. The coaches were always happy to oblige, and we got to soak up some of the local culture by working out with the football players.

If you're determined, you can find a place to work out virtually anywhere in the world. We even scouted out a remarkable gym in Bulawayo, Zimbabwe, called Muscle & Curves. The co-owner, 64-year-old Pete Karsten, had made all of the weight machines himself — welding them in his own garage with a couple of assistants — because he couldn't get hard currency to import equipment from the United States. Karsten's 58-year-old wife, Gwen, runs the health club. "As long as you know your basics, you don't have to have fancy equipment to build a strong body," she told us.

Some gyms let you work out for free, or they charge a token $2 fee; others charge you more for a single workout than you'd pay for an entire month of workouts at home. (One New York gym charges $50 for a guest pass.) A club is more likely to give you a break if you call ahead rather than just show up at the front desk with your gym bag in hand. By the way, some clubs have reciprocity agreements with other clubs around the country. If you're a member of one club, you can use all of the other affiliated clubs for free. Find out whether your gym at home has agreements with any other clubs.

Check the local yellow pages as soon as you hit town. Look under "health clubs" or "gymnasiums." If you travel a lot, it may be worth your while to purchase a list of local gyms throughout the country from American Business Directories. The book (which also comes on computer disk) has thousands of entries compiled from local yellow pages. The book tells you, for instance, that there are four gyms in Murray, Utah, and provides you with the street address and phone number of each club.

By the way, all of this makes a strong case for learning your fundamentals — basic routines for aerobic exercise, strength training, and stretching—before you hit the road. When you know what to do with a dumbbell and a treadmill, you feel comfortable walking into any health club, in any city. Make a special point of learning to use free weights; unlike machines, barbells and dumbbells are pretty much the same all over the world, even when they're welded in some guy's garage in southern Africa.

Take a Walk Outside

You don't need a fancy health club to work up a sweat — the great outdoors can be your gym away from home. When you go for a run or a walk, you not only burn calories but explore your surroundings. One of us was running along the beach at Florida's North Captiva Island and saw a whole host of sights that wouldn't be visible from a treadmill in your hotel room, including an osprey, a bald eagle, a whale, and two rather large humans going at it on the sand.

Many hotels have maps available at the concierge desk. During a recent stay in London, we were surprised to find that the hotel provided free, detailed maps of walking and running routes throughout the city's amazing park system. The maps were far better than any guide book we could have bought. If your hotel has a fitness center, a trainer (or even the concierge) may be able to offer the inside scoop on local running routes — where the water fountains are, where to find hilly terrain, and where you're least likely to get mugged. Some very fitness conscious hotels have guided walking tours in the mornings and evenings.

If your hotel can't help you, look up a running or walking club in the yellow pages, call the Chamber of Commerce, or call the local YMCA. Or just walk out the front door of your hotel and follow your instincts. But be careful — you don't want to accidentally wander into the red light district. Carry your hotel's address and phone number plus a quarter to make a call. Once we got lost while running in Atlanta, and it took us two hours to find our hotel. It didn't help that we were a little fuzzy on the name.

Other valuable references and sources: *Fitness on the Road,* a book that lists gyms, pools, and other fitness facilities in many major cities, and the Rado Watch Co., which publishes several guides to metropolitan health clubs and fitness facilities.

Bring Your Workout with You

If the hotel gym hours don't jibe with your schedule or you don't want to go running in a strange neighborhood, switch to Plan B: Bring your own workout equipment. You don't need to haul a trunk full of free weights and a treadmill through the airport. You can put together a travel exercise kit that fits in your carry-on bag or in a corner of your suitcase. A jump rope and a set of rubber exercise bands covers your aerobic and strength-training needs. Add a guest towel for a stretching mat, and you've covered all the fitness bases.

Skipping rope and pumping rubber in your hotel room may not be your idea of fun, but it's better than nothing. Some exercise bands come in their own travel bags and include a variety of snap-together bars and door attachments, so you can get pretty creative with your toning routine. Besides, periodically straying from your normal weight workout is a good idea. After a while, most of us do our workouts on autopilot; switching to bands might give you — and your muscles — a wake-up call. And a session with a jump rope can be an excellent cross-training alternative.

Call ahead and ask if your hotel room has a VCR. Many hotels do, especially those that cater to business travelers who make presentations in their room. If you're in luck, toss a couple of your favorite workout tapes into your suitcase. We know one organized and fanatically fit businesswoman who has a prepacked fitness kit complete with jump rope, bands, and exercise videos. She keeps it with her travel toiletries so that she's ready to go on a moment's notice. "I may forget my lipstick," she says, "but I always have my *Buns of Steel* tape."

If you're really ambitious or planning to be out of town for a few weeks, you may even want to bring along a step or a slide. For this purpose only, we recommend a step made of foam. A foam step is not sturdy enough to endure constant use, but it weighs far less than a wooden or plastic step, so you don't have to break your back lugging it from here to there. A foam step costs around $30, so it's not a bad investment to set one aside for emergencies.

Oh, and don't forget to pack up a gym bag with your exercise clothes, sneakers, radio headphones, and water bottle. It's no fun to get yourself ready for a jump rope workout and realize that the only pair of shoes you've brought along are your loafers.

Use Your Body as Equipment

When all else fails, you may have to go to Plan C: a workout that uses no equipment at all. We've spent more than a few nights jogging in place in a hotel room while flipping through TV channels. Actually, you have more options than you might think. To keep up your muscle strength, you can do abdominal crunches, low back exercises, push-ups, and tricep dips off the edge of the bed. Ask your trainer to teach you a travel routine sans equipment, so you have one less excuse to skip your workout. While you're at it, have your trainer jot down a gym routine plus a band and jump rope workout so that you're covered no matter what. Make sure that you get your workouts updated periodically to reflect changes in your fitness level and goals.

Dining Out on a Calorie Budget

When it comes to eating on the road, you're a captive audience. Although we recently received a catalog of cooking appliances that you can plug into your car's cigarette lighter (including a breadmaker), it's more likely that your options will be limited to restaurants, fast food joints, and the hotel snack shop. We hate to even mention plane food; at the less enlightened airlines, the idea of a balanced meal is a flight attendant carrying several trays at once. Still, you can eat healthfully just about anywhere. It just requires some advance planning and assertiveness. This section includes some tips to navigate your way through even the most treacherous menus.

Restaurant dining

Watch out for dish descriptions peppered with cooking terms, especially if they're in a foreign language; aloo gobi masala (our favorite Indian dish) can translate into extra fat and calories. *Sautéed* means pan fried in butter; *tempura* means batter-coated, *au gratin* means drenched in cheese sauce. Other terms to beware of: fried, deep fried, pan fried, crispy, braised, creamed, hollandaise, and scalloped.

Terms that signal healthy choices are steamed, poached, broiled (but not in butter or oil), in its own juice, garden fresh, roasted, lemon, and wine.

Order sauces, dressings, and gravies on the side. When you do this, be extra nice to the waiter. He may not be thrilled when you say, "I'll have the cobb salad with low-fat honey mustard dressing on the side, no bacon, and extra garbanzo beans — and could you go easy on the avocado and blue cheese?" Ask your waiter how dishes are prepared, and perhaps he can steer you toward the lightest choices on the menu. Also request that he not place butter or other fattening fare on the table.

If you have your heart set on a side of beef ribs or an Oreo cheesecake with chocolate fudge, consider eating half and doggy bagging the rest, or share with your dining partners. You can also save calories by ordering a la carte. This way, you won't feel obliged to eat a truckload of food simply because you paid for it.

Schedule your business meetings at times other than mealtimes. The longer you sit at the table kibitzing and drinking, the more you tend to eat, without even noticing. Watch it with the booze. Alcohol adds empty calories and stimulates your appetite.

Surviving fast food

A fast food joint isn't exactly a nutritional paradise, but sometimes you have absolutely no other choice. Here's how to survive these grease pits with your waistline intact.

Don't assume that a salad is the healthiest choice. At Taco Bell, a taco salad with ranch dressing, weighing in at 1,167 calories, has more calories than any other item on the menu. (61 percent of which come from fat.) Salad bars can be a danger zone, too. If you drown your lettuce in blue cheese dressing or pile on the marshmallow ambrosia and potato salad with olives, you may be even worse off than if you order a burger and fries. Fresh fruits and vegetables are great choices, naturally, but by themselves, they're not going to satisfy your appetite. Toss in some low-fat protein sources, like low-fat cottage cheese, beans, and tuna without mayo, and top off your salad with low-cal dressing. Also, keep your portions in control. Don't take the phrase "all you can eat" literally.

When you order burgers and sandwiches, look for words like "Junior" and "small." Order your burger without the cheese, special sauce, and mayo; lettuce, tomato, onion, mustard, ketchup, and pickles supply plenty of flavor. And avoid items with the words "double" or "super" in the description. We're fascinated by Taco Bell's new Double Decker Bacon Cheeseburger Taco, which includes not one but two taco shells and appears to be about four meals in one. This monster taco is an odd addition from a company that recently came out with an entire light menu.

If you can't resist those *two all-beef patties, special sauce, lettuce, cheese, pickles, and onions on a sesame-seed bun,* at least try to balance out the damage with exercise.

Fast-food facts

Here's a look at what you're eating at three popular fast-food restaurants. We have a feeling that you might order differently if this chart were posted in huge letters next to the counter or drive-through window. Stick to healthier fast-food choices such as grilled chicken sandwiches and low-fat salads. (To learn more about the significance of percent fat, fat grams, and saturated fat grams, see Chapter 4.)

Restaurant/Food Item	Calories	Percent Fat	Fat Grams	Saturated Fat Grams
McDonald's				
Hamburger	257	35	10	4
Cheeseburger	308	41	14	5
Quarter Pounder	414	46	21	8
Quarter Pounder, cheese	517	50	29	11
Big Mac	562	51	32	10
Filet-O-Fish	442	53	26	5
Chicken McNuggets	288	50	16	4
Regular Fries	220	49	12	5
Burger King				
Hamburger	275	39	12	5
Cheeseburger	317	43	15	7
Whopper	628	52	36	12
Whopper, Cheese	711	54	43	17
Bacon Double Cheeseburger	510	55	31	15
Whaler Fish Sandwich	488	54	27	6
Chicken Sandwich	688	52	40	8
Regular Fries	227	52	13	7
Taco Bell				
Bean Burrito	359	28	11	5
Beef Burrito	402	38	17	8
Burrito Supreme	422	41	19	9
Enchirito	382	47	20	10
Taco	184	54	11	4
Taco Salad with ranch dressing	1167	67	87	45
Taco Bellgrande Platter	1002	46	51	29
Nachos	346	47	18	6

Eating in the air

You may be a frequent flyer, but you don't want it to show, at least not on your waistline. Many airlines have cleaned up their act, switching from peanuts to pretzels, replacing croissants with multigrain muffins, and eliminating heavy cream sauces. But other airlines still don't get it. On a recent flight, one of us was served a bologna sandwich on white bread with mayo, potato chips, honey roasted peanuts, and ice cream. This might be your worst nightmare when you've been trying so hard to eat healthfully. Still, it is possible to beat the airlines at their own game.

Many airlines offer a long list of special meals. You can order vegetarian, all-fruit, low-calorie, low-fat, diabetic, kosher, or Hindu — you name it. Most airlines require at least 24 hours' notice, so get in the habit of reserving a special meal when you make your plane reservations. And around mealtime, be sure to watch the flight attendant like a hawk so he doesn't give your meal away to another passenger.

If you forget to preorder a special meal, choose judiciously from what's on your plate. Pass on the margarine, remove the skin from the chicken, and eat half of the cherry cheesecake. If you're worried that you'll be left with about ten calories on your plate, preempt the problem by bringing aboard some nutritious snacks of your own, like fruit, raisins, or whole-grain crackers — even a turkey sandwich.

Surviving airport layovers and unexpected flight delays takes some effort as well. Airports are notorious places for losing control, because you're surrounded by specialty ice cream shops, pizza stands, and donut displays — and you don't have much to do but sit around, read magazines, and eat. Many snack shops do offer fruit, but bananas and apples tend to lose their appeal when they're sitting on the counter next to glazed cinnamon rolls and fudge brownies. If you think that you're going to succumb to some fat-laden temptations, at least start by eating fruit, a low-fat chicken sandwich, or a soft pretzel with mustard. Wait a half hour, and if you still aren't satisfied, treat yourself to dessert, preferably something of the low-fat variety. By the way, don't think that we always follow these rules. One of us recently ate a Dove Bar at the Atlanta airport, a scoop of chocolate mint ice cream during a layover in Denver, and then two packages of peanuts on a flight back to Oakland.

Take Walking Breaks

Whatever your mode of transportation, get up at least once an hour and walk around for a few minutes. In a car, this might mean pulling off the interstate to a rest stop. On a plane, this might mean stepping over the guy who scored the aisle seat and navigating the obstacle course of flight attendants and food carts. It's worth the effort. You don't want to finish up a five-hour trip with rigormortis.

Moving around is especially important if you have back or neck problems. You don't want your muscles frozen in one position for too long; otherwise you're inviting hours of stiffness. Knees need to bend and straighten, especially if the airplane passenger in front of you has decided to recline his seat all the way back in your lap. Once you get to your destination, walk around for a while and then spend several minutes stretching out your muscles.

If, despite your efforts to move around in a restricted area, you feel a twinge of back pain coming on, shove a pillow under the small of your back or at the base of your neck. Or alternate tightening and relaxing those muscles so that you can at least get some blood flowing.

Drink Plenty of Water

It's very easy to become dehydrated when you're flying because the pressurized air in the plane cabin is short on humidity. You need to drink even more water than usual when you're traveling — a good guideline is one glass of water for every hour you spend in the air. Whenever possible, limit your caffeine, salt, and alcohol because they're notorious dehydrators.

While you're at it, take a multi-vitamin and a vitamin C supplement. You're more susceptible to sickness when you spend hours in the uncirculated air of an airplane cabin. Whenever anyone sneezes or coughs, the germs linger in the air for the rest of the flight. A supplement also can help compensate for nutritionally disastrous meals, like that bologna sandwich on white bread that we mentioned earlier.

Take a Fitness Vacation

Airline food might be an oxymoron, but fitness vacation is not. Vacation doesn't have to mean two weeks lying immobile on a lounge by the pool. An invigorating and satisfying alternative is to plan an active vacation. You'll feel so much better when you come home.

Active travel

Active travel is a booming industry, so you should have no trouble finding a trip that suits you. You can go snowshoeing in New Hampshire, take a walking tour of the British countryside, rope steer at a dude ranch, or hone your forehand at a tennis clinic. One world-wide active travel company, Backroads, offers a five-day smorgasbord in Northern California, where novices get to sample mountain biking, in-line skating, sailboarding, and rock climbing. (See Figure 26-1.)

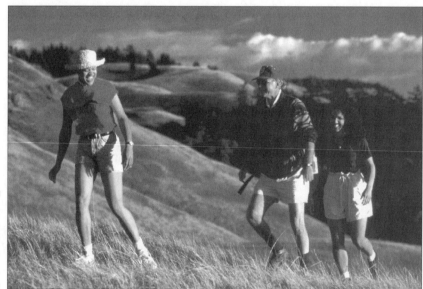

Figure 26-1:
Take a
walking tour
on your
vacation.

(Photo courtesy of Mountain Travel-Sobek.)

Tours last anywhere from a few days to a few months and are geared toward all fitness levels and budgets. Ask your travel agent for suggestions; your agent may be able to get you a better deal than you can get on your own. Many bicycling tours have a half-day option for novices. Some companies put you up in fancy hotels, fix you gourmet lunches on the road, and pump your bike tires for you; others hand you a map to your campsite 60 miles down the road, mention that there's a Dairy Queen at the halfway point, and say, "Have fun! Hope you learned how to fix a flat tire!"

If true indulgence is what you're looking for, consider a spa vacation. A group called Spa Finders can match you with a spa that's compatible with your personality. Or call the International Spa & Resort Association, a clearinghouse for spa resort information. These days most spas combine pampering with exercise and gourmet low-fat food. You can knock yourself out with step aerobics and weight lifting and then indulge yourself in those treatments that involve wax, mud, and seaweed. Just be aware that spa vacations can be pricey. For a four-day stay, you'll spend anywhere from $350 to upwards of $4,000 per person.

The real dilemma comes when you want an active vacation and your partner doesn't. Two solutions for the vacationally incompatible are cruises and Club Med. Many cruise ships have state-of-the-art gyms, walking programs, and a swimming pool. You can take the 4 p.m. aerobics class on the Lido deck while your spouse attends the napkin-folding demonstration in the Tahiti Lounge. Club Med, an all-inclusive hotel and airfare package, has dozens of locations worldwide. They offer a variety of activities throughout the day — from scuba diving to horseback riding to acrobatics — and nobody cares whether or not you show up. Make sure that you check with Club Med for a listing of activities that each location offers; some are better than others. Club Med vacations start at around $1,400 a week per person.

Adventure travel: the next step

If you're really ambitious, you can cross the line from active travel into adventure travel. You can go ice climbing in the Canadian Rockies, rappelling off cliffs in Borneo, dog sledding across the Alaskan tundra, spelunking (that's cave exploring), kayaking, white-water rafting, parasailing, and just about anything else you could possibly dream up. Excellent adventure travel companies include Mountain Travel-Sobek and Overseas Adventure Travel. (See Figure 26-2.)

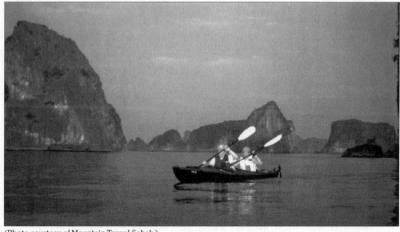

Figure 26-2:
Make your
vacation
an action
adventure.

(Photo courtesy of Mountain Travel-Sobek.)

Whatever trip you choose, pay close attention to the company's literature about how to get in shape for the trip. If the tour directors say that you need to be able to cycle 60 miles in a day or carry a 50-pound pack on your back at high altitudes, they're not kidding. We know a lawyer from Chicago who spent $4,000 on a two-week trek in the mountains of Nepal. Gasping for breath and overwhelmed by his pack, the guy had to turn back on the very first day. His training had consisted of a couple of aerobics classes a week — not exactly the kind of preparation you need to cover 15 miles a day at 16,000 feet.

Don't Sweat a Few Days Off

If your travel schedule is too hectic for even a short workout, don't stress out about it. Some rest may actually be good for you, and you can get back to your regular routine as soon as you come home. (Just make sure that you actually do this.)

One guy we know takes a lot of short-hop business trips that require him to fly out and back in one day. Between catching an early plane, racing from one appointment to the next, and then dashing to make the last flight home, he barely has time to catch his breath, let alone a workout at the gym. This used to really bother him. Now he arranges his workout schedule so that his travel day is his off day from exercise, and if he misses more than that, he doubles up on the weekend. He has learned to look forward to the plane trip as an opportunity to get off his feet for a few hours.

Chapter 27

Your Metabolism: Ten Burning Questions about Burning Calories

*P*oliticians go around promising to reform welfare, lock up criminals, and cut your taxes, but if they really want to get elected, they might try a new tactic: vowing to speed up your metabolism. If there's one goal that unites the American public, it seems to be burning extra calories without extra effort. Any promise — no matter how dubious — that includes the word "metabolism" seems to get plenty of attention.

Claims about metabolism are everywhere. "Hot, spicy foods can shift your metabolism into high gear so you burn off extra pounds without breaking a sweat!" one book advertisement maintains. One brand of diet pills claims to boost metabolism because it's made from bovine cartilage. Other claims about metabolism seem more plausible. According to one treadmill manufacturer, its new machine helps raise your metabolic rate, so even when you're not exercising, your body is burning more calories.

Is any of this true? What *can* you do to rev up your metabolism? What exactly does metabolism mean, anyway? This chapter addresses commonly asked questions about burning calories. The answers just might surprise you.

What's a Calorie, and How Do You Burn One?

Calories are what your body uses as fuel, just as a car runs on gas. In fact, it's not too farfetched to think of calories as miniature gallons of gas. Calories are the source of energy that your body uses to power your heart, expand your lungs, hug your aunt, and stand up and yell at the TV during "Monday Night Football" — in short, they're what your body uses to do every single physiological function it's capable of.

Calories come from food, but your body doesn't simply take that pork chop you just ate and toss it into some sort of biological furnace. First, your body must take the nutrients in your food and break them down into their most elemental form, a substance called glucose. If your body doesn't need the energy immediately, the calories get converted into body fat and stored for later use — like a savings account (but not one that you want to make too many deposits into).

Every 3,500 calories that you save for later becomes one pound of body fat. You can lose fat only by creating a calorie deficit — that is, either eating fewer calories than you burn up in a day or burning more calories than you eat. Once you take 3,500 calories out of your savings account, the scale will register a one-pound weight loss.

What Exactly Does Metabolism Mean?

Your metabolism — or metabolic rate — refers to the number of calories you're burning at any given moment, whether you're watching "The Weather Channel" or pedaling your heart out on a stationary bike. Naturally, your metabolic rate is higher when you're working out than when you're crashed out on the couch.

But when most people use the term metabolism — as in "I have a slow metabolism" or "This pill will increase your metabolism" — they're referring to your *resting metabolism,* the number of calories your body needs to maintain its vital functions. Your brain, heart, kidneys, liver, and other organs are cranking away 24 hours a day, and your muscle cells are constantly undergoing repair. All of these processes require energy in the form of calories simply to keep you alive. So when people say that a pill can speed up your metabolism, they're claiming that the pill can prompt your body to burn more calories without any extra exercise or effort on your part.

What Determines the Speed of Your Resting Metabolism?

The speed of your resting metabolism depends primarily on your amount of *fat-free mass* — everything in your body that's not fat, including muscle, bones, blood, organs, and tissue. The more fat-free mass you have — the bigger your muscles and the larger your bones — the more energy your body expends in order to keep going. Your weight also plays a role, and there's clearly a genetic component. Studies indicate that some babies are born with a revved-up metabolism, while other babies are off to a slow start from Day 1.

Generally, men have a faster resting metabolic rate than women, because they tend to have more muscle and larger bodies. Also, metabolism tends to slow with age. But scientists don't think that the decline (or at least most of it) is inevitable. It appears to be mostly due to a loss of muscle and a decrease in physical activity. If you don't exercise, you lose about 40 percent of your muscle from age 30 to age 70. But if you lift weights regularly, you probably can offset most of the decline. The sooner you start lifting, the better, because muscle is a lot easier to maintain than to build up.

Can You Determine How Many Calories You Burn in a Day?

The only way to accurately pin down your resting metabolism — or your metabolism during exercise, for that matter — is to get tested in a lab. A technician will hook you up to a great beast of a machine, place a plastic tube in your mouth, and then analyze the air you inhale and exhale to determine how efficiently you use fuel.

However, you can get a rough estimate of your resting metabolism by punching some numbers into your calculator. Typically, formulas for metabolism factor in only your weight, height, and sex (and sometimes your age). They can't take into consideration other key considerations, such as your fat-free mass and your genetics.

The formula we use in the following steps isn't necessarily the most accurate; it's just one of the easiest. We include calculations for a man who's 5-foot-10 and weighs 180 pounds and for a woman who's 5-foot-4 and weighs 132.

Step 1. **Change your weight from pounds to kilograms. To do, this divide your weight in pounds by 2.2.**

The man: $180 \div 2.2 = 82$
The woman: $132 \div 2.2 = 60$

Step 2. **If you're a man, don't do anything. If you're a woman, multiply the result of Step 1 by .9.**

The man: still at 82
The woman: $60 \times .9 = 54$

Step 3. **Multiply the result of Step 2 by 24. This calculation estimates your resting metabolic rate.**

The man: $82 \times 24 = 1,968$
The woman: $54 \times 24 = 1,296$

Now you've estimated the number of calories that your body would need if you did absolutely nothing but lie motionless in bed 24 hours a day. Naturally, you need to add calories to estimate a more typical day. To calculate your calorie needs for a relatively sedentary day — say, a day you spend lying on the beach — tack on 20 percent of your resting metabolic rate. That's another 394 calories for our sample guy, for a total of 2,362 calories. On days when you exercise, you may need to add 30 to 50 percent of your resting metabolism, depending on how long and hard you work out.

Does Exercise Increase Your Resting Metabolism?

Although you'd never know it from reading fitness product advertisements, this question hasn't yet been resolved. Also, the answer depends on what type of exercise you're talking about. Several studies have shown that aerobic exercise (like running and stairclimbing) does not boost metabolic rate.

Weight lifting, however, probably holds more promise. We know that muscle burns more calories than fat — your body requires more energy to maintain a pound of muscle than it does to maintain a pound of fat. And we know that lifting weights builds muscle. So it's only logical that, by building more muscle through weight lifting, you'll rev up your metabolism. That's a convincing theory, and it may ultimately be proven to be true. But studies have been so few and research results so mixed that, at this point, we can't say for sure whether weight lifting is guaranteed to increase your metabolic rate. However, we believe the odds are good, and we think a regular strength-training routine is well worth anybody's time.

After You Exercise, Does Your Metabolism Stay Elevated?

Yes. However, this *afterburn* effect depends on the type of exercise that you do and how hard and how long you work out. Weight lifting seems to have a greater afterburn effect than does aerobic exercise. In one study, subjects did an intense, 90-minute weight workout, performing 6 sets each of 10 different exercises with very little rest between sets. Two hours after the workout, their metabolic rate was 11 percent higher than normal. When the subjects were measured the next morning, 15 hours after the workout, their metabolism was still elevated by 9 percent, which would translate into about 150 extra calories burned.

These numbers are impressive, but the workouts were far longer and more strenuous than most of us would do. And the numbers become a lot less impressive when the workouts aren't so demanding. In general, we believe this afterburn concept has gotten too much hype. The calories that you burn after a workout are going to be negligible compared to what you burn *while* you're exercising.

As for aerobic exercise: Most studies have found that easy to moderate exercise — a pace that allows you to hold a conversation — elevates metabolic rate for only a few minutes to a few hours. The afterburn from a moderate aerobic workout probably won't account for more than 15 to 30 calories.

Can Drugs Boost Your Metabolism?

Yes, but don't take them. Amphetamines and over-the-counter appetite suppressants can raise your metabolic rate, but your body tends to adapt to these drugs, so the effect may be short-lived. Besides, these drugs can have harmful side-effects, including elevated heart rate and blood pressure.

Drugs that stimulate your thyroid also increase your metabolism. But they, too, have a few glitches, like increasing your chance of cardiac arrest. Interestingly, a woman back in the 1860s — who served as the first documented case of anorexia — died of complications from taking thyroid pills. Some disreputable diet doctors still prescribe them.

Anabolic steroids stimulate metabolism, but they come with a whole assort-ment of side-effects. Women on "the juice" take on many male characteristics, such as a deepened voice and facial hair. Males develop breasts and what we'll euphemistically call a shrunken steam pipe. Both sexes behave more aggres-sively and have increased risk of cardiovascular disease and some cancers. When you go off steroids, your metabolism may nearly grind to a halt.

We know one female bodybuilder who finally swore off steroids when her doctor warned her that her thyroid was about to explode. She gained about 50 pounds in three months and couldn't lose it no matter how hard she tried.

Finally, pass on those "fat-burning" supplements that have everyone all fired up. Research has not proven that chromium picolinate and its kind can boost metabolism.

Does Eating Frequent Meals Boost Your Metabolism?

Some scientists have suggested that you can boost your metabolism by eating several small meals each day rather than a few large ones. This theory is based on the fact that your metabolism rises after you eat. But very little research has been done on humans to prove this hypothesis. Also, eating a small snack really doesn't have much effect on your metabolic rate. However, if this sort of eating pattern suits your personality, it may cause you to eat less because you never get a chance to feel very hungry. People who go a long time between meals tend to get very hungry and eat everything in sight when they do eat.

Can a Low-Calorie Diet Affect Your Metabolism?

Absolutely. Your body will sense that it is being starved and will fight back by slowing down. Anorexic women, for instance, burn 40 percent fewer calories per day than women who eat normally. It's not clear how much of a calorie deficit triggers a drop in metabolism. But experts say that you can get into trouble by consuming fewer calories than required by your resting metabolic rate. If you want to lose weight, a good rule of thumb is to eat more calories than your resting metabolism requires but fewer calories than your total calorie expenditure. For instance, if your resting metabolism is 1,500 calories and you burn an additional 450 calories through daily activity and a short bike ride, try to eat between 1,500 and 1,950 calories.

How do you know whether you've inadvertently lowered your metabolism? Symptoms include fatigue, dry skin, constipation, a slow pulse, low blood pressure, and feeling cold. These symptoms also can indicate other conditions, so consult your doctor.

Yo-yo dieting — the phenomenon of repeatedly losing and regaining weight — has not been proven to lower resting metabolism. A recent review of 43 studies done on yo-yo dieting found that most of the studies do not show any effect on metabolism. However, researchers caution that the effects of yo-yo dieting are difficult to pinpoint and even the best studies were flawed. None of this, however, means that yo-yo dieting is a good thing. Some studies show that repeatedly losing and gaining weight can cause psychological trauma.

Can Hot Peppers Rev Up Your Metabolism?

No! When you eat something so hot that you break out in a sweat and your skin gets tingly, your blood vessels expand slightly and your metabolic rate jumps up briefly. But there is no reason to believe that the rise will be significant enough to help you lose an ounce, let alone pounds (see Figure 27-1). No food has special, magical, fat-burning powers — not even the long-revered grapefruit or the amino acid power shakes that bodybuilders gulp down by the gallon.

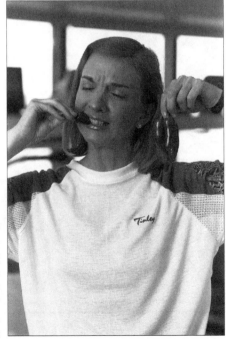

Figure 27-1: Eating hot peppers does not rev up your metabolism.

(Photo courtesy of Dan Kron.)

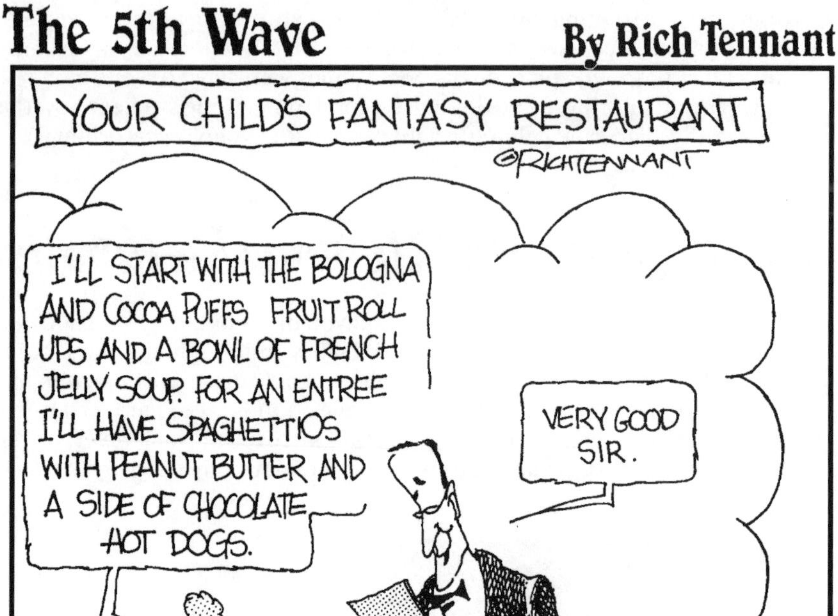
The 5th Wave
By Rich Tennant
YOUR CHILD'S FANTASY RESTAURANT
©RICHTENNANT
I'LL START WITH THE BOLOGNA AND COCOA PUFFS FRUIT ROLL UPS AND A BOWL OF FRENCH JELLY SOUP. FOR AN ENTREE I'LL HAVE SPAGHETTIOS WITH PEANUT BUTTER AND A SIDE OF CHOCOLATE HOT DOGS.
VERY GOOD SIR.

Appendix A

Resources

● ●

American Business Directories
5711 S. 86th Circle
P.O. Box 27347
Omaha, NE 68127
(402) 593-4600

AVIA Group International, Inc.
9605 SW Nimbus Ave.
Beaverton, OR 97008
(800) 345-2842
(503) 520-1500
Fax (503) 643-5599

Backroads
1516 Fifth Street
Berkeley, CA 94710
(510) 527-1555
Fax (510) 527-1444

Body Wrappers
Div. Attitudes in Dressing, Inc.
1350 Broadway, Ste. 304
New York, NY 10018
(212) 279-3492
(800) 323-0786
Fax (212) 564-3426

Bodyguard Fitness Corp.
2645 Rue Watt
Quebec City
Quebec, Canada G1P 3T2
(418) 657-2020
(800) 665-3407
Fax (418) 657-2157
Branch Office(s)
116 E. Park Avenue
(516) 889-1884
(800) 526-6667
Fax (516) 889-1186

Buns of Steel
Warnervision
1290 Avenue of the Americas
4th floor
New York, NY 10019
(212) 275-2900

Cal Gym Equipment Company
3140 E. Pico Ave.
Los Angeles, CA 90023
(213) 264-2715

CamelBak
FasTrak Systems, Inc.
P.O. Box 1029
901 West I-20
Weatherford, TX 76086
(817) 594-1000
Fax (817) 594-1030

Cat Eye Co. Ltd.
8-25, 2-chome
Kuwazu, Higashi
Sumiyoshi-ku
Osaka, Japan 546
(81-6-719-7781)
Fax (81-6-719-2362)

Collage Video Specialties, Inc.
The Complete Guide to Exercise Videos
5390 Main Street N.E.
Minneapolis, MN 55421
(800) 433-6769

Combi Corp.
3-16-9 Uchikanda
Chiyoda-Ku
Tokyo, Japan 101
(81-3-3256-8636)
Fax (81-3-3256-8529)

Concept II, Inc.
R.R. 1
Box 1100
Morrisville, VT 05661
(802) 888-7971
(800) 245-5676
Fax (802) 888-4791

CYCLEPLUS/Bioform Engineering Inc.
P.O. Box 1168
Ross, CA 94957
(415) 461-1747
(800) 535-5140
Fax (415) 461-4915

Dump Your Plump
P.O. Box 30
South Haven, MI 49090
(616) 639-1592
Fax (616) 637-2268

Dynaband
Fitness Wholesale
Div. Future Dynamics, Inc.
895-A Hampshire Road
Stow, OH 44224
(216) 929-7227
(800) 537-5512
Fax (800) 232-9348

Fitness on the Road
Shelter Publishing
P.O. Box 279
Bolinas, CA
(415) 868-0280

FreeForm
Integrated Health, Inc.
Div. Tyson & Assoc. Inc.
12832 Chadron Ave.
Hawthorne, CA 90250-5525
(310) 675-1164
(800) 367-7744

FreeForm
James Design Co., Inc.
3620 E. Landis Ave., #12
Vineland, NJ 08360
(609) 692-1128

Gerstung/Gym-Thing Inc.
6308 Blair Hill Lane
Baltimore, MD 21209-2102
(410) 337-0471
(800) 922-3575
Fax (410) 337-0471

Gym Source
40 E. 52nd Street
New York, NY 10022
(212) 688-4222
Fax (212) 750-2886

Health For Life
8033 Sunset Blvd., Ste. 483
Los Angeles, CA 90046
(310) 306-0777
(800) 874-5339
Fax (310) 305-7672

Hoist Fitness Systems
9990 Empire Street, #130
San Diego, CA 92126
(619) 578-7676
(800) 548-5438
Fax (619) 578-9558

Hydrafitness
Sprint/Rothhammer
P.O. Box 5579
Santa Maria, CA 93456-5579
(805) 481-2744
(800) 235-2156
Fax (805) 489-0360

International In-Line Skating Association
3720 Farragut Avenue, #400
Kensington, MD 20895
(301) 942-9770
Fax (301) 942-9771

Cynthia Kereluk
Lifetime Cable Everyday Workout
P.O. Box 75209
White Rock, B.C.
Postal #V4A9N4

Life Fitness
10601 Belmont Avenue
Franklin Park, IL 60131-1545
(708) 288-3300
(800) 735-3867
Fax (708) 288-3791
Branch Office(s)
10601 W. Belmont Avenue
Franklin Park, IL 60131-1545
(800) 351-3737

Life Measurement Instruments
1980 Olivera Road, Suite C
Concord, CA 94520
(510) 676-6002
Fax (510) 676-6005

Lifeline Int'l
1421 S. Park Street
Madison, WI 53715
(608) 251-4778
(800) 553-6633
Fax (608) 251-1870

Monark
Quinton Fitness Equipment
Div. Quinton Instrument Co.
3303 Monte Villa Parkway
Bothell, WA 98021-8906
(206) 402-2000
(800) 426-0337
Fax (206) 402-2001

Mountain Travel-Sobek
6420 Fairmount Avenue
El Cerrito, CA 94530
(510) 527-8100

NordicTrack
Training Camp Int'l
P.O. Box 0246
Merion Station, PA 19066-0246
(610) 664-5241
(800) 238-5241
Fax (610) 667-2931

Nutrition Action Newsletter
Center for Science in the Public
Interest
1875 Connecticut Ave. N.W., #300
Washington, DC 20009-5728
(202) 332-9110
Fax (202) 265-4594

Pacific Fitness Corp.
6600 W. Katella Ave.
Cypress, CA 90630-5104
(714) 373-5554
(800) 722-3482
Fax (714) 373-1226

Paramount Fitness Corp.
6450 E. Bandini Blvd.
Los Angeles, CA 90040-3185
(213) 721-2121
(800) 721-2121
Fax (213) 721-8841

PC Coach/Biometrics
637 S. Broadway, Suite B156
Boulder, CO 80303
(800) 522-6224
Fax (303) 494-9722

Physioballs
Resist-A-Ball
6435 Castleway West Drive
Ste. 130
Indianapolis, IN 46250
(317) 576-6571
(800) 843-3671
Fax (317) 576-6575

Pilates Studio, The
2121 Broadway, Ste. 210
New York, NY 10023
(800) 474-5283
Fax (212) 769-2368
Branch Office
8704 Santa Monica Blvd., Ste. 300
West Hollywood, CA 90069
(310) 659-1077
(800) 474-5283
Fax (310) 659-1163

PlateMate
Benoit Built Inc.
4 Factory Cove Road
Boothbay Harbor, ME 04538
(207) 633-5912
(800) 877-3322
Fax (207) 633-9729

Power Blocks
IntellBell, Inc.
2100 Austin Rd.
Owatonna, MN 55060
(507) 451-5152
(800) 446-5215
Fax (507) 451-5278

Precor Commercial Products Div.
Div. Precor, Inc.
20001 N. Creek Pkwy.
P.O. Box 3004
Bothell, WA 98041
(206) 486-9292
(800) 786-8404
Fax (206) 486-3856

ProStretch
82 Birch Ave.
Little Silver, NJ 07739
(908) 224-0900
(800) 535-3629
Fax (908) 224-0909

Quinton Fitness Equipment
Div. Quinton Instrument Company
3303 Monte Villa Parkway
Bothell, WA 98021-8906
(206) 402-2000
(800) 426-0337
Fax (206) 402-2001

Reebok Int'l Ltd.
100 Technology Center Drive
Stoughton, MA 02072
(617) 341-5000
(800) 435-7022
(800) 382-3823
Fax (617) 341-5087

Rollerblade Inc
5101 Shady Oak Road
Minnetonka, MN 55343
(800) 328-0171
Fax (612) 930-7030

Ropics, Inc.
P.O. Box 373
Greendale, WI 53129
(414) 423-1707
(800) 252-JUMP

Round Company, The
Canal Street Station
Box 885
New York, NY 10013-0885
(718) 789-9756

Schwinn Cycling & Fitness, Inc.
1690 38th Street
Boulder, CO 80301
(303) 939-0100
Fax (303) 939-0260

**SmartLock Adjustable
Dumbbell System**
Ultima Fitness, Inc.
2140 S. Ivanhoe Street, G-10
Denver, CO 80222
(303) 691-9610
Fax (303) 691-2805

Spalding Sports Rope
825 Riverside, Suite 2
Paso Robels, CA 93446
(800) 852-5567
Fax (805) 239-9016

Specialized Bicycle Components
15130 Concord Circle
Morgan Hill, CA 95037
(408) 779-6229
Fax (408) 778-1037

SPRI Products, Inc.
1554 Barclay Blvd.
Buffalo Grove, IL 60089
(708) 537-7876
(800) 222-7774
Fax (708) 537-4941

**Stairmaster Sports/Medical
Products, Inc.**
12421 Willows Road N.E.
Ste. 100
Kirkland, WA 98034
(206) 823-1825
(800) 635-2936
Fax (206) 823-9490

Step Co., The
400 Interstate N. Pkwy.
Ste. 1500
Atlanta, GA 30339
(404) 859-9292
(800) SAY-STEP
Fax (404) 952-6632

Super Rope Co.
P.O. Box 14051
West Allis, WI 53214
(414) 771-0849

Tectrix Fitness Equipment
Div. Laguna Tectrix, Inc.
68 Fairbanks
Irvine, CA 92718-1816
(714) 380-8710
(800) 767-8082
Fax (714) 380-8710

Total Gym/EFI
Div. Engineering Fitness Int'l Medical Systems
7766 Arjons Drive, Unit B
San Diego, CA 92126
(619) 586-6080
(800) 541-4900

Training Camp Int'l
P.O. Box 0246
Merion Stn., PA 19066-0246
(610) 667-2931
(800) 238-5241
Fax (610) 667-2931

Trotter
10 Trotter Drive
Medway, MA 02053-2275
(800) 677-6544
Fax (508) 533-5500
Branch Office
115 High Street
Sharpsville, PA 16150
(412) 962-3200
Fax (412) 962-0866

Tuff Stuff
Task Industries, Inc.
14829 E. Salt Lake Avenue
City of Industry, CA 91746-3131
(818) 961-6564
(800) 824-5210
Fax (818) 961-9094

Tunturi
Sta-Fit Gym Equipment
1004 S.W. 10th Street
Aledo, IL 61231-2353
(309) 582-5334

Ultimate Workout Log, The
Houghton Mifflin Co.
222 Berkeley St.
Boston, MA 02116
(800) 225-3362

VersaClimber
Heart Rate, Inc.
3188 Airway Ave., #E
Costa Mesa, CA 92626-6601
(714) 850-9716
(800) 237-2271
Fax (714) 755-4973

Vital Signs
Country Technology
P.O. Box 87
Gay Mills, WI 54631
(608) 735-4718
Fax (608) 735-4859

**Walk the Four Seasons Walking
and Cross-training Logbook**
Creative Walking, Inc.
P.O. Box 50296
Clayton, MO 63105
(800) 762-9255

WaterRower, Inc.
255 Armistice Blvd.
Pawtucket, RI 02860
(401) 728-1966
(800) 852-2210
Fax (401) 728-1968

Wintrainer
Abaco Software, Inc.
6 Trafalgar Square
Nashua, NH 03063
(603) 883-1818
(800) 859-1969
Fax (603) 883-2019

York Barbell
Box 1707
York, PA 17405
(717) 767-6481
(800) 358-YORK
Fax (717) 764-0044

Appendix B
Your Fitness Test Results

Write in the Name of Your Test Here ↓			Write in Your Goal Score Here ↓
Test	Your Score First Test	Your Score Second Test	Goal
Resting Heart Rate			
Resting Blood Pressure			
Aerobic Endurance			
Weight			
Body Fat Percentage			
Measurements			
Upper Body Strength			
Middle Body Strength			
Lower Body Strength			
Flexibility			

Index

common cold, 91, 92, 315
compression, for injuries, 289
computer(s). *See also* Internet
    computerized stationary bikes, 236
    computerized weight training, 159
    information kiosks, at health clubs, 190
    software, for workout logs, 31, 274
Cooking Light, 52
cool-down, 94, 95, 102
Cooper, Kenneth, 76
Copeland, Candice, 260, 261
copper, 65
copyrights, 255
Cosmopolitan, 41
cottage cheese, 61–62. *See also* dairy
    products
country-robics, 223
cramps, 58
credentials
    of dieticians, 284–285
    of exercise video instructors, 254
    of trainers, 280–281
cross-country skiing machines, 85,
    112–113, 239
cross-training, 119, 222, 267, 291
crunches, 20–21, 150, 175, 311
CYBEX, 156, 188
Cycle Plus, 107
cycling. *See also* stationary bicycles
    adding hills to, 90
    aerobic exercise and, 76
    basic recommendations for, 121–125
    burning calories through, 85
    choosing a bicycle for, 122–123
    correct posture for, 125
    as an endurance sport, 87
    fitness plans and, 26–28, 33, 35–36
    gear, 122–125, 294–295
    interval training and, 89
    listening to music while, 272
    maximum heart rates for, 77
    tips for rookies, 124–125
Cytomax, 58

• D •

dairy products, 50–53, 61, 64–69
dehydration, 17, 58, 64, 205, 300–301, 315.
    See also water, drinking
Delayed Onset Muscle Soreness, 203
deltoids, 142–144
Department of Agriculture, 64
depression, 91, 92
diabetes, 73
diarrhea, 63
dietary fat
    basic description of, 48–56
    calories from, cutting, 51–52
    different types of, 53–55
    how much you eat, finding out, 48–49
    monounsaturated/polyunsaturated, 54
    saturated, 53–54
    substitutes ("fake"), 55
    three strategies to trim, 48–52
    trans fatty acids (TFAs), 54
dieticians, 190, 284–285
dieting. *See also* nutrition
    diet centers and, 284–285
    fitness plans and, 27, 28, 33
    metabolic rates and, 38, 324–325
    "yo-yo," 325
dizziness, 304
doctors, 25, 77, 292
drinking
    alcohol, 38, 48, 56, 64
    water, 58, 63–64, 201, 272–273,
      300–301, 315
drugs
    amphetamines, 323
    anti-inflammatory drugs, 290, 291
    appetite suppressants, 323
    prescription drugs, 82
    steroids, 139, 323–324
dual action bikes, 107
Duke, Kacy, 262
dumbbells, 160, 243–245, 246. *See also* free
    weights
Dump Your Plump program, 34–35
DynaBand, 248

Notes

Notes

Notes

Notes

Notes

Notes